Clinical applications of artificial neural networks

Artificial neural networks provide a powerful tool to help doctors to analyse, model and make sense of complex clinical data across a broad range of medical applications. Their potential in clinical medicine is reflected in the diversity of topics covered in this cutting-edge volume. In addition to looking at new and forthcoming applications the book looks forward to exciting future prospects on the horizon. A section on theory looks at approaches to validate and refine the results generated by artificial neural networks. The volume also recognizes that concerns exist about the use of 'black-box' systems as decision aids in medicine, and the final chapter considers the ethical and legal conundrums arising out of their use for diagnostic or treatment decisions. Taken together, this eclectic collection of chapters provides an exciting overview of current and future prospects for harnessing the power of artificial neural networks in the investigation and treatment of disease.

Richard Dybowski is a Research Fellow in the Division of Medicine, King's College London. His main research interest is the application of statistics (including data visualization) and formal logics to medical informatics and bioinformatics.

Vanya Gant is Consultant and Senior Lecturer in Microbiology and Clinical Director in Infection at University College London Hospitals Trust. His particular interests are the application of emerging technologies to microbial diagnosis, and the interpretation and clinical decision-making that flow from complex high-dimensional datasets of either clinical or machine origin.

Clinical applications of artificial neural networks

Edited by

Richard Dybowski
King's College London

and

Vanya Gant
University College London Hospitals NHS Trust

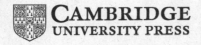
CAMBRIDGE
UNIVERSITY PRESS

CAMBRIDGE UNIVERSITY PRESS
Cambridge, New York, Melbourne, Madrid, Cape Town, Singapore, São Paulo

Cambridge University Press
The Edinburgh Building, Cambridge CB2 8RU, UK

Published in the United States of America by Cambridge University Press, New York

www.cambridge.org
Information on this title: www.cambridge.org/9780521662710

First published 2001
This digitally printed version 2007

A catalogue record for this publication is available from the British Library

Library of Congress Cataloguing in Publication data

Clinical applications of artificial neural networks/edited by Richard Dybowski & Vanya Gant.
    p.   ; cm.
Includes bibliographical references and index.
ISBN 0 521 66271 0 (hardback)
1. Medicine – Research – Data processing. 2. Neural networks (Computer science).
3. Clinical medicine – Decision making – Data processing. I. Dybowski, Richard, 1951–
II. Gant, Vanya.
[DNLM: 1. Neural Networks (Computer). 2. Automatic Data Processing. W 26.55.A7 C641 2001]
R853.D37 C535 2001
616′.00285′632 – dc21   00-046796

ISBN 978-0-521-66271-0 hardback
ISBN 978-0-521-00133-5 paperback

Contents

Contributors

Charles W. Anderson
Dept of Computer Science
Colorado State University
Fort Collins, CO 80523-1873
USA

Robert Andrews
Faculty of Information Technology
Queensland University of Technology
PO Box 2434
Brisbane, QLD 4000
Australia

Mathilde E. Boon
Leiden Cytology and Pathology Laboratory
PO Box 16084
2301 GB Leiden
The Netherlands

Emma A. Braithwaite
Oxford Biosignals
Magdalen Centre
Oxford
Oxfordshire OX4 4GA
UK

Simon S. Cross
Department of Pathology
Division of Genomic Medicine
University of Sheffield Medical School
Beech Hill Road
Sheffield S10 2UL
UK

Joachim Diederich
Faculty of Information Technology
Queensland University of Technology
PO Box 2434
Brisbane, QLD 4000
Australia

Joseph Downs
Dept of Automatic Control and Systems
Engineering
University of Sheffield
Mappin Street
Sheffield S1 3JD
UK

Jimmy Dripps
Integrated Systems Group (ISG)
Electronics and Electrical Engineering
Edinburgh University
Mayfield Road
Edinburgh EH9 3JL
UK

Richard Dybowski
Envisionment
143 Village Way
Pinner
Middlesex HA5 5AA
UK

David B. Fogel
Natural Selection Inc.
3333 N. Torrey Pines Ct
Suite 200
La Jolla, CA 92037
USA

Vanya Gant
Dept of Clinical Microbiology
University College Hospital
London WC1E 6DB
UK

Richard M. Golden
Applied Cognition and Neuroscience
Program
School of Human Development, GR 41
University of Texas at Dallas
Richardson, TX 75086-0688
USA

Royston Goodacre
Institute of Biological Sciences
Cledwyn Building
The University of Wales
Aberystwyth
Ceredigion SY23 3DD
UK

Robert F. Harrison
Dept of Automatic Control and Systems
Engineering
University of Sheffield
Mappin Street
Sheffield S1 3JD
UK

R. Lee Kennedy
Dept of General Internal Medicine
Sunderland Royal Hospital
Kayll Road
Sunderland SR4 7TP
UK

Lambrecht P. Kok
Dept of Biomedical Engineering
University of Groningen
Nijenborgh 4
9747 AG Groningen
The Netherlands

Chee Peng Lim
Dept of Automatic Control and Systems
Engineering
University of Sheffield
Mappin Street
Sheffield S1 3JD
UK

Andrew J. Lyon
Neonatal Unit
Simpson Memorial Maternity Pavilion
Edinburgh EH3 9EF
UK

Alan Murray
Integrated Systems Group
Electronics and Electrical Engineering
Edinburgh University
Mayfield Road
Edinburgh EH9 3JL
UK

Craig S. Niederberger
Dept of Urology M/C 955
University of Illinois at Chicago
840 South Wood Street
Chicago, IL 60612
USA

James Pardey
Oxford Instruments Medical Ltd
Manor Way
Old Woking
Surrey GU22 9JU
UK

David A. Peterson
Dept of Computer Science
Colorado State University
Fort Collins, CO 80523-1873
USA

V. William Porto
Natural Selection Inc.
3333 N. Torrey Pines Ct
Suite 200
La Jolla, CA 92037
USA

Brian D. Ripley
Dept of Statistics
University of Oxford
1 South Parks Road
Oxford OX1 3TG
UK

Ruth M. Ripley
Dept of Statistics
University of Oxford
1 South Parks Road
Oxford OX1 3TG
UK

Stephen J. Roberts
Dept of Engineering Science
University of Oxford
Parks Road
Oxford OX1 3PJ
UK

Susan Rodway
12 King's Bench Walk
London EC4Y 7EL
UK

Lionel Tarassenko
Dept of Engineering Science
University of Oxford
Parks Road
Oxford OX1 3PJ
UK

Alan B. Tickle
Faculty of Information Technology
Queensland University of Technology
PO Box 2434
Brisbane, QLD 4000
Australia

Jeremy Wyatt
School of Public Policy
University College London
29/30 Tavistock Square
London WC1H 9EZ
UK

Mayela Zamora
Dept of Engineering Science
University of Oxford
Parks Road
Oxford OX1 3PJ
UK

Introduction

Richard Dybowski and Vanya Gant

In this introduction we outline the types of neural network featured in this book and how they relate to standard statistical methods. We also examine the issue of the so-called 'black-box' aspect of neural network and consider some possible future directions in the context of clinical medicine. Finally, we overview the remaining chapters.

A few evolutionary branches

The structure of the brain as a complex network of multiply connected cells (*neural networks*) was recognized in the late 19th century, primarily through the work of the Italian cytologist Golgi and the Spanish histologist Ramón y Cajal.[1] Within the reductionist approach to cognition (Churchland 1986), there appeared the question of how cognitive function could be modelled by artificial versions of these biological networks. This was the initial impetus for what has become a diverse collection of computational techniques known as *artificial neural networks* (ANNs).

The design of artificial neural networks was originally motivated by the phenomena of learning and recognition, and the desire to model these cognitive processes. But, starting in the mid-1980s, a more pragmatic stance has emerged, and ANNs are now regarded as non-standard statistical tools for pattern recognition. It must be emphasized that, in spite of their biological origins, they are not 'computers that think', nor do they perform 'brain-like' computations.

The 'evolution' of artificial neural networks is divergent and has resulted in a wide variety of 'phyla' and 'genera'. Rather than examine the development of every branch of the evolutionary tree, we focus on those associated with the types of ANN mentioned in this book, namely multilayer perceptrons (Chapters 2–8, 10–13), radial basis function networks (Chapter 12), Kohonen feature maps (Chapters 2, 5), adaptive resonance theory networks (Chapters 2, 9), and neuro-fuzzy networks (Chapters 10, 12).

We have not set out to provide a comprehensive tutorial on ANNs; instead, we

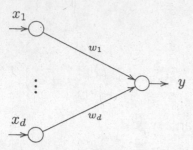

Figure 1.1. A graphical representation of a McCulloch–Pitts neuron, and also of a single-layer perceptron. In the former, a discontinuous step function is applied to the weighted sum
$w_0 + w_1 x_1 + \cdots + w_d x_d$ to produce the output y; in the latter, the step function is replaced by a
continuous sigmoidal function.

have suggested sources of information throughout the text, and we have provided
some recommended reading in Appendix 1.1.

Multilayer perceptrons

At the start of the 20th century, a number of general but non-mathematical
theories of cognition existed, such as those of Helmholtz and Pavlov. At the
University of Pittsburgh in the 1920s, Nicolas Rashevsky, a physicist, began a
research programme to place biology within the framework of mathematical
physics. This involved a number of projects, including an attempt to mathematically model Pavlovian conditioning in terms of neural networks (Rashevsky
1948). He continued his work at the University of Chicago, where he was joined by
Warren McCulloch, a neuroanatomist, and then, in 1942, by a mathematical
prodigy called Walter Pitts. Together, McCulloch & Pitts (1943) devised a simple
model of the neuron. In this model (Figure 1.1), the input signals $x_1, \ldots, x_d$ to a
neuron are regarded as a weighted sum $w_0 + w_1 x_1 + \cdots + w_d x_d$. If the sum exceeds a
predefined threshold value, the output signal y from the neuron equals 1; otherwise, it is 0. However, a McCulloch–Pitts neuron by itself is capable only of simple
tasks, namely discrimination between sets of input values separable by a (possibly
multidimensional) plane. Furthermore, the weights required for the neurons of a
network had to be provided as no method for automatically determining the
weights was available at that time.

Rosenblatt (1958) proposed that the McCulloch–Pitts neuron could be the basis
of a system able to distinguish between patterns originating from different classes.
The system, which he dubbed a *perceptron*, was a McCulloch–Pitts neuron with
preprocessed inputs.[2] Motivated by Hebb's (1949) hypothesis that learning is
based on the reinforcement of active neuronal connections, Rosenblatt (1960,

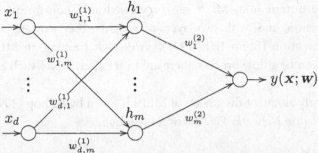

Figure 1.2. A multilayer perceptron with two layers of weights. The first layer of nodes, which receive the inputs $x_1, \ldots, x_d$, is called the *input layer*. The layer of nodes producing the output values is called the *output layer*. Layers of nodes between the input and output layers are referred to as *hidden layers*. The weighted sum h_j at the j-th hidden node is given by $w_{0,j}^{(1)} + w_{1,j}^{(1)} + \cdots w_{d,j}^{(1)} x_d$. The value from the j-th hidden node to the output node is a function f_{hid} of h_j, and the output $y(x; w)$ is a function of f_{out} of the weighted sum $w_0^{(2)} + w_1^{(2)} f_{hid}(h_1) + \cdots + w_m^{(2)} f_{hid}(h_m)$. Functions f_{hid} and f_{out} are typically sigmoidal. Note that a multilayer perceptron can have more than one layer of hidden nodes and more than one node providing output values.

1962) developed the *perceptron learning rule* and its associated convergence theorem. This solved the problem of a McCulloch–Pitts neuron 'learning' a set of weights. A number of workers (e.g. Block 1962) proved that the learning rule, when applied to a perceptron consisting of only a single layer of weights, would always modify the weights so as to give the optimal planar decision boundary possible for that perceptron.

Multilayer perceptrons (MLPs) are perceptrons having more than one layer of weights (Figure 1.2), which enables them to produce complex decision boundaries. Unfortunately, as pointed out by Minsky & Papert (1969), the perceptron learning rule did not apply to MLPs,[3] a fact that severely limited the types of problem to which perceptrons could be applied. This caused many researchers to leave the field, thereby starting the 'Dark Ages' of neural networks, during which little research was done. The turning point came in the mid-1980s when the back-propagation algorithm for training multilayer perceptrons was discovered independently by several researchers (LeCun 1985; Parker 1985; Rumelhart et al. 1986).[4] This answered the criticisms of Minsky & Papert (1969), and the Renaissance of neural networks began.

Multilayer perceptrons with sigmoidal hidden node functions are the most commonly used ANNs, as exemplified by the contributions to this book and the reviews by Baxt (1995) and Dybowski & Gant (1995). Each hidden node in Figure 1.2 produces a hyperplane boundary in the multidimensional space containing the input data. The output node smoothly interpolates between these boundaries to give decision regions of the input space occupied by each class of interest. With a single logistic output unit, MLPs can be viewed as a non-linear extension of logistic regression, and, with two layers of weights, they can approximate any continuous function (Blum & Li 1991).[5] Although training an MLP by back-propagation can be a slow process, there are faster alternatives such as *Quickprop* (Fahlman 1988).

A particularly eloquent discussion of MLPs is given by Bishop (1995, Chap. 4) in his book *Neural Networks for Pattern Recognition*.

A statistical perspective on multilayer perceptrons

The genesis and renaissance of ANNs took place within various communities, and articles published during this period reflect the disciplines involved: biology and cognition, statistical physics, and computer science. But it was not until the early 1990s that a probability-theoretic perspective emerged, with Bridle (1991), Ripley (1993), Amari (1993) and Cheng & Titterington (1994) being amongst the first to regard ANNs as being within the framework of statistics. The statistical aspect of ANNs has also been highlighted in textbooks by Smith (1993), Bishop (1995) and Ripley (1996).

A recurring theme of this literature is that many ANNs are analogous to, or identical with, existing statistical techniques. For example, a popular statistical method for modelling the relationship between a binary response variable y and a vector (an ordered set) of covariates x is *logistic regression* (Hosmer & Lemeshow 1989; Collett 1991), but consider the single-layer perceptron of Figure 1.1:

$$y(x; w) = f_{out}\left(w_0 + \sum_{i=1}^{d} w_i x_i\right).$$ (1.1)

If the output function f_{out} of Eq. (1.1) is logistic,

$$f_{out}(r) = 1 + \exp[-(r)]^{-1},$$

(where r is any value) and the perceptron is trained by a cross-entropy error function, Eq. (1.1) will be functionally identical with a main-effects logistic regression model

$$\hat{p}(y=1 \mid x) = \left\{1 + \exp\left[-(\beta_0 + \sum_{i=1}^{d} \beta_i x_i)\right]\right\}^{-1}.$$

Using the notation of Figure 1.2, the MLP can be written as

$$y(x; w) = f_{out}\left(w_0^{(2)} + \sum_{j=1}^{m} w_j^{(2)} f_{hid}\left(w_{0,j}^{(1)} + \sum_{i=1}^{d} w_{i,j}^{(1)} x_i\right)\right),$$ (1.2)

but Hwang et al. (1994) have indicated that Eq. (1.2) can be regarded as a particular type of projection pursuit regression model when f_{out} is linear:

$$y(x; w) = v_0 + \sum_{j=1}^{m} v_j f_j \left(u_{0,j} + \sum_{i=1}^{d} u_{i,j} x_i \right).$$ (1.3)

Projection pursuit regression (Friedman & Stuetzle 1981) is an established statistical technique and, in contrast to an MLP, each function f_j in Eq. (1.3) can be different, thereby providing more flexibility.[6] However, Ripley and Ripley (Chapter 11) point out that the statistical algorithms for fitting projection pursuit regression are not as effective as those for fitting MLPs.

Another parallel between neural and statistical models exists with regard to the problem of overfitting. In using an MLP, the aim is to have the MLP generalize from the data rather than have it fit to the data (*overfitting*). Overfitting can be controlled for by adding a *regularization function* to the error term (Poggio et al. 1985). This additional term penalizes an MLP that is too flexible. In statistical regression the same concept exists in the form of the *Akaike information criterion* (Akaike 1974). This is a linear combination of the deviance and the number of independent parameters, the latter penalizing the former. Furthermore, when regularization is implemented using weight decay (Hinton 1989), a common approach, the modelling process is analogous to ridge regression (Montgomery & Peck 1992, pp. 329–344) – a regression technique that can provide good generalization.

One may ask whether the apparent similarity between ANNs and existing statistical methods means that ANNs are redundant within pattern recognition. One answer to this is given by Ripley (1996, p. 4):

> The traditional methods of statistics and pattern recognition are either *parametric* based on a family of models with a small number of parameters, or *non-parametric* in which the models used are totally flexible. One of the impacts of neural network methods on pattern recognition has been to emphasize the need in large-scale practical problems for something in between, families of models with large but not unlimited flexibility given by a large number of parameters. The two most widely used neural network architectures, *multi-layer perceptrons* and *radial basis functions* (RBFs), provide two such families (and several others already in existence).

In other words, ANNs can act as *semi-parametric* classifiers, which are more flexible than parametric methods (such as the quadratic discriminant function (e.g. Krzanowski 1988)) but require fewer model parameters than non-parametric methods (such as those based on kernel density estimation (Silverman 1986)). However, setting up a semi-parametric classifier can be more computationally intensive than using a parametric or non-parametric approach.

Another response is to point out that the widespread fascination for ANNs has attracted many researchers and potential users into the realm of pattern recognition. It is true that the neural-computing community rediscovered some statistical concepts already in existence (Ripley 1996), but this influx of participants has created new ideas and refined existing ones. These benefits include the *learning of sequences* by time delay and partial recurrence (Lang & Hinton 1988; Elman 1990) and the creation of powerful visualization techniques, such as *generative topographic mapping* (Bishop et al. 1997). Thus the ANN movement has resulted in statisticians having available to them a collection of techniques to add to their repertoire. Furthermore, the placement of ANNs within a statistical framework has provided a firmer theoretical foundation for neural computation, and it has led to new developments such as the Bayesian approach to ANNs (MacKay 1992).

Unfortunately, the rebirth of neural networks during the 1980s has been accompanied by hyperbole and misconceptions that have led to neural networks being trained incorrectly. In response to this, Tarassenko (1995) highlighted three areas where care is required in order to achieve reliable performance: firstly, there must be sufficient data to enable a network to generalize effectively; secondly, informative features must be extracted from the data for use as input to a network; thirdly, balanced training sets should be used for underrepresented classes (or *novelty detection* used when abnormalities are very rare (Tarassenko et al. 1995)). Tarassenko (1998) discussed these points in detail, and he stated:

It is easy to be carried away and begin to overestimate their capabilities. The usual consequence of this is, hopefully, no more serious than an embarrassing failure with concomitant mutterings about black boxes and excessive hype. Neural networks cannot solve every problem. Traditional methods may be better. Nevertheless, neural networks, when they are used wisely, usually perform at least as well as the most appropriate traditional method and in some cases significantly better.

It should also be emphasized that, even with correct training, an ANN will not necessarily be the best choice for a classification task in terms of accuracy. This has been highlighted by Wyatt (1995), who wrote:

Neural net advocates claim accuracy as the major advantage. However, when a large European research project, StatLog, examined the accuracy of five ANN and 19 traditional statistical or decision-tree methods for classifying 22 sets of data, including three medical datasets [Michie et al. 1994], a neural technique was the most accurate in only one dataset, on DNA sequences. For 15 (68%) of the 22 sets, traditional statistical methods were the most accurate, and those 15 included all three medical datasets.

But one should add the comment made by Michie et al. (1994, p. 221) on the results of the StatLog project:

With care, neural networks perform very well as measured by error rate. They seem to provide either the best or near best predictive performance in nearly all cases . . .

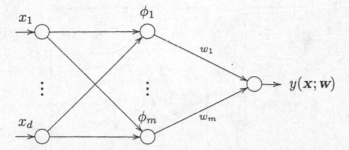

Figure 1.3. A radial basis function network. The network has a single layer of basis functions between the input and output layers. The value of ϕ_j produced by the j-th basis function is dependent on the distance between the 'centre' $x^{[j]}$ of the function and the vector of input values $x_1, ..., x_d$. The output $y(x; w)$ is the weighted sum $w_0 + w_1\phi_1 + \cdots + w_m\phi_m$. Note that a radial basis function network can have more than one output node, and the functions $\phi_1, ..., \phi_m$ need not be the same.

Nevertheless, when an ANN is being evaluated, its performance must be compared with that obtained from one or more appropriate standard statistical techniques.

Radial basis function networks

Unlike MLPs, a number of so-called 'neural networks' were not biologically motivated, and one of these is the radial basis function network. Originally conceived in order to perform multivariate interpolation (Powell 1987), *radial basis function networks* (RBFNs) (Broomhead & Lowe 1988) are an alternative to MLPs. Like an MLP, an RBFN has input and output nodes; but there the similarity ends, for an RBFN has a middle layer of radially symmetric functions called *basis functions*, each of which can be designed separately (Figure 1.3). The idea of using basis functions originates from the concept of potential functions proposed by Bashkirov et al. (1964) and illustrated by Duda & Hart (1973).

Each basis function can be regarded as being centred on a prototypic vector of input values. When a vector of values is applied to an RBFN, a measure of the proximity of the vector to each of the prototypes is determined by the corresponding basis functions, and a weighted sum of these measures is given as the output of the RBFN (Figure 1.3).

The basis functions define *local responses* (*receptive fields*) (Figure 1.4). Typically, only some of the hidden units (basis functions) produce significant values for the final layers. This is why RBFNs are sometimes referred to as *localized receptive field networks*. In contrast, all the hidden units of an MLP are involved in determining the output from the network (they are said to form a *distributed representation*). The receptive field approach can be advantageous when the

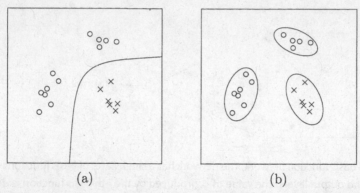

Figure 1.4.   Schematic representation of possible decision regions created by (a) the hyperplanes of a multilayer perceptron, and (b) the kernel functions of a radial basis function network. The circles and crosses represent data points from two respective classes.

distribution of the data in the space of input values is multimodal (Wilkins et al. 1994). Furthermore, RBFNs can be trained more quickly than MLPs (Moody & Darken 1989), but the number of basis functions required can grow exponentially with the number of input nodes (Hartman et al. 1990), and an increase in the number of basis functions increases the time taken, and amount of data required, to train an RBFN adequately.

Under certain conditions (White 1989; Lowe & Webb 1991; Nabney 1999), an RBFN can act as a classifier. An advantage of the local nature of RBFNs compared with MLP classifiers is that a new set of input values that falls outside all the localized receptor fields could be flagged as not belonging to any of the classes represented. In other words, the set of input values is novel. This is a more cautious approach than the resolute classification that can occur with MLPs, in which a set of input values is always assigned to a class, irrespective of the values. For further details on RBFNs, see Bishop (1995, Chap. 5).

A statistical perspective on radial basis function networks

A simple linear discriminant function (Hand 1981, Chap. 4) has the form

$$g(x) = w_0 + \sum_{i=1}^{d} w_i x_i. \tag{1.4}$$

with x assigned to a class of interest if $g(x)$ is greater than a predefined constant. This provides a planar decision surface and is functionally equivalent to the McCulloch–Pitts neuron. Equation (1.4) can be generalized to a linear function of functions, namely a *generalized linear discriminant function*

$$g(x) = w_0 + \sum_{i=1}^{m} w_i f(x), \tag{1.5}$$

which permits the construction of non-linear decision surfaces. If we represent an RBFN by the expression

$$g(x) = w_0 + \sum_{i=1}^{m} w_i \phi_i(\| x - x^{[i]} \|),$$ (1.6)

where $\| x - x^{[i]} \|$ denotes the distance (usually Euclidean) between input vector x and the 'centre' $x^{[i]}$ of the i-th basis function ϕ_i, comparison of Eq. (1.5) with Eq. (1.6) shows that an RBFN can be regarded as a type of generalized linear discriminant function.

Multilayer perceptrons and RBFNs are trained by *supervised learning*. This means that an ANN is presented with a set of examples, each example being a pair (x, t), where x is a vector of input values for the ANN, and t is the corresponding target value, for example a label denoting the class to which x belongs. The training algorithm adjusts the parameters of the ANN so as to minimize the discrepancy between the target values and the outputs produced by the network.

In contrast to MLPs and RBFNs, the ANNs in the next two sections are based on unsupervised learning. In *unsupervised learning*, there are no target values available, only input values, and the ANN attempts to categorize the inputs into classes. This is usually done by some form of clustering operation.

Kohonen feature maps

Many parts of the brain are organized in such a way that different sensory inputs are mapped to spatially localized regions within the brain. Furthermore, these regions are represented by *topologically ordered maps*. This means that the greater the similarity between two stimuli, the closer the location of their corresponding excitation regions. For example, visual, tactile and auditory stimuli are mapped onto different areas of the cerebral cortex in a topologically ordered manner (Hubel & Wiesel 1977; Kaas et al. 1983; Suga 1985). Kohonen (1982) was one of a group of people (others include Willshaw & von der Malsburg (1976)) who devised computational models of this phenomenon.

The aim of Kohonen's (1982) *self-organizing feature maps* (SOFMs) is to map an input vector to one of a set of neurons arranged in a lattice, and to do so in such a way that positions in input space are topologically ordered with locations on the lattice. This is done using a training set of input vectors $\xi(1), \ldots, \xi(m)$ and a set of prototype vectors $w(1), \ldots, w(n)$ in input space. Each prototype vector $w(i)$ is associated with a location $S(i)$ on (typically) a lattice (Figure 1.5).

As the SOFM algorithm presents each input vector ξ to the set of prototype vectors, the vector $w(i^*)$ nearest to ξ is moved towards ξ according to a learning

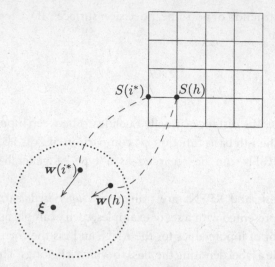

Figure 1.5.   A graphical depiction of Kohonen's self-organizing feature map. See pp. 9–10 for an explanation. The lattice is two-dimensional, whereas data point (input vector) ξ and prototype vectors $w(i^*)$ and $w(h)$ reside in a higher-dimensional (input) space.

rule. In doing so, the algorithm also 'drags' towards ξ (but to a lesser extent) those prototype vectors whose associated locations on the lattice are closest to $S(i^*)$, where $S(i^*)$ is the lattice location associated with $w(i^*)$. For example, $w(h)$ in Figure 1.5 is dragged along with $w(i^*)$ towards ξ. Hertz et al. (1991) likened this process to an elastic net, existing in input space, which wants to come as close as possible to $\xi(1), \ldots, \xi(m)$. The coordinates of the intersections of the elastic net are defined by the prototype vectors $w(1), \ldots, w(n)$. If successful, two locations $S(j)$ and $S(k)$ on the lattice will be closer to each other the closer their associated prototype vectors $w(j)$ and $w(k)$ are positioned in input space.

The SOFM algorithm provides a means of visualizing the distribution of data points in input space, but, as pointed out by Bishop (1995), this can be weak if the data do not lie within a two-dimensional subspace of the higher-dimensional space containing the data. Another problem with SOFM is that the 'elastic net' could twist as it moves towards the training set, resulting in a distorted visualization of the data (e.g. Hagan et al. 1996).

For those wishing to know more about SOFMs, we recommend the book *Neural Computation and Self-Organizing Maps* by Ritter et al. (1992).

Adaptive resonance theory networks

A feature of cognitive systems is that they can be receptive to new patterns (described as *plasticity*) but remain unchanged to others (described as *stability*).

The vexing question of how this is possible was referred to as the *stability/plasticity dilemma* (Grossberg 1976), but Carpenter & Grossberg (1987) developed a theory called *adaptive resonance theory* (ART) to explain this phenomenon.

In terms of design, ART networks are the most complex ANN given in this book, yet the principle is quite straightforward. Caudill & Butler (1990) regard the process as a type of hypothesis test. A pattern presented at an input layer is passed to a second layer, which is interconnected to the first. The second layer makes a guess about the category to which the original pattern belongs, and this hypothetical identity is passed back to the first layer. The hypothesis is compared with the original pattern and, if found to be a close match, the hypothesis and original pattern reinforce each other (*resonance* is said to take place). But if the hypothesis is incorrect, the second layer produces another guess. If the second layer cannot eventually provide a good match with the pattern, the original pattern is learned as the first example of a new category.

Although ART provides unsupervised learning, an extension called ARTMAP (Carpenter et al. 1991) combines two ART modules to enable supervised learning to take place.

In spite of resolving the stability/plasticity dilemma, the ART algorithms are sensitive to noise (Moore 1989). Furthermore, Ripley (1996) questions the virtue of the ART algorithms over adaptive *k*-means clustering, such as that of Hall & Khanna (1977).

Details of the ART concept are provided by Beale & Jackson (1990, Chap. 7) and Hertz, Krogh & Palmer (1991, pp. 228–32).

Neuro-fuzzy networks

Although probability theory is the classic approach to reasoning with uncertainty, Zadeh (1962) argued that there exist linguistic terms, such as 'most' and 'approximate', which are not describable in terms of probability distributions. He then set about developing a mathematical framework called *fuzzy set theory* (Zadeh 1965) to reason with such qualitative expressions. In classical set theory, an object is either a member of a set or it is not; in fuzzy set theory, grades of membership are allowed, the degree of membersship being defined by a *membership function*.

At a time when representation of knowledge was a focal point in artificial intelligence research, Zadeh (1972) suggested that control expertise could be represented using a set of linguistic if–then rules acquired from an operator. In his scheme, execution of the resulting *fuzzy controller* would be based on the formal rules of fuzzy set theory. But this left the problem of defining the membership functions incorporated in a fuzzy system.

A *neuro-fuzzy system* determines the parameters of the membership functions of a fuzzy system from examples by means of a neural network. Either the fuzzy system and the neural network are two distinct entities (*collaborative neuro-fuzzy systems*; e.g. Nomura et al. 1992) or the fuzzy system has a neural-net-like architecture (a *hybrid neuro-fuzzy system*). The various types of hybrid neuro-fuzzy system include systems analogous to MLPs (Berenji 1992), to RBFNs (Dabija & Tschichold-Gürman 1993), and to Kohonen feature maps (Pedrycz & Card 1992).

More information on neuro-fuzzy networks can be found in the textbook *Foundations of Neuro-Fuzzy Systems* by Nauck et al. (1997).

The 'black-box' issue

A criticism levelled against neural networks is that they are 'black-box' systems (Sharp 1995; Wyatt 1995). By this it is meant that the manner in which a neural network derives an output value from a given feature vector is not comprehensible to the non-specialist, and that this lack of comprehension makes the output from neural networks unacceptable. This issue is encountered several times in this book, namely in Chapters 9, 12, and 14.

There are a number of properties that we desire in a model, two of which are accuracy (the 'closeness' of a model's estimated value to the true value) and interpretability. By *interpretability*, we mean the type of input–output relationships that can be extracted from a model and are comprehensible to the intended user of the model. At least three types of interpretation can be identified:

1. A summary of how a change in each input variable affects the output value. This type of interpretation is provided by the regression coefficients of a main-effects logistic regression model (Hosmer & Lemeshow 1989), a virtue of additive models in general (Plate 1998).
2. A summary of all possible input–output relationships obtainable from the model as a finite set of if–then rules. This sort of interpretation is provided by all the root-to-leaf paths present in a tree-structured classifier (Breiman et al. 1984; Buntine 1992).
3. A sequential explanation that shows how the output value provided by a model was obtained from a given input vector. The explanation uses a chain of inference with steps that are meaningful to the user of the model. Such an explanation is provided by a most probable configuration in Bayesian belief networks (Jensen 1996, pp. 104–107).

An interpretable model is advantageous for several reasons:

It could be educational by supplying a previously unknown but useful input–output summary. This, in turn, can lead to new areas of research.

It could disclose an error in the model when an input–output summary or explanation contradicts known facts.

Does the lack of interpretability, as defined above, make a model unacceptable? That depends on the purpose of the model. Suppose that the choice of a statistical model for a given problem is reasonable (on theoretical or heuristic grounds), and an extensive empirical assessment of the model (e.g. by cross-validation and prospective evaluation) shows that its parameters provide an acceptable degree of accuracy over a wide range of input vectors. The use of such a model for prediction would generally be approved, subject to a performance-monitoring policy. Why not apply the same reasoning to neural networks, which are, after all, non-standard statistical models?

But suppose that we are interested in *knowledge discovery* (Brachman & Anand 1996); by this we mean the extraction of previously unknown but useful information from data. With a trained MLP, it is very difficult to interpret the mass of weights and connections within the network, and the interactions implied by these. The goal of *rule extraction* (Chapter 12) is to map the (possibly complex) associations encoded by the functions and parameters of an ANN to a set of comprehensible if–then rules. If successful, such a mapping would lead to an interpretable collection of statements describing the associations discovered by the ANN.

New developments and future prospects

What have ANNs got to offer medicine in the future? The answer is not so much whether they can, but how far they can be used to solve problems of clinical relevance – and whether this will be considered acceptable. Medicine is a complex discipline, but the ability of ANNs to model complexity may prove to be rewarding. Complexity in this context can be broken down into three elements, each with very different parameters and requirements.

The first is in many ways the 'purest' and yet the most impenetrable, and concerns the complexity of individual cells. After the initial flush of enthusiasm, and the perceived empowerment and promise brought about by the revolution of molecular biology, it soon became apparent that a seemingly endless stream of data pertaining to genetic sequence was of little avail in itself. We have begun to come to terms with the extraordinary number of genes making up the most basic of living organisms. Added to this is the growing realization that these genes, numbered in their thousands in the simplest of living organisms, interact with each other both at the level of the genome itself, and then at the level of their protein products. Therefore, a fundamental difficulty arises in our ability to understand such processes by 'traditional' methods. This tension has generated amongst others the discipline of reverse genomics (Oliver 1997), which attempts to impute function to individual genes with known and therefore penetrable sequences in the context of seemingly impenetrable complex living organisms. At the time of writing, the potential of such mathematical methods to model these interactions at the level of the single cell remains unexplored. ANNs may allow complex biological systems to be modelled at a higher level, through thoughtful experimental design and novel data derived from increasingly sophisticated techniques of physical measurement. Any behaviour at the single cell level productively modelled in this way may have fundamental consequences for medicine.

The second level concerns individual disease states at the level of individual human beings. The cause for many diseases continues to be ascribed (if not understood) to the interaction between individuals and their environment. One example here might be the variation in human response to infection with a virulent pathogen, where one individual whose (genetically determined) immune system has been programmed by his environment (Rook & Stanford 1998), may live or die depending on how the immune system responds to the invader. Complex data sets pertaining to genetic and environmental aspects in the life-or-death interaction may be amenable to ANN modelling techniques. This question of life or death after environmental insult has already been addressed using ANNs in the 'real' context of outcome in intensive care medicine (e.g. Dybowski et al. 1996). We see no reason why such an approach cannot be extended to questions of epidemiology. For example, genetic and environmental factors contributing to the impressive worldwide variation in coronary heart disease continue to be identified (Criqui & Ringel 1994), yet how these individual factors interact continues to elude us. An ANN approach to such formally unresolved questions, when coupled with rule extraction (Chapter 12), may reveal the exact nature and extent of risk-factor interaction.

The third level concerns the analysis of clinical and laboratory observations and disease. Until we have better tools to identify those molecular elements responsible for the disease itself, we rely on features associated with them whose relationship to disease remains unidentified and, at best, 'second hand'. Examples in the real world of clinical medicine include X-ray appearances suggestive of infection rather than tumour (Medina et al. 1994), and abnormal histological reports of uncertain significance (PRISMATIC project management team 1999). Until the discipline of pathology reveals the presence or absence of such abnormality at the molecular level, many pathological findings continue to be couched in probabilistic terms; however, ANNs have the potential of modelling the complexity of the data at the supramolecular level. We note some progress in at least two of these areas: the screening of cytological specimens, and the interpretation of flow-cytometric data.

Clinical pathology laboratories are being subjected to an ever-increasing workload. Much of the data received by these laboratories consists of complex figures, such as cytological specimens – objects traditionally interpreted by experts – but experts are a limited resource. The success of using ANNs to automate the interpretation of such objects has been illustrated by the PAPNET screening system (Chapter 3), and we expect that the analysis of complex images by ANNs will increase with demand.

We now switch to a different channel in our crystal ball and consider three relatively new branches on the evolutionary tree of neural computation, all of which could have an impact on clinically oriented ANNs. The first of these is Bayesian neural computation, the second is support vector machines, and the third is graphical models.

Bayesian neural computation

Whereas classical statistics attempts to draw inferences from data alone, *Bayesian statistics* goes further by allowing data to modify prior beliefs (Lee 1997). This is done through the Bayesian relationship

$$p(\xi \mid D) \propto p(\xi)p(D \mid \xi),$$

where $p(\xi)$ is the prior probability of a statement ξ, and $p(\xi \mid D)$ is the posterior probability of ξ following the observation of data D. Another feature of Bayesian inference, and one of particular relevance to ANNs, is that unknown parameters such as network weights w can be integrated out, for example

$$p(C \mid x, D) = \int_{w} p(C \mid x, w)p(w \mid D)dw,$$

where $p(C \mid x, w)$ is the probability of class C given input x and weights w, and $p(w \mid D)$ is the posterior probability distribution of the weights.

The Bayesian approach has been applied to various aspects of statistics (Gelman et al. 1995), including ANNs (MacKay 1992). Advantages to neural computation of the Bayesian framework include:

a principled approach to fitting an ANN to data via regularization (Buntine & Weigend 1991),

allowance for multiple solutions to the training of an MLP by a *committee* of networks (Perrone & Cooper 1993),

automatic selection of features to be used as input to an MLP (*automatic relevance determination* (Neal 1994; MacKay 1995)).

Bayesian ANNs have not yet found their way into general use, but, given their capabilities, we expect them to take a prominent role in mainstream neural computation.

Because of its intrinsic mathematical content, we will not give a detailed account of the Bayesian approach to neural computation in this introduction; instead, we refer the interested reader to Bishop (1995, Chap. 10).

Support vector machines

Although the perceptron learning rule (see p. 3) is able to position a planar decision boundary between two linearly separable classes, the location of the boundary may not be optimal as regards the classification of future data points. However, if a single-layer perceptron is trained with the iterative *adatron algorithm* (Anlauf & Biehl 1989), the resulting planar decision boundary will be optimal.

It can be shown that the optimal position for a planar decision boundary is that which maximizes the Euclidean distance between the boundary and the nearest exemplars to the boundary from the two classes (the *support vectors*) (see e.g. Vapnik 1995).

One way of regarding an RBFN is as a system in which the basis functions collectively map the space of input values to an auxiliary space (the *feature space*), whereupon a single-layer perceptron is trained on points in feature space originating from the training set. If the perceptron can be trained with a version of the adatron algorithm suitable for points residing in feature space then the perceptron will have been trained optimally. Such an iterative algorithm exists (the *kernel adatron algorithm*; Friess & Harrison 1998), and the resulting network is a *support vector machine*. Vapnik (1995) derived a non-iterative algorithm for this optimization task, and it is his algorithm that is usually associated with support vector machines. A modification of the procedure exists for when the points in feature space are not linearly separable.

In order to maximize the linear separability of the points in feature space, a basis function is centred on each data point, but the resulting support vector machine effectively uses only those basis functions associated with the support vectors and ignores the rest. Further details about support vector machines can be found in the book by Cristianini & Shawe-Taylor (2000).

Neural networks as graphical models

Within mathematics and the mathematical sciences, it can happen that two disciplines, developed separately, are brought together. We are witnessing this type of union between ANNs and graphical models.

A (*probabilistic*) *graphical model* is a graphical representation (in the graph-theoretic sense (Wilson 1985)) of the joint probability distribution $p(X_1, \ldots, X_n)$

over a set of variables $X_1, \ldots, X_n$ (Buntine 1994).[7] Each node of the graph corresponds to a variable, and an edge between two nodes implies a probabilistic dependence between the corresponding variables.

Because of their structure, graphical models lend themselves to modularity, in which a complex system is built from simpler parts. And through the theorems developed for graphical models (Jensen 1996), sound probabilistic inferences can be made with respect to the structure of a graphical model and its associated probabilities. Consequently, graphical models have been applied to a diversity of clinical problems (see e.g. Kazi et al. 1998; Nikiforidis & Sakellaropoulos 1998). An instructive example is the application of graphical models to the diagnosis of 'blue' babies (Spiegelhalter et al. 1993).

The nodes of a graphical model can correspond to hidden variables as well as to observable variables; thus MLPs (and RBFNs) can be regarded as directed graphical models, for both have nodes, hidden and visible, linked by directed edges (Neal 1992). An example of this is Bishop's work on latent variable models, which he has regarded from both neural network and graphical model viewpoints (Bishop et al. 1996; Bishop 1999). But graphical models are not confined to the layered structure of MLPs; therefore, the structure of a graphical model can, in principle, provide a more accurate model of a joint probability distribution (Binder et al. 1997), and thus a more accurate probability model in those situations where the variables dictate such a possibility.

In the 1970s and early 1980s, knowledge-based system were the focus of applied artificial intelligence, but the so-called 'knowledge-acquisition bottleneck' shifted the focus during the 1980s to methods, such as ANNs, in which knowledge could be extracted directly from data. There is now interest in combining background knowledge (theoretical and heuristical) with data, and graphical models provide a suitable framework to enable this fusion to take place. Thus a unification or integration of ANNs with graphical models is a natural direction to explore.

Overview of the remaining chapters

This book covers a wide range of topics pertaining to artificial neural networks for clinical medicine, and the remaining chapters are divided into four parts: I Applications, II Prospects, III Theory and IV Ethics and Clinical Practice. The first of these, Applications, is concerned with established or prototypic medical decision support systems that incorporate artificial neural networks. The section begins with an article by Cross (Chapter 2), who provides an extensive review of how artificial neural networks have dealt with the explosion of information that has taken place within clinical laboratories. This includes hepatological, radiological and clinical-chemical applications, amongst others.

The PAPNET system for screening cervical carcinoma was one of the first neural computational systems developed for medical use. Boon and Kok (Chapter 3) give an update on this system, and they do this from the viewpoints of the various parties involved in the screening process, such as the patient, pathologist and gynaecologist.

QUESTAR is one of the most successful artificial neural network-based systems developed for medicine, and Tarassenko et al. (Chapter 4) describe how QUESTAR/BioSleep analyses the sleep of people with severe disorders such as obstructive sleep apnoea and Cheyne–Stokes respiration.

Chapter 5 by Braithwaite et al. describes *Mary*, a prototypic online system designed to predict the onset of respiratory disorders in babies that have been born prematurely. The authors have compared the performance of the multilayer perceptron incorporated within *Mary* with that of a linear discriminant classifier, and they also describe some preliminary findings based on Kohonen self-organizing feature maps.

Niederberger and Golden (Chapter 6) describe another application based on multilayer perceptrons, namely, the neUROn urological system. This predicts stone recurrence following extracorporeal shock wave lithotripsy, a non-invasive procedure for the disruption and removal of renal stones. As with Chapter 5, they compare the performance of the MLP with a linear discriminant classifier. They also describe the use of Wilk's generalized likelihood ratio test to elect which variables to use as input for the multilayer perceptron. An interesting adjunct to their work is the availability of a demonstration of neUROn via the World Wide Web.

This section closes with a review by Goodacre (Chapter 7) on the instrumental approaches to the classification of microorganisms and the use of multilayer perceptrons to interpret the resulting multivariate data. This work is a response to the growing workload of clinical microbiology laboratories, and the need for rapid and accurate identification of microorganisms for clinical management purposes.

In the section entitled Prospects, a number of feasibility studies are presented. The first of these is by Anderson and Peterson (Chapter 8), who provide a description of how feedforward networks were used for the analysis of electroencephalograph waveforms. This includes a description of how independent components analysis was used to address the problem of eye-blink contamination.

ARTMAP networks are one of the least-used ANN techniques. These networks provide a form of rule extraction to complement the rule-extraction techniques developed for multilayer perceptrons, and Harrison et al. (Chapter 9) describe how ARTMAP and fuzzy ARTMAP can be used to automatically update a knowledge base over time. They do so in the context of the electrocardiograph (ECG) diagnosis of myocardial infarction and the cytopathological diagnosis of breast lesions.

Like neural computation, evolutionary computation is an example of computer science imitating nature. A solution given by Porto and Fogel (Chapter 10) to the problem of finding a near-optimal structure for an artificial neural network is to 'evolve' a network through successive generations of candidate structures. They explain how evolutionary computation has been used to design fuzzy min–max networks that classify ECG waveforms and multilayer perceptrons that interpret mammograms.

The first of the papers in the Theory section is by Ripley and Ripley (Chapter 11), who compare the performance of linear models of patient survival analysis with their neural network counterparts. This is done with respect to breast cancer and melanoma survival data.

A response to the 'black-box' issue is to extract comprehensible sets of if–then rules from artificial neural networks. Andrews et al. (Chapter 12) examine extensively how relationships between clinical attributes 'discovered' by ANNs can be made explicit, thereby paving the way for hitherto unforeseen clinical insight, and possibly providing a check on the clinical consistency of a network. They discuss rule extraction with respect to MLPs, RBFNs, and neuro-fuzzy networks. Rule extraction via fuzzy ARTMAP is also mentioned, and this chapter places the earlier chapter by Harrison et al. in a wider context. The authors also look at rule refinement, namely the use of ANNs to refine if–then rules obtained by other means. ·

By definition, some degree of uncertainty is always associated with predictions, and this includes those made by multilayer perceptrons. In the last chapter of this section, Dybowski and Roberts review the various ways in which prediction uncertainty can be conveyed through the use of confidence and prediction intervals, both classical and Bayesian.

Finally, this book addresses some issues generated by combining these apparently disparate disciplines of mathematics and clinical medicine. In the section entitled Ethics and clinical practice, Gant et al. (Chapter 14) present a critique on the use of 'black-box' systems as decision aids within a clinical environment. They also consider the ethical and legal conundrums arising out of the use of ANNs for diagnostic or treatment decisions, and they address issues of which every practitioner must be aware if they are to use neural networks in a clinical context.

NOTES

1. In the year that Golgi and Ramón y Cajal were jointly awarded the Nobel Prize for physiology and medicine, Sherrington (1906) proposed the existence of special areas (synapses) where neurons communicate, but it was not until the early 1950s (Hodgkin & Huxley 1952) that the

basic electrophysiology of neurons was understood.

2. The preprocessing was analogous to a hypothesis that the mammalian retina was composed of receptive fields. Each field was a limited area of the retina, the activation of which excited a neuron associated with that field (Hubel & Wiesel 1962).

3. To avoid ambiguity, the number of layers of a perceptron should refer to the layers of weights, and not to the layers of units (nodes), as this avoids a single-layer perceptron also being regarded as a two-layer perceptron (Tarassenko 1998).

4. It was later found that the first documented description of the back-propagation algorithm was contained in the doctoral thesis of Werbos (1974).

5. With a single hidden layer, the number of hidden nodes required to approximate a given function may be very large. If this is the case, a practical alternative is to insert an additional hidden layer into the network.

6. Another non-linear statistical technique with flexibility comparable to that of an MLP is *multivariate adaptive regression splines* (Friedman 1991).

7. *Graphical models* are also known as *belief networks, Bayesian networks* and *probabilistic networks.* Heckerman (1997) has written a good tutorial on this topic.

Appendix 1.1. Recommended reading

Recommending material to read is not easy. A suitable recommendation is dependent upon a reader's background knowledge, the topics on which he or she wants to focus, and the depth to which he or she wishes to delve.

The only book of which we know that has attempted to introduce neural networks without resorting to a single equation is that by Caudill & Butler (1990), with the unfortunate title of *Naturally Intelligent Systems.* The book does manage to convey a number of concepts to a certain extent; however, in order to learn more about neural computation, some mathematical literacy is required. The basic tools of linear algebra, calculus, and probability theory are the prerequisites, for which there are many suitable publications (e.g. Salas & Hille 1982; Anton 1984; Ross 1988).

The ideas encountered in Caudill & Butler's (1990) *Naturally Intelligent Systems* (Chaps. 1–3, 8–10, 13, 14, 16) can be expanded upon by a visit to Beale & Jackson's (1990) *Neural Computing* (Chaps. 1–5, 8). Although somewhat mathematical, this book is by no means daunting and is worthy of attention. After Beale & Jackson, the next step is undoubtedly Bishop's (1995) *Neural Networks for Pattern Recognition,* a clear and comprehensive treatment of a number of neural networks, with an emphasis on their statistical properties – a landmark textbook.

For those wishing to go more deeply into the theory, there are a number of routes from which to choose. These include taking a statistical perspective (e.g. Ripley 1996) and the statistical physics approach (e.g. Hertz et al. 1991; Haykin 1994). On the other hand, those seeking examples of medical applications can find a diverse collection in the book *Artificial Neural Networks in Biomedicine* (Lisboa et al. 2000). We should also mention *A Guide to Neural*

Computing Applications (Tarassenko 1998), a useful guide to the practicalities of neural-network development.

MATLAB (MathWorks 1997) is a powerful software package for performing technical computations, and a useful adjunct to Bishop's (1995) book is *Netlab* (Nabney & Bishop 1999), a library of MATLAB files based on his book. These files can be downloaded from http://www.ncrg.aston.ac.uk/netlab/ and they provide implementations of the concepts given in Bishop's text. The MATLAB connection is also a feature of *Neural Network Design* by Hagan et al. (1996). This well-written book provides a clear survey of neural networks (but not RBFNs), and is accompanied by many detailed examples and numerous solved problems. The book comes with a disc of MATLAB demonstration files for the user to experiment with whilst studying the text.

The book *Neural and Adaptive Systems* by Principe, Euliano & Lefebvre (2000) is also worth reading, and includes a description of support vector machines. This book is accompanied by an interactive version of the book on CD, along with a copy of the NeuroSolutions ANN simulator. However, unlike Bishop's (1995) *Neural Networks for Pattern Recognition*, neither this book nor *Neural Network Design* describe the Bayesian approach.

REFERENCES

Akaike, H. (1974). A new look at statistical model identification. *IEEE Transactions on Automatic Control* **AU-19**, 195–223.

Amari, S.-I. (1993). Mathematical methods of neurocomputing. In O. Barndor-Nielsen, J. L. Jensen & W. Kendell, eds., *Networks and Chaos – Statistical and Probabilistic Aspects.* Chapman & Hall, London, pp. 1–39.

Anlauf, J. K. & Biehl, M. (1989). The adatron: an adaptive perceptron algorithm. *Europhysics Letters* **10**, 687–692.

Anton, H. (1984), *Elementary Linear Algebra,* 4th edn. John Wiley, New York.

Bashkirov, O. A., Braveman, E. M. & Muchnik, I. B. (1964). Potential function algorithms for pattern recognition learning machines. *Automation and Remote Control* **25**, 629–631.

Baxt, W. G. (1995). Application of artificial neural networks to clinical medicine. *Lancet* **346**, 1135–1138.

Beale, R. & Jackson, T. (1990). *Neural Computing: An Introduction.* IOP Publishing, Bristol.

Berenji, H. R. (1992). A reinforcement learning-based architecture for fuzzy logic control. *International Journal of Approximate Reasoning* **6**, 267–292.

Binder, J., Koller, D., Russel, S. & Kanazawa, K. (1997). Adaptive probabilistic networks with hidden variables. *Machine Learning* **29**, 213–244.

Bishop, C. M. (1995). *Neural Networks for Pattern Recognition.* Clarendon Press, Oxford.

Bishop, C. M. (1999). Latent variable models. In M. Jordan, ed., *Learning in Graphical Models.* MIT Press, Cambridge, MA, pp. 371–403.

Bishop, C. M., Svensen, M. & Williams, C. K. I. (1996). EM optimization of latent-variable density models. In D. Touretzky, M. Mozer & M. Hasselmo, eds., *Advances in Neural Information Processing Systems,* vol. 8. MIT Press, Cambridge, MA, pp. 465–471.

Bishop, C. M., Svensen, M. & Williams, C. K. I. (1997). GTM: the generative topographic mapping. *Neural Computation* **10**(1), 215–234.

Block, H. D. (1962). The perceptron: a model for brain functioning. *Reviews of Modern Physics* **34**, 123–135.

Blum, E. K. & Li, L. K. (1991). Approximation theory and feedforward networks. *Neural Networks* **4**, 511–515.

Brachman, R. J. & Anand, T. (1996). The process of knowledge discovery in databases. In U. Fayyad, G. Piatetsky-Shapiro, P. Smyth & R. Uthurusamy, eds. *Advances in Knowledge Discovery and Data Mining.* AAAI Press and MIT Press, Menlo Park, CA, Chap. 2.

Breiman, L., Friedman, J. H., Olshen, R. A. & Stone, C. J. (1984). *Classification and Regression Trees.* Chapman & Hall, New York.

Bridle, J. S. (1991). Probabilistic interpretation of feedforward classification network outputs, with relationships to statistical pattern recognition. In F. Fogleman-Soulié & J. Herault, eds.. *Neurocomputing: Algorithms, Architectures, and Applications.* Springer-Verlag, Berlin, pp. 227–236.

Broomhead, D. S. & Lowe, D. (1988). Multivariable functional interpolation and adaptive networks. *Complex Systems* **2**, 321–355.

Buntine, W. L. (1992). Learning classification trees. *Statistics and Computing* **2**, 63–73.

Buntine, W. L. (1994). Operations for learning with graphical models. *Journal of Artificial Intelligence Research* **2**, 159–225.

Buntine, W. L. & Weigend, A. S. (1991). Bayesian back-propagation. *Complex Systems* **5**, 603–643.

Carpenter, G. A. & Grossberg, S. (1987). A massively parallel architecture for a self-organizing neural pattern recognition machine. *Computer Vision, Graphics, and Image Processing* **37**, 54–115.

Carpenter, G., Grossberg, S. & Reynolds, J. (1991). ARTMAP: supervised real-time learning and classification of nonstationary data by a self-organizing neural network. *Neural Networks* **4**, 565–588.

Caudill, M. & Butler, C. (1990). *Naturally Intelligent Systems.* MIT Press, Cambridge, MA.

Cheng, B. & Titterington, D. M. (1994). Neural networks: a review from a statistical perspective. *Statistical Science* **9**, 2–54.

Churchland, P. S. (1986). *Neurophilosophy: Toward a Unified Science of the Mind/Brain.* MIT Press, Cambridge, MA.

Collett, D. (1991). *Modelling Binary Data.* Chapman & Hall, London.

Criqui, M. H. & Ringel, B. L. (1994). Does diet or alcohol explain the French paradox? (with commentary). *Lancet* **344**, 8939–8940, 1719–1723.

Cristianini, N. & Shawe-Taylor, J. (2000). *An Introduction to Support Vector Machines.* Cambridge University Press, Cambridge.

Dabija, V. G. & Tschichold-Gürman, N. (1993). A framework for combining symbolic and connectionist learning with equivalent concept descriptions. In *Proceedings of the 1993 International Joint Conference on Neural Networks* (IJCNN-93), Nagoya, pp. 790–793.

Duda, R. O. & Hart, P. E. (1973). *Pattern Classification and Scene Analysis.* Wiley, New York.

Dybowski, R. & Gant, V. (1995). Artificial neural networks in pathology and medical laboratories. *Lancet* **346**, 1203–1207.

Dybowski, R., Weller, P., Chang, R. & Gant, V. (1996). Prediction of outcome in critically ill patients using artificial neural network synthesised by genetic algorithm. *Lancet* **347**, 1146–1150.

Elman, J. L. (1990). Finding structure in time. *Cognitive Science* **14**, 179–211.

Fahlman, S. E. (1988). Faster-learning variations on back-propagation: an empirical study. In D. Touretzky, G. Hinton & T. Sejnowski, eds., *Proceedings of the 1988 Connectionist Models Summer School*. Morgan Kaufmann, San Mateo, CA, pp. 38–51.

Friedman, J. H. (1991). Multivariate adaptive regression splines (with discussion). *Annals of Statistics* **19**(1), 1–141.

Friedman, J. H. & Stuetzle, W. (1981). Projection pursuit regression. *Journal of the American Statistical Association* **76**, 817–823.

Friess, T. & Harrison, R. (1998). Support vector neural networks: the kernel adatron with bias and soft margin. Technical report ACSE-TR-752. Department of Automatic Control and Systems Engineering, University of Sheffield.

Gelman, A., Carlin, J. B., Stern, H. S. & Rubin, D. B. (1995). *Bayesian Data Analysis*. Chapman & Hall, London.

Grossberg, S. (1976). Adaptive pattern classification and universal recording. I. Parallel development and coding of neural feature detectors. *Cybernetics* **23**, 121–134.

Hagan, M. T., Demuth, H. B. & Beale, M. (1996). *Neural Network Design*. PWS Publishing, Boston.

Hall, D. J. & Khanna, D. (1977). The ISODATA method of computation for relative perception of similarities and differences in complex and real computers. In K. Enslein, A. Ralston & H. Wilf, eds., *Statistical Methods for Digital Computers*. Wiley, New York, pp. 340–373.

Hand, D. J. (1981). *Discrimination and Classification*. John Wiley, Chichester.

Hartman, E. J., Keeler, J. D. & Kowalski, J. M. (1990). Layered neural networks with Gaussian hidden units as universal approximations. *Neural Computation* **2**, 210–215.

Haykin, S. (1994). *Neural Networks: A Comprehensive Foundation*. Macmillan, New York.

Hebb, D. (1949). *Organization of Behaviour*. Wiley, New York.

Heckerman, D. (1997). Bayesian networks for data mining. *Data Mining and Knowledge Discovery* **1**, 79–119.

Hertz, J., Krogh, A. & Palmer, R. G. (1991). *Introduction to the Theory of Neural Computation*. Addison-Wesley, Reading, MA.

Hinton, G. E. (1989). Connectionist learning procedures. *Artificial Intelligence* **40**, 185–234.

Hodgkin, A. L. & Huxley, A. F. (1952). A quantitative description of membrane current and its application to conduction and excitation in nerves. *Journal of Physiology* **117**, 500–544.

Hosmer, D. W. & Lemeshow, S. (1989). *Applied Logistic Regression*. Wiley, New York.

Hubel, D. H & Wiesel, T. N. (1962). Receptive fields, binocular interaction and functional architecture of the cat's visual cortex. *Journal of Physiology* **160**, 106–154.

Hubel, D. H & Wiesel, T. N. (1977). Functional architecture of macaque visual cortex. *Proceedings of the Royal Society of London (Series B)* **198**, 1–59.

Hwang, J. N., Lay,, S. R., Maechler, M., Martin, R. D. & Schimert, J. (1994). Regression modelling in back-propagation and projection pursuit learning. *IEEE Transactions on Neural Networks* **5**, 342–353.

Jensen, F. V. (1996). *An Introduction to Bayesian Networks.* UCL Press, London.

Kaas, J. H., Merzenich, M. M. & Killackey, H. P. (1983). The reorganization of somatosensory cortex following peripheral nerve damage in adult and developing mammals. *Annual Review of Neurosciences* **6**, 325–356.

Kazi, J. I., Furness, P. N. & Nicholson, M. (1998). Diagnosis of early acute renal allograft rejection by evaluation of multiple histological features using a Bayesian belief network. *Journal of Clinical Pathology* **51**(2), 108–113.

Kohonen, T. (1982). Self-organizing formation of topologically correct feature maps. *Biological Cybernetics* **43**, 59–69.

Krzanowski, W. J. (1988). *Principles of Multivariate Analysis.* Oxford University Press, Oxford.

Lang, K. L. & Hinton, G. E. (1988). The development of the time-delay neural network architecture for speech recognition, Technical report CMU-CS-88-152, Carnegie-Mellon University, Pittsburgh, PA.

LeCun, Y. (1985). 'Une procédure d 'apprentissage pour réseau à seuil asymétrique. *Cognitiva* **85**, 599–604.

Lee, P. M. (1997). *Bayesian Statistics: An Introduction,* 2nd edn. Edward Arnold, London.

Lisboa, P. J. G., Ifeachor, E. C. & Szczepaniak, P. S. eds. (2000). *Artificial Neural Networks in Biomedicine.* Springer, London.

Lowe, D. & Webb, A. R. (1991). Opimized feature extraction and the Bayes decision in feed-forward classifier networks. *IEEE Transactions on Pattern Analysis and Machine Intelligence* **13**, 355–364.

MacKay, D. J. C. (1992). A practical Bayesian framework for back-propagation networks. *Neural Computation* **4**, 448–472.

MacKay, D. J. C. (1995). Bayesian non-linear modeling for the 1993 energy prediction competition. In G. Heidbreder, ed., *Maximum Entropy and Bayesian Methods, Santa Barbara, 1993.* Kluwer Academic, Dordrecht, pp. 221–234.

MathWorks (1997). *Using MATLAB Version 5.* The MathWorks, Natick, MA.

McCulloch, W. & Pitts, W. (1943). A logical calculus of the ideas imminent in nervous activity. *Bulletin of Mathematical Biophysics* **5**, 115–133.

Medina, L. S., Siegel, M. J., Glazer, H. S., Anderson, D. J., Semenkovich, J. & Bejarano, P. A. (1994). Diagnosis of pulmonary complications associated with lung transplantation in children: value of CT vs histopathologic studies. *American Journal of Roentgenology* **162**, 969–974.

Michie, D., Spiegelhalter, D. J. & Taylor, C. C., eds. (1994). *Machine Learning, Neural and Statistical Classification.* Ellis Horwood, New York.

Minsky, M. L. & Papert, S. A. (1969). *Perceptrons.* MIT Press, Cambridge, MA.

Montgomery, D. C. & Peck, E. A. (1992). *Introduction to Linear Regression Analysis,* 2nd edn. John Wiley, New York.

Moody, J. & Darken, C. (1989). Fast learning in networks of locally-tuned processing units. *Neural Computation* **1**, 281–294.

Moore, B. (1989). ART1 and pattern clustering In D. Touretzky, G. Hinton & T. Sejnowski, eds., *Proceedings of the 1988 Connectionist Models Summer School*, Morgan Kaufmann, San Mateo, CA, pp. 174–185.

Nabney, I. T. (1999). Efficient training of RBF networks for classification In *Proceedings of the Ninth International Conference on Artificial Neural Networks* (ICANN 99). IEEE, London, pp. 210–215.

Nabney, I. T. & Bishop, C. M. (1999). *Netlab Neural Network Software* [online]. Available from: http://www.ncrg.aston.ac.uk/netlab/index.html [Accessed 4 May 1999].

Nauck, D., Klowonn, F. & Kruse, R. (1997). *Foundations of Neuro-Fuzzy Systems*. John Wiley, Chichester.

Neal, R. (1992). Connectionist learning in belief networks. *Artificial Intelligence* **56**, 71–113.

Neal, R. M. (1994). Bayesian learning for neural networks. PhD thesis, University of Toronto.

Nikiforidis, G. C. & Sakellaropoulos, G. C. (1998). Expert system support using Bayesian belief networks in the prognosis of head-injured patients of the ICU. *Medical Informatics* **23**, 1–18.

Nomura, H., Hayashi, I. & Wakami, N. (1992). A learning method of fuzzy inference rules by descent method. In *Proceedings of the IEEE International Conference on Fuzzy Systems*. IEEE Press, San Diego, CA, pp. 203–210.

Oliver, S. G. (1997). From gene to screen with yeast. *Current Opinion in Genetics & Development* **7**, 405–409.

Parker, D. B. (1985). Learning-logic: casting the cortex of the human brain in silicon. Technical report TR-47. Center for Computational Research in Economics and Management Science, MIT, Cambridge, MA.

Pedrycz, W. & Card, H. C. (1992). Linguistic interpretation of self-organizing maps. In *Proceedings of the IEEE International Conference on Fuzzy Systems*. IEEE Press, San Diego, CA, pp. 371–378.

Perrone, M. P. & Cooper, L. N. (1993). When networks disagree: ensemble methods for hybrid neural networks. In R. Mammone, ed., *Artificial Neural Networks for Speech and Vision*. Chapman & Hall, London, pp. 126–142.

Plate, T. A. (1998). Accuracy versus interpretability in flexible modeling: implementing a tradeoff using Gaussian process models. Technical report. School of Mathematical and Computing Sciences, Victoria University of Wellington.

Poggio, T., Tore, V. & Koch, C. (1985). Computational vision and regularization theory. *Nature* **317**, 314–319.

Powell, M. J. D. (1987). Radial basis functions for multivariable interpolation: a review. In J. Mason & M. Cox, eds., *Algorithms for the Approximation of Functions and Data*. Clarendon Press, Oxford, Chapter 19.

Principe, J. C., Euliano, N. R. & Lefebvre, W. C. (2000). *Neural and Adaptive Systems*. John Wiley, New York.

PRISMATIC project management team (1999). Assessment of automated primary screening on PAPNET of cervical smears in the PRISMATIC trial. *Lancet* **353**, 1381–1385.

Rashevsky, N. (1948). *Mathematical Biophysics*. University of Chicago Press, Chicago, IL.

Ripley, B. D. (1993). Statistical aspects of neural networks. In O. Barndorff-Nielsen, J. L. Jensen

& W. Kendell, eds., *Networks and Chaos – Statistical and Probabilistic Aspects*. Chapman & Hall, London, pp. 40–123.

Ripley, B. D. (1996). *Pattern Recognition and Neural Networks*. Cambridge University Press, Cambridge.

Ritter, H., Martinetz, T. & Schulten, K. (1992). *Neural Computation and Self-Organizing Maps: An Introduction*. Addison-Wesley, Reading, MA.

Rook, G. A. & Stanford, G. A. (1998). Give us this day our daily germs. *Immunology Today* **19**, 113–116.

Rosenblatt, F. (1958). The perceptron: a probabilistic model for information storage and organization in the brain. *Psychological Review* **65**, 386–408.

Rosenblatt, F. (1960). On the convergence of reinforcement procedures in simple perceptrons, Technical Report VG-1196-G-4. Cornell Aeronautical Laboratory, Buffalo, NY.

Rosenblatt, F. (1962). *Principles of Neurodynamics: Perceptrons and the Theory of Brain Mechanisms*. Spartan Books, New York.

Ross, S. (1988). *A First Course in Probability*, 3rd edn. Macmillan, New York.

Rumelhart, D. E., Hinton, G. E. & Williams, R. J. (1986). Learning internal representations by error propagation. In D. Rumelhart & J. McCelland, eds., *Parallel Distributed Processing*. MIT Press, Cambridge, MA, Chap. 8.

Salas, S. L. & Hille, E. (1982). *Calculus: One and Several Variables*, 4th edn. John Wiley, New York.

Sharp, D. (1995). From 'black-box' to bedside, one day?. *Lancet* **346**, 1050.

Sherrington, C. S. (1906). *The Integrative Action of the Nervous System*. Yale University Press, New Haven, CT.

Silverman, B. W. (1986). *Density Estimation for Statistics and Data Analysis*. Chapman & Hall, London.

Smith, M. (1993). *Neural Networks for Statistical Modelling*. Van Nostrand Reinhold, New York.

Spiegelhalter, D. J., Dawid, A. P., Lauritzen, S. L. & Cowell, R. G. (1993). Bayesian analysis in expert systems. *Statistical Science* **8**, 219–283.

Suga, N. (1985). The extent to which bisonar information is represented in the bat auditory cortex. In G. Edelman, W. Gall & W. Cowan, eds., *Dynamic Aspects of Neocortical Function*. Wiley, New York, pp. 653–695.

Tarassenko, L. (1995). Neural networks. *Lancet* **346**, 1712.

Tarassenko, L. (1998). *A Guide to Neural Computing Applications*. Edward Arnold, London.

Tarassenko, L., Hayton, P., Cerneaz, N. & Brady, M. (1995). Novelty detection for the identification of masses in mammograms. In *Proceedings of the 4th IEE International Conference on Artificial Neural Networks*. Cambridge Univeristy Press, Cambridge, pp. 442–447.

Vapnik, V. (1995). *The Nature of Statistical Learning Theory*. Springer-Verlag, New York.

Werbos, P. J. (1974). Beyond regression: new tools for prediction and analysis in the behavioral sciences. PhD thesis, Harvard University.

White, H. (1989). Learning in neural networks: a statistical perspective. *Neural Computation* **1**, 425–464.

Wilkins, M. F., Morris, C. W. & Boddy, L. (1994). A comparison of radial basis function and backpropagation neural networks for identification of marine phytoplankton from multivariate flow cytometry data. *Computer Applications in the Biosciences* **10**, 285–294.

Willshaw, D. J. & von der Malsburg, C. (1976). How patterned neural connections can be set up by self-organization. *Proceedings of the Royal Society (London)* **B194**, 431–445.

Wilson, R. J. (1985). *Introduction to Graph Theory*, 3rd edn. Longman, New York.

Wyatt, J. (1995). Nervous about artificial neural networks? *Lancet* **346**, 1175–1177.

Zadeh, L. A. (1962). From circuit theory to system theory. *Proceedings of the Institute of Radio Engineers* **50**, 856–865.

Zadeh, L. A. (1965). Fuzzy sets. *Information and Control* **8**, 338–353.

Zadeh, L. A. (1972). A rationale for fuzzy control. *Journal of Dynamic Systems, Measurement and Control (Series 6)* **94**, 3–4.

Part I

Applications

2

Artificial neural networks in laboratory medicine

Simon S. Cross

Introduction

Laboratory medicine is the prime generator of objective data on patients in the medical system. The development of automated analysers in haematology and clinical chemistry has led to the generation of huge amounts of numerical data for each patient and increased sophistication in radiology and histopathology have produced concomitant increases in the informational content of reports (Cross & Bull 1992). This informational explosion in laboratory medicine has led to a great need for intelligent decision support systems to assist the laboratory physicians in formulating their reports and for the clinicians who have to integrate all the laboratory information in the context of an individual patient. It is likely that neural networks will play an increasing role in such support systems given their advantages of model-free estimation, generalization and ability to process non-linear data (Alvager et al. 1994; Baxt 1994; Su 1994; Dybowski & Gant 1995; Kattan & Beck 1995).

Cytology

Cytological examination entails the examination of preparations, obtained by scraping or fine needle aspiration, in which the predominant feature is the individual cell rather than the whole tissue architecture seen in histological samples. The nature of cytological specimens, with mainly separate cells distributed on a background of plain glass, lend themselves to digitization and thresholding in image analysis systems with semi-automated measurement of features such as nuclear area or densitometry measurements. The interpretation of cytological specimens may be more difficult for humans than histological diagnosis, since the visual interpretation systems of the brain are better evolved for dealing with whole scenes rather than individual objects. All these factors combine to make cytological diagnosis a rich field for the development of intelligent decision support systems in which neural networks may feature (Weid et al. 1990).

Cervical cytology

Cervical cytology is used as a screening test for the detection of carcinoma, and dysplasia, of the uterine cervix. It has been shown to be effective with reductions in mortality from cervical carcinoma in all countries that have a well-organized screening programme. These screening programmes generate an enormous number of tests (73 million a year in the USA) and until very recently all these tests were performed by human observation. Human observation of cervical cytology is a difficult task – a typical slide will contain around 300 000 cells, all of which have to be observed. Around 90% of tests in most screening programmes are negative so there is a psychological accustomization to negativity. There is a relatively high false negative rate in the human screening of cervical cytology and this has the unfortunate consequence of allowing cases of cervical carcinoma to go untreated in that screening interval, which is around 3–5 years in most countries. The problems of false negatives are compounded by the biology of some tumours in young women that often produce very few abnormal cells in a smear and these cells are often small in size; however, these tumours behave biologically more aggressively than usual cervical carcinoma so the penalty for a false negative test is greater. For all these reasons there have been attempts to devise automated systems of screening cervical cytology from the 1940s onwards but until recently these have not been successful. One of the major problems in interpretation of the slides is the fact that many of the cells overlap in a conventionally prepared smear, there being problems in separating single cells from the background. Some systems have used specially prepared monolayers of cells prepared from cells scraped from the cervix and put into transport fluid but it has proved very difficult to get the smear-takers to change their working practices. With the advent of neural networks a few systems have appeared that do appear to offer a reasonable promise of automation, or at least semi-automation, of the screening of cervical cytology.

Foremost amongst these systems is PAPNET (Boon & Kok 1993; Boon et al. 1994, 1995a,b; Husain et al. 1994; Koss 1994; Koss et al. 1994, 1997; Ouwerkerk et al. 1994; Sherman et al. 1994, 1997; Keyhani-Rofagha et al. 1996; Kok & Boon 1996; Mango 1996, 1997; Rosenthal et al. 1996; Schechter 1996; Cenci et al. 1997; Denaro et al. 1997; Doornewaard et al. 1997; Halford et al. 1997; Jenny et al. 1997; Michelow et al. 1997; Mango & Valente 1998; Mitchell & Medley 1998; Sturgis et al. 1998) a commercially available system produced by Neuromedical Systems in New York, USA; this system is described in Chapter 3. Another system for cervical cytology has been developed by Mehdi et al. (1994). The published reports on this system are still at the stage of using individual cell images rather than automated scanning of slides but the neural network system used has some interest. The investigators used a standard multilayer perceptron with 57 measured parameters as input data from the image analysis of each cell. Initially they used a single network with four output neurons for the relevant diagnostic categories (normal, mild, moderate and severe dyskaryosis) but found that this system did not produce acceptable results. They then developed a system of three networks used in a hierarchical process: the first network distinguishes between normal/mild dyskaryosis and moderate/severe dyskaryosis and then one of two networks is used to make the further subdivision to a single diagnostic category. They used large numbers of cells (with expert cytopathological opinion as the 'gold standard') to train the relevant networks (e.g. 600-item training set and 300-item test set for the first network). The overall performance gave a false negative rate (the key parameter in this domain) of 1.4% and a false positive rate of 4.8%; this was not compared with human performance on these images but performed as well as other automated machines overall, with a lower false negative rate. One possible criticism of the study is rigid use of the mild, moderate and severe categories of dyskaryosis. Biologically the important distinction is between (a) those cells that signal a process that will progress to invasive carcinoma with a high degree of probability and (b) those that are very unlikely to progress to carcinoma. It is possible that this information was present in their 57 measured parameters on each cell but, because of rigid adherence to the somewhat arbitrary grading system used in most cytopathology laboratories, this was distorted. It would have been interesting to take the image analysis data and use an unsupervised neural network to see whether there was any distinct cluster formation that could suggest a more biologically valid division of the data.

Brouwer & MacAuley have used a Hopfield type of neural network to classify cervical cells (Brouwer & MacAuley 1995). They used either measurements from image analysis or direct digitized images as input data, with relatively small numbers of training and test sets (25). The system gave good results for distinctions between ends of the spectrum (e.g. 94% accuracy for normal/severe dyskaryosis distinction) but less impressive results for other classifications (e.g. 58% for moderate/severe). The method was much quicker than using the back-propagation method of training multilayer perceptrons with only two or three training epochs required for the network that contained only 25 neurons. The authors recognize that much larger training and test sets are required to validate these initial results. Further studies from this group (Kemp et al. 1997a,b) have used much larger numbers of images and have produced a correct classification rate of 61.6%.

Breast cytology

The cytological diagnosis of lesions of the breast presents a contrasting problem to cervical cytology. Whereas cervical cytology involves searching through a huge number of normal cells to find a few abnormal ones, in breast cytology the majority of the cells in the specimen will come from the lesion. The diagnostic process is thus mainly an interpretative problem rather than a searching vigilance task. In cervical cytology sensitivity is the key parameter, since the penalty for missing carcinoma in a screening programme is large but definitive treatment (such as loop excision) is not initiated until further investigations have been made (e.g. colposcopy), so the penalty for false positive tests is not great. In breast cytology specificity is the key parameter, since definitive treatment (e.g. mastectomy) will be performed if the cytological test is reported as malignant and this is supported by clinical and radiological suspicion of malignancy. The false positive rate in breast cytology should be as close to zero as possible whilst retaining a reasonably high sensitivity (above 80% on adequate specimens). Many countries are introducing national breast screening programmes with mammography as the screening modality but using cytology as the diagnostic method for radiographic abnormalities, leading to an increased number of these specimens.

Wolberg & Mangasarian (1993) have used a multilayer perceptron to diagnose breast cytology. Their study conforms to almost all the best principles for such studies using a large training set, a prospectively collected test set, a rigorous validation of outcome and comparison with other statistical methods (the only deficiency is statistical comparison between the different methods). The input data were nine defined human observations each rated on a scale of 1 to 10, for example cellular dyshesion clumps in which all marginal cells were adherent and not deformed were rated as 1 and those with little cohesion were rated as 10. All observations were made by a single experienced observer who was blind to the outcome at the time of observation. The multilayer perceptron had nine input neurons, a single hidden layer of five neurons and single output neuron for the dichotomous (benign/malignant) prediction. The network was trained on 420 cases and tested on a further 163. On the test set the trained network produced only one false positive (thus a rate of 0.6%) and one false negative. One of the stated advantages of neural networks is their ability to produce classifiers with good generalization and this is illustrated in this report. In the 215 carcinomas in the study there were only two that shared the same scalar values for the nine input variables. Among the benign cases (total 368) there was more duplication, with 175 cases having four or more identical input vectors, but there were still 146 with unique combinations of the scalar values. Therefore all but one of the cancers, and many of the benign cases, occurred as new combinations of scalar values for the nine input variables that were not encountered in the training set but were still classified correctly. In this study the neural network system was compared with a data-derived decision tree with dichotomous branchings and a multisurface separation method. The decision tree gave a performance inferior to that of the neural network, with nine false positives in the test set, which is an unacceptably

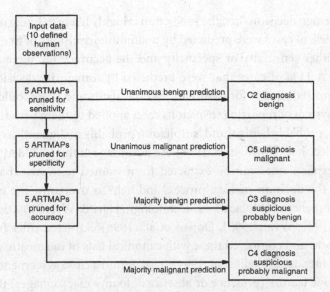

Figure 2.1.   The cascaded network of differently optimized ARTMAPs used by Downs et al. (1996) in the cytological diagnosis of fine needle aspirates of the breast.

high rate (5.5%); but the multisurface separation method was superior, with completely correct classification of the test set although the statistical significance of this was not reported.

Downs et al. (1995a,b, 1996, 1998) have reported similar studies on breast cytology using defined human observations but using the adaptive resonance theory mapping (ARTMAP) neural network architecture (Carpenter & Grossberg 1987a,b; Carpenter et al. 1991, 1992; Carpenter & Tan 1993; Carpenter & Markuson 1998). In their studies there were 10 observations, each coded in binary fashion, for example cellular dyshesion coded as 0 if the majority of epithelial cells were adhesive and 1 if the majority were dyshesive. These data are therefore less information rich than those used by Wolberg & Mangasarian (1993) but are more suitable for some biologically dichotomous variables such as the presence or absence of intracytoplasmic lumina. The networks were trained on 313 cases and tested on a further 100. ARTMAP networks cluster the input data in an unsupervised learning stage before these clusters are linked to the outcome (in this case a diagnosis of benignity or malignancy) and the formation of the input clusters is dependent on the order in which the data are presented. Downs et al. (1996) exploited this property to produce multiple networks trained on different orders of the training data and then either selected the best performers or combined them into majority voting systems and finally into a cascaded voting system (Figure 2.1). The cascaded voting system gives an indication of the confidence in the neural network prediction, since if five networks optimized for sensitivity give a unanimous benign decision then the prediction is highly likely to be correct. Using this system, 89% of cases were predicted by unanimous decisions of five networks pruned for either sensitivity or specificity and the accuracy for these cases was 100%. This left 11% of cases that were predicted by a majority decision of five networks optimized equally for sensitivity and specificity and these could have the Nottingham system of reporting suspicious cases applied to them with the reports of 'suspicious, probably benign' and 'suspicious, probably malignant' according to the majority decision (Downs et al. 1998). An advantage of the ARTMAP architecture is that explicit rules can be extracted from trained networks that give an indication of the decision-making process and help to overcome the user resistance to the impenetrable 'black-box' technology (Hart & Wyatt 1990a; Wyatt & Spiegelhalter 1991; Wyatt 1995). Downs et al. (1996) extracted rules from their trained networks and compared these with canonical lists of diagnostic criteria in the published literature (Wells et al. 1994). They found a close agreement, with the exception of one feature (presence or absence of foamy macrophages) that in the published literature was said to favour a benign diagnosis but in the network rules appeared with an equal frequency in benign and malignant extracted rules.

The same investigators have also published a study using image analysis parameters from fine needle aspirates of the breast to train a multilayer perceptron (Cross et al. 1997). The measured parameters included integrated optical density, fractal textural dimension, number of cellular objects, distance between cellular objects and derivatives (e.g. kurtosis and skewness) of these. The training set contained 200 cases and the test set 162 cases, the perceptron had a 15–12–1 architecture. The neural network produced a sensitivity of 83%, specificity of 85% and a positive predictive value of a malignant result of 85%. Logistic regression produced a virtually identical performance with no statistical difference. These performance values are well below what would be acceptable in a diagnostic situation but all the image analysis was performed automatically on a single low-power field of view of each specimen. At this magnification, nuclear detail was not resolvable (a single nucleus would be represented as a single pixel) and most of the features cited as being important in the diagnosis of breast cytology are related to nuclear detail. It is thus possible that the reported system would give much better results if combined with an analysis of nuclear images.

Cytological diagnosis of pleural and peritoneal effusions

Truong et al. (1995) have used measurements from image analysis as input data for a multilayer perceptron to classify lymphocyte-rich pleural and peritoneal effusions into malignant or reactive categories. They used data from 112 cases in a jack-knife method of training and testing, with a final neural network architecture of seven input neurons, one hidden layer of 10 neurons and a single output neuron. Measurements had been made on 200 nuclei from each case. The network gave an overall accuracy of 89% with a sensitivity of 77% and a specificity of 93%; there was no comparison with conventional statistical methods.

Cytological diagnosis of oral epithelial lesions

A study with a similar design, but applied to cells from oral smears, has been reported by Brickley et al. (1996). They made measurements of nuclear and cytoplasmic areas on 50 cells from each of 348 specimens that represented a mixture of normal, dysplastic and cancerous oral epithelium. They used patient age, patient gender, mean nuclear area, mean cytoplasmic area and mean nuclear/ cytoplasmic ratio as the inputs to a multilayer perceptron of unspecified architecture. They used two-thirds of the cases for training and the remaining one-third for testing to give discrimination between normal and dysplastic/malignant epithelium with a specificity of 82% and a sensitivity of 76%. This performance was not compared with conventional statistical analysis or human performance (the 'gold standard' outcome measure was the histological, rather than cytological, diagnosis of the excised tissue).

Cytological diagnosis of thyroid lesions

Karakitsos et al. (1996a) have used image analysis measurements of cytological specimens from thyroid lesions to train a multilayer perceptron classifier. One methodological weakness of this study is that they use single nuclei as individual items in the training and test sets. Each nucleus has 26 measurements made on it and, since 100 nuclei were measured from each of 51 patients, the investigators describe a training set of 2770 items with a test set of 11 080 items. However, within the 51 cases there were only two cases of follicular carcinoma of the thyroid and three cases of oncocytic carcinoma so the data could well have an 'oligoclonal' artefact. The authors also preprocessed the training set data, excluding any similar input vectors that had disparate outcomes. The optimal neural network had 26 input neurons, a single hidden layer of 22 neurons and one output neuron. This gave correct classification in 98% of cases, which was statistically better than the original human cytological diagnosis ($p = 0.03$).

Cytological diagnosis of gastric lesions

Karakitsos et al. (1996b) have also made a similar study of diagnosis of gastric lesions by image analysis measurements on cell nuclei. Again individual nuclei were taken as the unit item in training and test sets but in this case the possibility of 'oligoclonal' artefact was reduced, since there were 23 cases of carcinoma in the total study population of 100. Twenty-six image analysis parameters were again presented as the input data: there was a single hidden layer of 32 neurons and one output neuron. This trained system gave an overall accuracy of 98% but was not compared with human performance or conventional statistical methods. Molnar et al. (1993) have also used image analysis data (such as DNA content from Feulgen-stained preparations) from gastric cytology specimens to train a neural network classifier of multilayer perceptron type with an architecture of eight input neurons, two hidden layers each with 25 neurons, and three output neurons. Fifty-nine cases in total were used in a cross-validation training/testing method using 53 cases to train and six cases to test in each cycle. This system gave 100% accuracy of classification of benign and malignant cases and 98% accuracy for dysplastic cases (one incorrectly classified) but the huge size of the network (15 000 connections) for the small sample size suggests that there may be an element of overtraining in this study and that the classifier might not generalize to any entirely separate test set with a large number of cases. The PAPNET system has also been applied to the domain of oesophageal cytology (Koss et al. 1998) and abnormal cells were selected by the system in all cases of oesophageal cancer.

Cytological diagnosis of urothelial lesions

Hurst et al. (1997) have published a study in which they use a number of different input data sets to train multilayer perceptrons to discriminate between benign and malignant urothelial cells. The cells were all stained using a fluorescent dye linked to an antibody directed against a bladder cancer tumour-associated antigen but artefacts such as autofluorescene still produced non-cancerous cells that stained positive, but in a pattern different from that of the true tumour antigen staining. The investigators employed low and high magnification views of the cells and used both raw digitized images and image analysis measurements as input data. At high power the raw digitized images presented in a 60 × 60 pixel array as grey scale values and trained the networks using human interpretation of each cell as the 'gold standard' with a jack-knife ('leave one out') training and testing process on the 20 images. This system produced 100% agreement with the human classification but there is a huge (144 000) number of network connections compared with the size of the sample population, so overtraining may be a problem. At lower magnifications much larger training and test sets were used (216 in each) and the overall accuracy was 75%. Using image analysis measurements derived from low magnification images in a network with four input neurons, four hidden neurons and two output neurons, an accuracy of 69% was obtained. The PAPNET system has also been applied to urine cytology with good results (Hoda et al. 1997).

Histopathology

Histopathology is a discipline that is based almost entirely on subjective human interpretation of visual images; only in a very few specialist areas (such as the diagnosis of partial hydatidiform mole by flow cytometry) have quantitative techniques found routine use in histopathology. The dominant role of human interpretation is explained by the complexity of the images seen down the microscope and the very efficient processing of this information by the human brain. A single binary image at a resolution of 256×256 pixels contains over 65 000 bits of information, which places an enormous computational burden on a neural network if this is presented as raw input data, but which is a very crude representation of a microscopic image. Images at a resolution of 1024×1024 pixels and 64 000 colours are closer to the appearances seen down the microscope but still have less resolution and finer detail, which may be important diagnostically but is not visible. Neural networks have been proposed as tools that may be used in the pattern recognition and machine vision areas of histopathology (Dytch & Wied 1990; Becker 1994; Cohen 1996) and some of these potentials are being realized, but at present many neural network applications are using parameters measured from image analysis as the input data rather than the raw digitized images.

Histological diagnosis of breast carcinoma

O'Leary et al. (1992) have used data from image analysis of histological slides to train a neural network to distinguish between sclerosing adenosis (a benign process) and tubular carcinoma of the breast. They used an image analysis system to measure 18 morphological parameters and then used modified Bonferroni analysis to select those features that were significant in discriminating between the two diagnoses. These two parameters (glandular surface density and the coefficient of variation of luminal form factor) were used as the input data to a multilayer perceptron with a single hidden layer of four neurons and one output neuron. The network was trained on 36 cases and tested on a separate set of 19 cases. It classified 33 out of 36 of the training cases correctly and all 19 in the test set. Comparison was not made with conventional statistical methods or human performance but the authors comment that they would have expected a pathologist exposed to the 36 training cases to be able to correctly assign the test cases, and the 'gold standard' in this study was expert human diagnosis. The preselection of input variables is worthy of comment, since one of the postulated advantages of neural networks is that noisy or irrelevant input data is ignored as the weighting on the routes from those neurons will be adjusted during training to give no overall effect. In this study the authors could have submitted all 18 measurements on each case to the network and it is possible that subtle interactions between these variables, not revealed by the Bonferroni analysis, could have acted to improve the performance. However, since the training set was small, 36 cases, using 18 input variables would risk overtraining, with each case occupying a unique location in

18-dimensional space and a consequent loss of generalization and poor performance on independent test sets. Although the results of this study appear promising,
they would need to be validated on much larger data sets and a problem with the
overall system is that generation of the image analysis data is extremely time-
consuming, requiring tracing of glandular profiles with a light pen after some
image preprocessing and selection.

Naguib et al. (1996, 1997; Naguib & Sherbet 1997; Albertazzi et al. 1998) have
used neural networks to predict axillary lymph node metastasis using features
derived from the histopathological features of the primary tumours. The study
contained 81 unselected patients with breast cancer who had had mastectomies
and axillary lymph node sampling and these were split into a training set of 50 and
a test set of 31. The histopathology features used included grade, tumour size,
oestrogen receptor status, progesterone receptor status, nm23 oncogene protein
staining, and RB1-RB3 oncogene protein staining. They used a multilayer percep-
tron-type neural network with training by back-propagation of errors. The results
on the test set gave a sensitivity of 73% and specificity of 90%. Since the presence
of axillary lymph node metastases means that a patient should receive adjuvant
chemotherapy the sensitivity would need to be increased before axillary lymph
node sampling could be discontinued and the system used as a substitute.

Automated segmentation of renal biopsies

Neural networks have found several applications in the field of image processing
and quantification in histopathology. Applications that focus on a particular
histopathological problem are reviewed in the relevantly titled section below; this
section deals with technique-led studies. Serón et al. (1996) have used a multilayer
perceptron to segment automatically images from renal biopsies into tubules and
interstitium (the ratio of these two areas correlates with renal function measured
as the glomerular filtration rate). In digitized images they applied a local
granulometry method to each pixel to derive eight numerical values, which were
input to the neural network together with the grey scale value of that pixel. The
network had nine input neurons, two hidden layers of 10 and three neurons and a
single output neuron. One hundred and sixty pixels were selected randomly from
images of eight biopsies and the pixel visually classified as tubule or interstitium by
a human observer; these values were used to train the network. The trained
network was applied to all pixels in 202 images (a total of more than 13 million
pixels) and the output (interstitium or tubule) was used to create a visual image
and to calculate the ratio of area of tubule to area of interstitium. The images
produced had different qualitative appearances from a simple grey scale thresholded image but the correlation of both methods with the subject's glomerular
filtration rate was the same ($r = 0.73$). The neural network method showed very

close correlation with a manual point-counting method ($r = 0.92$), so it is possible that this could be implemented as an automated method of measuring these parameters.

Histological diagnosis of parathyroid lesions

Einstein et al. (1994) have used quantitative measurements of nuclear diffuseness and nuclear profile area to train a multilayer perceptron (neuron number/architecture 2–10–3) to distinguish between normal parathyroid tissue, parathyroid adenoma and parathyroid carcinoma. They used a jack-knife system of training and testing but had a very small study population of 16 cases (for a network with 50 weighted connections). The network classified 15 of the 16 cases correctly but clearly many more cases need to be examined to be able to evaluate the performance of this system.

Histological diagnosis of hepatocellular carcinoma

Erler et al. (1994) have used measurements from an image analysis system to train a neural network to discriminate between well-differentiated hepatocellular carcinoma and dysplastic hepatocytes. An image analysis system was used to measure 35 nuclear morphometric and densitometric parameters of 100 nuclei from each of 90 cases (56 hepatocellular carcinomas, 34 normal or dysplastic). Stepwise discriminant analysis was used to identify the parameters that gave the lowest classification error rates, which were then used as input data. The morphometric variables used were area, skewness of area, length of major axis, nuclear roundness factor and circularity factor. The network was a multilayer perceptron with an architecture of five input neurons, a single hidden layer of five neurons and one output neuron that was trained with 45 cases and then tested with a further 45. On the test set the neural network gave a positive predictive value of 100% and a negative predictive value of 85%, which compared favourably with 86% and 81%, respectively, for linear discriminant analysis and 86% and 77% for quadratic discriminant analysis. The criticisms that can be made of this study are similar to those of the breast carcinoma study reviewed above (O'Leary et al. 1992) that the image analysis process is too time-consuming to be used in routine practice and that the validation of the outcome (by expert human diagnosis) is open to some doubt, since this diagnostic area has been identified as too problematic to justify the undertaking of the study.

Histological grading of astrocytomas

The histological grading of astrocytomas is important for the selection of appropriate therapies, disease prognosis and a standardization of disease for comparison of trials of different therapies. Studies using the World Health Organization

(WHO) classification have shown a large amount of inter- and intra-observer variation in assigning tumours to one of the four grades, especially in the two intermediate grades. Kolles et al. (1995) have developed an automated image analysis grading system based on neural networks. From previous studies they selected four morphometric parameters – the relative nuclear area of all cells per field of vision, the relative volume-weighted mean nuclear volumes of proliferating (i.e. proliferating cellular nuclear antigen, MIB1, positive) nuclei and the mean value and variation coefficient of the secant lengths of the minimal spanning trees per field of vision. They used these parameters on a set of 68 tumours and applied cluster analysis to derive their own quantitative system of grading astrocytomas into three grades. They then used neural networks (multilayer perceptron with a 4–30–10–3 neuron/layer architecture) and discriminant analysis on training and testing sets to classify the tumours using their own unique grading system. The neural networks showed a 60% accuracy of assigning tumours to the WHO grades (as subjectively assessed by a neuropathologist) and a 99% accuracy of assigning tumours to the authors' cluster analysis-derived grades. By comparison, discriminant analysis gave overall accuracies of 62% and 92%, respectively. The main defect of this study is that the authors derived their own grading system by cluster analysis, which the neural network could reproduce very well. This shows merely that neural networks are efficient at approximating the technique of cluster analysis that the authors used. In a follow-up study Kolles et al. (1996) used a number of different neural networks on a data set similar to the first study. As well as standard multilayer perceptrons they used Kohonen and self-editing nearest neighbour networks (SEN[3]). All the employed neural networks showed similar performances in classifying the astrocytomas into grades of the three different systems examined (WHO, St Anne-Mayo system and the authors' own morphometric grading system (HOM)) and again the accuracy of classification was highest with the morphometric cluster-derived HOM system (about 90%). The SEN[3] network was much less computer intensive (1 hour of Sun SPARC2 processing time versus 1 day for the Kohonen networks) and has the advantages of incremental learning and possible rule extraction. An important follow-up to these studies would be a prospective collection of tumours and then investigation of the relationship between tumour prognosis and the automated tumour grade.

Prediction of staging in testicular teratomas

Moul et al. (Moul 1995; Moul et al. 1995; Douglas & Moul 1998) have used histological features of testicular teratomas to predict the stage of the tumour at presentation. The seven histological features used included vascular invasion in the primary tumour and percentage of tumour composed of embryonal carcinoma component and they predicted stage with an accuracy of 92%.

Histological grading of prostate cancer

The grading of prostate carcinoma is important for prognosis and associated therapeutic decisions. As is common with all tumour-grading systems, the grading of well and poorly differentiated tumours is quite reliable between observers but there is wide intra- and inter-observer variability on intermediate grades. Stotzka et al. (1995) have published a comprehensive study of a sophisticated image analysis-based system of grading prostatic carcinomas. The basic data structure used in the study was a 64×64 binary pixel array representing the spatial position of the nuclei in an area of prostatic carcinoma. When viewed alongside the photographic image of the same area this array is an enormous simplification of the original image that would be viewed down the microscope by a histopathologist but it still contains 4096 items of information, which requires an immense amount of computation if this is input into an artificial neural network in its raw unprocessed form. In one part of this paper the investigators reduced the size of the binary pixel array to 45×45 and presented this to a multilayer perceptron with 2025 input neurons, a single layer of 35 neurons and one output neuron (Figure 2.2). Training of this network required 3 weeks of computing time on a Sun SPARC workstation! Using as outcome a dichotomous grading system derived from quadratic Bayes classifiers applied to features extracted from image analysis this trained network classified the training set with an accuracy of 82% and 65% for the test set. The authors then developed an interesting hybrid system with a partially trained multilayer perceptron used to preprocess the binary image before presentation of outputs from the hidden layer of neurons to a set of statistical classifiers. This system produced an accuracy of classification of 96% on a training set and 77% on a test set but this was an improvement of only 2% on test set performance when compared with a pure Bayes classifier. This well-written paper contains much useful discussion for any investigators contemplating using image analysis systems and artificial neural networks as classifiers.

Microbiology

Rapid identification of bacteria and fungi by pyrolysis mass spectroscopy

Curie-point pyrolysis mass spectrometry is becoming a popular technique for identifying microorganisms. In this technique, pyrolysis fragments are derived from the thermal degradation of whole organisms in an inert atmosphere and these are then detected and quantified by mass spectrometry. The output data thus form a spectrum of integrated ion counts at unit mass intervals that in the past has been analysed using conventional multivariate statistical analysis. There are now several published studies (Chun et al. 1993; Goodacre et al. 1996a–c; Nilsson et al. 1996) that describe the use of artificial neural networks to interpret the mass

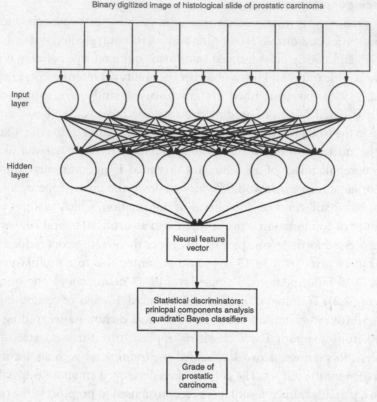

Binary digitized image of histological slide of prostatic carcinoma

Input layer

Hidden layer

Neural feature vector

Statistical discriminators:
prinicpal components analysis
quadratic Bayes classifiers

Grade of prostatic carcinoma

Figure 2.2.   The hybrid classifier system with neural network processing and statistical classifiers used by Stotzka et al. (1995) to grade prostatic carcinoma.

spectra. Chun et al. used multilayer perceptrons, trained by the back-propagation method, to identify novel species of *Streptomyces* and to discriminate between these and unknown organisms (Chun et al. 1993). They used a network with 150 input neurons entering scaled and normalized integrated ion counts at unit mass intervals from 51 to 200. The network contained a hidden layer of 10 neurons and, in its final version, four output neurons. Initially the network was trained with just the *Streptomyces* species groups A, B and C and testing of this showed complete accuracy of classification of these species but misclassification of unknown species (e.g. mycobacteria). A revised network was developed which was trained with *Streptomyces* species and other species, with the latter being given the global outcome of 'unknown'. Using a cascaded output classification this network gave 100% accuracy in identifying the individual *Streptomyces* species and classifying other species as unknown (Figure 2.3) (Chun et al. 1993). The authors suggest that clusters of neural networks could be developed and used for the sequential identification of diverse taxa. Goodacre et al. (1996b) have extended this technique to provide quantitative analysis of mixtures of bacteria such as *Staphylococ-*

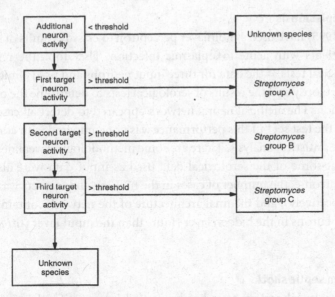

Figure 2.3. The cascaded output system used by Chun et al. (1993) to classify *Streptomyces* from
pyrolysis mass spectra.

cus aureus and *Escherichia coli*. After appropriate development and training the
authors have produced a multilayer perceptron that will provide quantitative
estimates from pyrolysis data in less than 2 minutes. Goodacre et al. (1996a) have
also used a different neural network architecture, of the Kohonen type, for
unsupervised learning of pyrolysis data from *Propionibacterium acnes* isolated
from human skin. The neural network analysis was compared with canonical
variates analysis and hierarchical cluster analysis and all three methods gave
similar results, showing that three of the human hosts examined had more than
one strain of *P. acnes* (Goodacre et al. 1996a). Neural network analysis of pyrolysis
data has also been used in the classification of *Penicillium* species (Nilsson et al.
1996). In this study conventional statistical analyses – such as principal components analysis, canonical variates analysis and hierarchical cluster analysis – could
not discriminate between the closely related species *P. commune* and *P. palitans*,
despite inclusion of data from more isolates and limiting the analysis to five
species. Use of a suitably trained multilayer perceptron resulted in correct classification of all species in the test set (Nilsson et al. 1996). Another technique that
produces spectra as output data is diffuse reflectance–absorbance Fourier transform infrared spectroscopy, which has the advantage of using intact cells without
destruction by pyrolysis. Goodacre et al. (1996c) have used neural networks
applied to the output data from this technique to identify *Streptococcus* and
Enterococcus species, again with complete accuracy, which principal components
analysis failed to match.

Diagnosis of acute toxoplasmosis

Afifi et al. (1995) have used a multilayer perceptron to classify results of serological tests on patients with acute toxoplasmic infection. They took the results from three serological tests as the data for three input neurons and used clinical history, lymph node biopsy and the results of serological tests to determine the outcome of acute infection. The artificial neural network appeared to detect all cases of acute infection in the test set but this performance was not compared with conventional multivariate statistical analysis. There are some methodological weaknesses in this study in that some of the serological data used as input data were also used to verify the outcome, the number of cases in the training and test sets was small (65 and 61, respectively), and the final architecture of the network contains a greater number of neurons in the hidden layer (four) than the input layer (three) (Afifi et al. 1995).

Prediction of outcome in septic shock

Input data from laboratory tests has been used in an artificial neural network system to predict survival in patients with septic shock (Warner et al. 1996). The input data consisted of septic shock factors interleukin-6 level, interleukin-6 soluble receptor level and a composite score derived from physiological measurements including temperature and blood pressure. The neural network was of the multilayer perceptron architecture with four input neurons, five neurons in a single hidden layer and a single output neuron. A training set of 50 patients and a test set of 18 patients were used. The best performance correctly classified 16 of the 18 patient test set into surviving and non-surviving groups. The rationale for developing the classification was to allow allocation of resources to patients who would most benefit from them, with the implication that some expensive new treatment might be withheld from those predicted to have a negligible chance of survival. However, this whole concept is flawed, since a new treatment could alter the prognosis for all the patients and this will not be taken into account during the initial training of the neural network; all new treatments require randomized controlled trials to evaluate their potential benefit.

Prediction of outcome in pneumonia

Cooper et al. (1997) have produced a paper that could be used as an exemplar for all studies examining the efficacy of neural network classifiers. The study concerns prediction of mortality from pneumonia with the aim of selecting patients for inpatient or outpatient care. The data come from a large set covering patients discharged from 78 hospitals in 23 states of the USA allowing a training set of 9847 cases and a separate test set of 4352 cases. Using these data the authors employ a wide range of different statistical classifiers: neural networks, a rule-learning

technique, two casual discovery methods, a simple Bayesian classifier, a generalized decision tree induction method, logistic regression and a k-nearest neighbour
method. The artificial neural network system was a multilayer perceptron with 67
input neurons, a single hidden layer of eight neurons and one output neuron. The
authors compared all these methods by calculating the error rate when predicting
that a given fraction of patients will survive and at a 30% survival rate all the
methods had an error rate of less than 1.5%. Over a wide range of survival
fractions each method's error rate was within 1% of the error rate of every other
model. Since there was no statistically significant difference between the methods
the usefulness of particular models was more related to the number of input
variables used and the ease with which they could be implemented. In this respect
the neural network used all 67 available input neurons and required a computer to
implement it. In contrast a hybrid learning belief network/logistic regression
method required only nine variables and 10 parameters, and could be implemented as a paper-based model. The authors comment that no attempt was made to
minimize the number of input variables for techniques such as neural networks
and that it is likely that a restricted subset of input variables could maintain the
levels of performance.

Modelling viral epidemics

Cristea & Zaharia (1994) have used neural networks to model the course of viral
epidemics in a closed community. They have used the activation thresholds of the
artificial neurons to represent the immune status of the individual to the specific
virus and the overall activation state of the neuron to represent the contagiousness
of that person. The model is most easily constructed for viruses that confer a
persistent immunity after infection and do not induce a healthy carrier state: the
mumps or hepatitis A viruses are natural examples of such agents. Using this
model implemented in a multilayer perceptron the authors have demonstrated the
different patterns that may occur with viruses with different levels of contagiousness (Cristea & Zaharia 1994).

Prediction of gentamicin concentration

Gentamicin is an antibiotic used in intravenous form to treat some serious
infections. It is nephrotoxic and monitoring its peak concentration (to prevent
nephrotoxicity) and its trough concentration (to ensure a continuing adequate
antimicrobial level) is required. Dosage may vary widely from patient to patient
owing to many factors, including size and pre-existing renal function. Corrigan et
al. (1997) have used a neural network to predict gentamicin levels at peak and
trough concentrations. They used a multilayer perceptron (with architecture of
8–5–1) inputing age, sex, height, dose, dosing interval, serum creatinine level and

time of sampling; there were 220 training cases and 20 test cases. The linear correlation coefficients for observed versus predicted concentrations were 0.90 for peak concentration and 0.89 for trough concentrations. These results appear promising and could be used to produce a system that would predict the correct initial dosage for a patient but they were not compared with conventional statistical methods that are well-developed in this area.

Radiology

The advent of digital storage of radiographs and the vast amounts of data from magnetic resonance imaging (MRI) and computed axial tomography (CT) provide an enormous amount of material that could be input into artificial neural networks in the diagnostic setting (El-Deredy 1997).

Mammography

Mammography is the primary screening modality for breast carcinoma and recent years have seen a huge increase in the number of mammograms performed (and hence radiologists required to interpret them) as a result of the introduction of breast screening programmes in many Western countries. Two approaches to the use of artificial neural networks in assisting interpretation of mammograms have been reported; one method uses human observations as the input data (Wu et al. 1993; Floyd et al. 1994; Baker et al. 1996), while an alternative method is to use direct information from digitized mammograms as input data (Giger et al. 1994; Zhang et al. 1994). Wu et al. (1993) used human observations of 43 defined features as input data for a three-layer perceptron trained by the back-propagation of errors method. A training set of 133 cases was generated from a textbook of mammographic images and a test set of 60 clinical cases with known outcome. If a neural network is to be used in a real clinical situation then its training and testing should represent that situation as closely as possible so possible criticisms of this study are the use of a textbook to derive training cases and the use of a test set that contained a considerably higher number of malignant cases than is indicated by the prior probabilities for the usual clinical context. The performance of the neural network was not compared with any conventional statistical methods but it was compared with the performance of experienced and trainee radiologists. It was found that a reduced set of 14 input features produced a larger area under the receiver operator characteristic (ROC) curve than all 43 features (0.89 versus 0.84) and this network was used in the comparisons with human performance. The performance of the artificial neural network using features extracted by an experienced radiologist was better than that of the radiologist alone (0.89 versus 0.84), but this difference was not statistically significant. The neural network was significantly better than trainee radiologists (0.89 versus 0.80) but no comparison is given for the neural network using features extracted by the trainees so it may be that the quality of feature extraction is the most important factor in making the correct diagnosis. A similar study has been performed by Floyd et al. (1994) using eight observed features on 260 cases. The neural network gave an area of 0.94 under the ROC curve compared with 0.91 for unassisted radiologists, which was statistically significant at $p = 0.08$. A follow-up study to this (Baker et al. 1996) used a separate prospectively collected set of 60 cases to test a modified version of the original network (Floyd et al. 1994). The artificial neural network gave a sensitivity for a malignant diagnosis of 100%, with a positive predictive value of 66%. Since mammography is a screening test, the result of which is confirmed by subsequent cytology or histology, then this performance is acceptable and was statistically better than that of unassisted human observers. The study also examined the effect of human inter-observer variation on the performance of the neural network and showed that the output from the network was virtually identical with all observer input data despite there being variations in this input data. This illustrates the potential advantages of neural networks over conventional statistical methods in generalization and error tolerance. In a further study this group of investigators (Lo et al. 1997) used an artificial neural network to predict whether a lesion was in situ or invasive carcinoma on mammography, since these categories require different therapies (i.e. axillary lymph node dissection for invasive carcinomas) that could be performed as a one-step procedure if mammographic prediction was accurate. Ninety-six malignant lesions (68 invasive, 28 in situ were used with seven defined human observations of mammographic features, presence/absence of axillary lymphadenopathy and asymmetric breast tissue and the patient's age. A multilayer perceptron with a 10–15–1 architecture was trained by a jack-knife procedure to produce an area of 0.91 under the ROC curve, with a specificity of 100% for carcinoma in situ and a sensitivity of 71% for invasive carcinoma. These results appear promising but the total data set contained 96 cases for a network with 165 connections so overtraining could be a problem and the effect of individual parameters is not assessed (e.g. did the vast majority of invasive carcinomas have axillary lymphadenopathy?). Another study in a similar vein by Lo et al. (1995) used only four features extracted by radiologists to produce an area under the ROC of 0.96, which was significantly better than the radiologist's unassisted performance of 0.90.

Giger et al. (1994) have used features extracted from digitized mammograms as input data for a multilayer perceptron network. The two features assess the spiculation of the edge of discrete lesions seen on mammography, one summating margin fluctuations and the other a normalized area difference. Using these features on a jack-knifed data set of 53 cases produced an area of 0.82 under an

ROC curve, which was significantly better than either feature alone (0.66 and 0.63, respectively) but similar to the subjective rating of spiculation by a radiologist (0.83). A follow-up study (Zhang et al. 1994) used a shift-invariant multilayer perceptron to detect clustered microcalcifications in mammograms using a jack-knifed study population of 168 cases. The area under the ROC was 0.91; that was significantly better than the previous neural network performance (0.81).

Sahiner et al. (1996) have used a genetic algorithm to select parameters from a wide range (587 variables) generated by image analysis of digitized mammograms and then used these to train a multilayer perceptron (with a 16–4–1 architecture). They used separate training and test sets of adequate size (504 and 168, respectively) and compared the performance of the neural network with linear discriminant analysis using ROC curves. The area under the curve for the neural network was 0.90 and it was 0.89 for the discriminant analysis, with no significant difference between the two. This suggests that in this domain it is selection of the input features that has a greater effect on the performance than the type of classifier that is used.

Wu et al. (1995b) have used convolution neural networks to analyse the pattern of microcalcification on radiographs of excised samples of breast tissue that were known to have pathological lesions within them. They used digital images as the input features and achieved an area under the ROC of 0.90 for classification of clusters of microcalcifications into benign or malignant categories. These results are impressive, but since the tissue had been excised much background noise would have been removed from the images and, unless this study leads to a system that works on mammograms of the intact breast, it will not be useful since histopathology examination of the excised tissue would provide the definitive diagnosis on such samples.

Diagnosis of pulmonary embolism

The diagnosis of pulmonary embolism is important, since immediate treatment by anticoagulation is required but this treatment has a significant morbidity and mortality so a test with high sensitivity and high specificity is required. The definitive method of diagnosing pulmonary embolism is by pulmonary angiography but this is an invasive procedure with an associated morbidity. Ventilation–perfusion (VQ) scanning is used as the initial investigation in patients with suspected pulmonary embolism because it is non-invasive. The interpretation of these scans is made by subjective human assessment and the criteria for assessing them has not reached a satisfactory consensus. Tourassi et al. (1993) have used semiquantitative data from VQ scans and a multilayer perceptron to diagnose pulmonary embolism. Their study has many exemplary features: the outcome was validated by the definitive method of diagnosis (pulmonary angiography) in all cases, the training and test sets were large (532 cases in each), performance was assessed using ROC curves, and comparison was made with unassisted human diagnosis at the time of the VQ scan. Twenty-one input features were used that represented the presence and size of a defect in a particular lung zone on ventilation scan, perfusion scan or chest radiograph. When the network was trained with 532 cases for 50 iterations, the area under the ROC curve was 0.80, which was similar to that of the human diagnosis (0.81). With 500 iterations an overtraining effect appeared, with the area under the curve reduced to 0.78, which was worse than the human performance. In a jack-knife method training and testing (so now with 1063 cases in the training set), the performance improved to give an area of 0.91 under the ROC curve, which was significantly better than the human performance ($p < 0.01$). This result emphasizes the need for large numbers of cases in the training sets for most medical applications of artificial neural networks. A follow-up study by Tourassi et al. (1995) is also exemplary in that it is testing the established neural network model on a prospectively collected data set. The data set consisted of a further 104 patients who had VQ scans and then went on to have pulmonary angiography. The area under the ROC curve for these patients was 0.80, which is similar to the non-jack-knife results from their previous study (Tourassi et al. 1993) and was not significantly better than the results of two experienced clinicians whose diagnoses were used for comparison (0.81). In a further study, using optimally selected clinical and chest radiographic findings, Tourassi et al. (1996) produced a trained neural network with an area of 0.77 under the ROC curve, which was significantly better than the human performance on the same data (0.72). The human performance in this study was from all clinicians participating in a large prospective study rather than the two experienced clinicians in the smaller prospective study (Tourassi et al. 1995). Using data from the same large study of pulmonary embolism, Patil et al. (1993) used clinical and laboratory data (e.g. arterial blood gas analysis) together with VQ scan assessment to train a multilayer perceptron to predict whether or not pulmonary embolism was present. The network had 54 input variables, a four neuron hidden layer and a single output neuron, it was trained with 606 cases and tested on a further 607. The ROC curve area was 0.82, which was not significantly different from the performance of experienced physicians (0.85) and the authors; the trained network could therefore be a useful decision support system for less experienced clinicians.

Positron emission tomography scans and the diagnosis of dementia

Positron emission tomography (PET) scans of the brain can show many abnormalities of brain metabolism and in Alzheimer's-type dementia typical patterns of abnormality have been described. However, the patterns are not totally characteristic in all cases, particularly early dementia, and interpretation is currently made subjectively. Kippenhan et al. have published two studies (Kippenhan et al. 1992, 1994) that used objective measurements from PET scans as input data for multilayer perceptrons. The data related to the metabolic activity of defined areas of the brain and the number of input neurons varied according to the resolution of the PET cameras. In the earlier study (Kippenhan et al. 1992) there were eight input neurons, a single layer of two neurons and a single output neuron (dementia/not dementia). A total of 130 cases was used (50 normal, 41 Alzheimer's dementia, 39 probable Alzheimer's dementia) in a jack-knife training/ testing methodology. For probable cases of dementia the area under the ROC curve was 0.85 for the neural network and 0.89 for subjective assessment by an expert interpreter, for possible cases the area under both curves was 0.81. In the later study, with more input data from a higher resolution PET camera, the area increased to 0.95.

Diagnosis of liver disease by ultrasound examination

Ultrasonic examination of the liver is a useful test for the diagnosis of hepatic disease, particularly the differentiation of hepatic tumours into primary hepatic tumours (which may be amenable to surgical resection) and multiple deposits of metastatic tumour (which are usually not amenable to surgical resection). The images seen on ultrasound are usually viewed in conjunction with biochemical tests of liver function when a diagnosis is made. Maclin & Dempsey (1992) have coded features (such as size of mass, whether single or multiple, hyper- hypo- or anechoic) from liver ultrasound scans and used these, in conjunction with the results of liver enzyme studies, to train a multilayer perceptron to diagnose hepatic masses. The training outcomes were validated by histological or cytological samples from the masses, 64 cases were used with a jack-knife technique of training and testing. Several different architectures were used but the most successful had the unusual configuration of 35 input neurons, two hidden layers each of 35 neurons and five output neurons. The overall accuracy of classification was 75%, which was better than that of radiologists in training (50%) but far short of the performance by board-certified radiologists (90%). A follow-up paper by the same authors (Maclin & Dempsey 1994) presents the same data but discusses improvements that could be made to the system, including using digitized images of the ultrasound examination as raw input data. Gebbinck et al. (1993) have used parameters calculated directly from ultrasound data that describe texture and other features to train both a multilayer perceptron and a non-supervised self-organizing feature map. They used a jack-knife training/test technique on a study population of 163 cases, of which 79% were normal, but they increased the data set to 1000 cases by statistical generation of more 'cases'. In discriminating between diseased liver and normal the multilayer perceptron produced specificities of 87–99%, the self-organizing network 82–95% and linear discriminant analysis 90–96%; no statistical tests were used to investigate the significance of the different performances. Analysis of the performance for assigning diseased liver to different diagnostic categories is difficult to extrapolate from the paper but the multilayer perceptron did appear to have a performance superior to that of linear discriminant analysis.

Interpretation of chest radiographs

Plain chest radiographs are used for many purposes in medicine, including the detection and diagnosis of lung infections, lung tumours and other pulmonary abnormalities; interpretation of the radiographs is made by well trained radiologists. There are several studies in the literature where artificial neural networks have been used to assist the interpretation of chest radiographs, the largest category centres on the detection and interpretation of nodules in the lung fields. Lo et al. (1993) have developed an automated system of detecting lung nodules using digitized chest radiographs, some image preprocessing and then direct use of the digitized image as input data for a multilayer perceptron neural network. The digitized radiographs were processed to enhance nodules using median filters and Fourier transforms. Areas of 32 × 32 pixels were then used as the input data for a three-layer perceptron with 1024 input neurons, 200 neurons in a single hidden layer and two output neurons. The network was trained with 60 images and tested with 153, giving an area under the ROC curve of 0.78, which appears promising but it was not formally compared with other statistical methods or human performance. A similar system has been developed by Chiou & Lure (1994) that also used 32 × 32 pixel blocks as input data to a multilayer perceptron with two hidden layers of 128 and 64 neurons and two output neurons. They divided the image blocks into eight classes, which includes true nodules and known causes of false positives (rib crossing, vessel cluster, etc.). A total of 157 blocks was used to train the network and 235 to test it. The overall accuracy of the system was 97.5%, with a 6.7% false positive rate and a 1.3% false negative rate but no comparisons were made with other statistical methods or human performance. Another study using 32 × 32 pixel blocks of digitized radiographs has been reported by Lin et al. (1993). Again some preprocessing of the image was made using ring-background subtraction before submission to a two-layer convolution neural network with 1024 input neurons, five groups in the hidden layer and five output neurons. There were 92 image blocks in the training set (40 true nodules, 52 false positive nodules) and 554 image blocks in the test set. This network gave an area of 0.80 under the ROC curve, which was equivalent to a sensitivity of 80% with two or three false detections per chest radiograph; there was no comparison with other methods. A further example of this type of methodology is that of Wu et al. (1995a) again using preprocessed digitized images presented to a multilayer perceptron. This study investigated several aspects of the system, including the effect of different numbers of pixels in the input data (blocks of 8×8 pixels were found to be most effective but this may have been due to the small numbers of cases, 32, in the whole study) and the effects of different methods of presentation of this information to the network (line by line presentation of the image was more effective than a 'square spiral' approach). The area under the ROC curve for 'obvious' nodules was 0.93 but the performance was much less impressive for 'subtle' nodules. A system using human observations of chest radiographs as input data has been reported (Gurney & Swensen 1995); it used a multilayer perceptron with seven input neurons, three neurons in a single hidden layer and one output neuron to give a dichotomous benign/malignant prediction. A jack-knife training/ testing method was used on the 320 cases that all had a proven histological diagnosis. The area under the ROC curve was 0.87, which was significantly less than the 0.89 for Bayesian analysis on the same data. One study on chest radiographs that did not look at pulmonary nodules is that of Gross et al. (1990), which used 21 defined observations on neonatal chest radiographs to train a multilayer perceptron to diagnose 12 possible cases, including amniotic fluid aspiration and respiratory distress syndrome. Seventy-seven cases were used to train the network and 103 cases were used in testing. The network had 21 input neurons, a single hidden layer of 15 neurons and 12 output neurons. Since there was no 'gold standard' by which outcome could be validated, the performance of the network was only compared in terms of agreement with the observations of two experienced radiologists. The results showed that the agreement between the network and each of the radiologists was greater than between the radiologists but it is difficult to draw any conclusions about absolute performance.

Ultrasound diagnosis of gallbladder disease

Rinast et al. (1993) have extracted 19 image analysis parameters from digitized ultrasound images of the gallbladder in 90 cases and used these to train a multilayer perceptron using human interpretation of the image as the 'gold standard' of outcome. They used a jack-knife method of training and validation and compared the artificial neural network performance with that of nearest neighbour analysis and linear discriminant analysis. The neural network gave the best performance, with 99% accuracy, but linear discriminant analysis produced 97% accuracy and no formal tests were made to compare the relative performance of these methods.

Diagnosis of dementia and cocaine abuse using cerebral perfusion scans

The cerebral perfusion scan, where a radiolabelled agent that remains in the blood is injected, is another radiological test subjectively interpreted by trained observers. Chan et al. (1994) have used quantitative data from such scans to train a multilayer perceptron to distinguish between normal and demented subjects and between normal and chronic cocaine polydrug abusers. They used quantitative measures of cerebral perfusion (i.e. the count of radiolabel) in 120 identified volume units (voxels) for each scan and then trained a network with 120 input neurons, eight neurons in a single hidden layer and one output neuron (for the normal/dementia distinction) and 120 input neurons, two hidden layers with 28 and four neurons, and a single output neuron (for the normal/cocaine abuse distinction). They used separate training and test sets with a total of 81 cases for the dementia study and 61 cases for the cocaine abuse limb. The area under the ROC curve for the dementia diagnosis was 0.93 and it was 0.89 for the diagnosis of chronic cocaine abuse, but the network performance was not compared with conventional statistical methods or human interpretation.

ID number recognition

An apparently trivial (in the sense of use of technology) problem for which artificial neural networks have been used is the recognition of identification (ID) numbers on radiographs (Itoh 1994). The justification for this use is that if automated analysis of radiographs is to be possible then automatic recognition of ID numbers will be required and these will be subject to some distorting processes during the exposure and processing of the radiographs. Itoh (1994) used 550 characters on radiographs (10 arabic numbers and the alphabetic characters S and M in the distribution of usual prior probabilities) to train a two-layer perceptron and then tested this with a further 575 characters. The network failed to recognise three characters in the test set but identified all the others correctly.

Focal bone lesions

Reinus et al. (1994) have used a multilayer perceptron to diagnose focal bone lesions (both benign and malignant) using 95 input variables that ranged from measurements made by human observers (e.g. maximal diameter of the lesion) to subjective human observations (e.g. degree of edge definition). They used a jack-knife training and test strategy on 709 lesions. There were no comparisons with other statistical methods but comparison with human performance was implicit (though not comparable), since the outcome used to train the network was human diagnosis. The network diagnosed 56% of lesions correctly if its first choice was taken and included the correct diagnosis in a differential of three in 72% of cases. This rather poor performance is not surprising if the human diagnoses used as outcome in training are examined, since nine diagnoses were represented by single cases and 24 diagnoses by fewer than 10 cases each. The cases were split into four groups and three-quarters used to train each network and a quarter to test it so it is very likely that some diagnoses were not represented in the test set but were present in the training set. Since focal bone lesions represent discrete diagnostic categories with little overlap, and not continuous spectra, it is very unlikely that such training deficiencies would be compensated for by the inherent generalization properties of neural networks.

Magnetic resonance imaging of astrocytomas

Christy et al. (1995) have used defined human observations of features of magnetic resonance images (MRI) of astrocytomas to train a multilayer perceptron to predict whether the astrocytoma would have a low or high histological grade when biopsied and examined histologically. A problem with the design of this study is that the 'gold standard' for histological grade is taken as the subjective grading of the tumour by a neuropathologist into one of four categories without examination of the intra- or inter-observer variability of this process. The study also uses defined human observations of features on the MRI images as input data without testing the reproducibility of the data. The accuracy of the artificial neural network in a dichotomous division of the tumours into low and high grade was 61%, which compared with 59% for multivariate linear regression and 57% for subjective assessment by a radiologist and there was no statistically significant difference between any of these results.

A more sophisticated study has been carried out by Usenius et al. (1996) and has the immediate advantage of using raw objective data as the input material to the neural network. The study used in vivo nuclear magnetic resonance spectro-scopy with a water-suppressed ^1H scanning technique. The data were preprocessed to remove residual water-associated spectra and then 207 points from the spectra were presented to the input neurons of a multilayer perceptron that had two hidden layers of 60 and 30 neurons and four output neurons. Data from 33 tumours and 28 normal controls were used with a jack-knife technique of training and testing. The neural network gave 100% accuracy in discriminating between normal and abnormal tissue and 82% accuracy for the histological type of tumour but there were some misdiagnoses across the benign/malignant classification boundary. This study shows considerable promise as a non-invasive means of classifying human brain tumours. The results might be improved just by expansion of the training set, since six diagnostic categories were represented only by a single case, which by definition would be excluded from the training set by the jack-knife technique used in this study.

Brain ventricular size on computed tomography

Fukuda et al. (1995) have made linear measurements from computed tomographic (CT) scans of brains and used these, together with patient age, as input data for an artificial neural network to assess ventricular size. The main defect of this study is the outcome measure used for training, which was a consensus subjective grading of the scans into three categories – normal, slightly enlarged or definitely enlarged. Since CT scans provide three-dimensional data it would have been possible to use a reconstruction method that would have provided an accurate objective estimate of ventricular volume as the outcome measure. The study used a multilayer perceptron with a training set of 38 patients and a test set of 47 patients with relatively small numbers of cases of definite enlargement (12% of the total population). The neural network misclassified only one case in the test set but there was no comparison with other statistical methods.

Skeletal age

The determination of skeletal maturity is often performed in paediatric practice and if it differs significantly from the subject's chronological age this indicates skeletal growth abnormality. Skeletal maturity is usually performed by a paediatric radiologist, who compares the appearances of a radiograph of the subject's hand with those in a specialist atlas. Gross et al. (1995) have taken seven linear measurements from hand radiographs and calculated four parameters that they have used as input data for a multilayer perceptron. They used a population of 521 subjects with a jack-knifing training and test strategy. The results from the neural network were compared with observations of a consultant radiologist. There was no difference between human and artificial neural network performance, with a mean difference from the chronological age of −0.23 years for the radiologist and −0.26 for the neural network so the neural network could only have a potential advantage if less experienced human observers produced less reliable results.

Isotope scans

Isotope scans, in which a patient ingests or is injected with a radiolabelled substance that is then distributed according to some aspect of function, provide relatively low resolution images that could be used as direct input data for artificial neural networks. Ikeda (1996) has used data from isotopic liver scans to train a multilayer perceptron but the data were linear measurements from the images such as the ratio of sizes of the left and right lobes. Thirty-six patients were included with a histopathological diagnosis (chronic hepatitis, severe fibrosis, frank cirrhosis) from liver biopsy as validation of the outcome. Fifteen cases were used for training and 21 for testing. The overall accuracy of assignment to the diagnostic categories was 77%, which was better than the fuzzy inference method also used, but statistical comparison of the methods was not made.

Clinical chemistry

Clinical chemistry is now a specialty dominated by massive parallel analysers capable of producing thousands of results each hour and it is natural that investigators have applied artificial neural networks to the data produced by these machines (Winkel 1994; Shultz 1996). Whether this application has been an indiscriminant search for relationships between unconnected data or a more considered approach to diagnosis is discussed in the reviews of individual studies under specific headings below.

Diagnosis of cancer from blood tests

Astion & Wilding (1992) conducted a study of the utility of nine parameters measured in patient serum to discriminate between patients with malignant and benign breast disease. The study is interesting because none of the parameters (triglycerides, cholesterol, high-density lipoprotein (HDL)-cholesterol, apolipo-protein A, apolipoprotein B, albumin, 'tumour marker' CA15-3, nuclear magnetic resonance linewidth and age) are a direct measurement of a product of a malignant breast tumour and only two showed a univariate statistical difference between the benign and malignant groups. Any discrimination between the two groups must therefore be due to differences in patterns of these nine paraneoplastic markers. The authors used a multilayer perceptron with training by back-propagation of errors in an architecture with nine input neurons, one hidden layer of 15 neurons and two output neurons. The training set contained 57 cases and the test set 20 cases; comparison was made with quadratic discriminant function analysis.

The neural network correctly classified all cases in the training set and 80% of cases in the test set, which was better than the performance of the discriminant function analysis (84% correct classification on the training set, 75% on the test set). The numbers in the study are small but show encouraging results and, although the diagnosis of the primary breast carcinoma will always be by direct means (e.g. fine needle aspiration cytology), this may be a method of detecting metastatic disease after resection of the primary tumour. A follow-up study by Wilding et al. (1994) using larger numbers of cases gave rather lower performance, with a sensitivity of 56% and specificity of 73% for breast cancer patients, which was little better than the tumour marker CA15-3 alone (61% and 64%, respectively). Results on ovarian cancer patients gave a sensitivity of 81% and a specificity of 86%, but the performance of CA15-3 alone was again close to these levels (78% and 82%). A similar study (Dwarakanath et al. 1994) used the methyl and methylene regions of nuclear magnetic resonance spectra of patient's blood to distinguish between those with and those without colorectal carcinoma. A multilayer perceptron with 27 input neurons, two neurons in a single hidden layer and one output neuron was used and produced complete discrimination on a 37-case training set, but no separate test set was reported in this study.

Prediction of ischaemic events due to coronary artery atherosclerosis from serum lipid profiles

Several different serum lipids have proven associations with the development of coronary artery atherosclerosis and subsequent ischaemic events in the myocardium but measurement of these gives a population-based statistical risk rather than an individual prediction. Lapuerta et al. (1995) have used a multilayer perceptron neural network to predict ischaemic events (e.g. myocardial infarction) from measurement of seven different serum lipids. The data they used came from a randomized placebo-controlled clinical trial evaluating the effects of lipid-lowering drugs on clinical outcomes in patients with known coronary artery disease. The study highlights many of the problems that can arise when using artificial neural networks to predict temporally related events. The main problem is how to deal with censored data, i.e. patients who do not have complete follow-up for the whole trial. Such patients may have follow-up with no disease for a year but are then lost to follow-up and no further data are available. If such patients are excluded then this can introduce selection bias into a study, since those without further disease are more likely to be lost to follow-up (those with further disease, in this study myocardial infarction, are likely to re-present to medical services even if they do not attend regular follow-up appointments). The study of Lapuerta et al. (1995) uses an unusual strategy to deal with censored data by imputing the outcome for patients lost to follow-up using neural networks trained on the uncensored data for that time period. They divided the study into three time periods and then trained multilayer perceptrons for each period using patients on whom complete data were available. If a patient was lost to follow-up during the second period then the input data for that patient was put into the trained network for the second period and the prediction of the network was used as the outcome in the final complete analysis. Since the authors also used a modified jack-knife approach to segregation of training and test sets this appears to be a rather circular way of dealing with censored data and not as secure as other methods proposed for tackling this problem (Burke 1994; Clark et al. 1994; De Laurentiis & Ravdin 1994a,b; Liestol et al. 1994; Ohno-Machado et al. 1995; Burke et al. 1996). The performance of the final network was relatively modest, with a 66% accuracy of prediction, but this was statistically better than a Cox regression model developed on the same data (56%, $p = 0.005$) (Lapuerta et al. 1995). This study has another methodological problem because the data were taken from a randomized trial of lipid-lowering drugs but the data used appear to be for all patients in the trial rather than just those on the placebo, which may well distort the relationship between serum lipids and ischaemic events.

Prediction of acute myocardial infarction from serum myoglobin measurements

Kennedy et al. (1997) have used serum myoglobin measurements, in combination with clinical features, to diagnose acute myocardial infarction in accident and emergency departments. They used a multilayer perceptron with training by back-propagation of errors. Ninety cases were used to train the network and 200 cases to test it. The sensitivity and specificity on the test set were 91.2% and 90.2%, which were significantly better than linear discriminant analysis (77.9% and 82.6%, respectively). Myoglobin measurements on their own were highly specific but relatively insensitive (38%) but when combined with the clinical features in the neural network system the results are good enough to be used in the working environment.

Prediction of the activity of hepatitis from isoforms of serum alkaline phosphatase

Wallace et al. (1996) have used a multilayer perceptron neural network to predict whether or not a hepatitic process was active employing data of the isoforms of serum alkaline phosphatase and other liver-associated enzymes. They used a training set of 34 patients and a test set of 34 and constructed various network architectures by varying the number and selection of input variables. It is interesting that the best performance was achieved with either four selected input variables (alkaline phosphatase, aspartate aminotransferase, alanine aminotransferase and total bilirubin) or all 11 measured variables. From theoretical considerations it is thought that most artificial neural network architectures should ignore noisy or irrelevant input data during the training period with no decrease in performance (or subsequent improvement in performance if noisy input data is excluded), which this study confirms in contrast to other studies (Narayanan & Lucas 1993).

Haematology

Control of anticoagulation with warfarin

Warfarin is a drug widely used for anticoagulation but it is often difficult to titrate the dose to produce the desired degree of effect. This is because of the complex pharmacodynamics of warfarin, which include a long biological half-life and complex interactions with other drugs including alcohol. Narayanan & Lucas (1993) have developed multilayer perceptrons that predict the degree of anticoagulation, using the information of the dosage of warfarin on the preceding 7 days, the degree of anticoagulation when last measured and the time since anticoagulation was last measured. The method of developing trained neural networks was complex, using a genetic algorithm to select five out of the nine possible input data and an architecture that included two hidden layers. Networks were developed for individual patients and then its prediction performance was compared with actual measurements of anticoagulation. The performance of the artificial neural networks was not compared with any conventional statistical techniques. It is difficult to assess the utility of these networks given the lack of comparison with other techniques but it appears that the use of the genetic algorithm in selecting input variables reduced the error to 25% of that found when using all the variables (Narayanan & Lucas 1993). This in itself may be an anomalous result, since one of the postulated theoretical advantages of neural networks over conventional statistical techniques is a resistance to noise in the input data.

Molecular biology

The advent of rapid methods of sequencing DNA and RNA have led to an explosion of information in the field of molecular biology and one direct use of neural networks is in the interpretation of output from automated sequencers into one of the four specific base types (Golden et al. 1993). The Human Genome Project has completed the sequencing of the human genome and the data on mutations in disease are proliferating at an ever-increasing rate. There is thus a huge requirement for software that can assist in the interpretation of the data. Much of the requirement is for database software that allows the comparison and alignment of newly sequenced nucleotides with known sequences and artificial neural networks have been used as associative memory in such software (Wu et al. 1993) but the main areas of use have been the detection of coding regions in DNA and the prediction of protein structure (Rawlings & Fox 1994; Wu 1997).

Gene classification from DNA sequences

Eukaryotic DNA is made of genes and intervening lengths of DNA whose function is currently uncertain (so-called 'junk' DNA). Within each gene there are regions that code for proteins (exons) and non-coding regions called introns. The code at the start and finish of a gene, or the start and finish of an exon, has some statistical similarity with the start and stop regions of other genes but there are no unique combinations of base-pairs that can be used to find these points with 100% accuracy. This poses obvious problems for those who are sequencing unknown regions of DNA that may, or may not, contain genes with coding regions. Several systems with artificial neural networks have been developed to assist in the identification and classification of genes.

A problem with the use of neural networks in classification of DNA sequences is the coding of the input vectors for the network. DNA consists of chains of nucleotide bases of four types – adenosine (A), thymine (T), guanine (G) and cytosine (C) – but there is no logical ordinal sequence for these bases. This means that they cannot be coded directly as four digits (e.g. 0,1,2,3) for one input neuron. If direct coding of the sequence is required, it is usually done as binary coding for four input neurons (e.g. 0,0,0,1 represents adenosine; 0,1,0,0 represents thymine, etc.) but whilst an improvement on the numerical coding for a single neuron it attributes some artificial positional data to the different bases. Direct coding also produces a huge input vector, since a single gene can be composed of thousands of base-pairs. An alternative strategy is to use some statistical condensation of the information in the DNA as input data that reduces the size of the input vector but could be losing some unknown information during this preprocessing phase. Wu (1996) has used the latter approach to produce a neural network-based gene classification system. She has used an n-gram hashing method of coding the sequence. This extracts and counts the occurrence of patterns of n consecutive bases using a sliding window across the entire sequence producing frequency, rather than positional, data that is length invariant. This method still produced input vectors that were too large to present to the neural network (sometimes 8000 items) so a singular value decomposition method was used to extract the semantics from the patterns and reduce the overall size. Wu used conventional back-propagation three-layer perceptrons and a more sophisticated counter-propagation network with an input layer, hidden Kohonen layer and a Grossberg outstar conditioning layer. From existing sequence databases, 12 572 examples were used to train the network to make predictions as to which protein superfamily the sequence was coding (training took 1.4 hours of Cray central processor unit (CPU) time). At a low threshold for fit, 81% of sequences were classified correctly, at a more stringent threshold only 52% were correctly classified but incorrectly classified sequences were reduced to 0.23%.

Cai & Chen (1995) developed a neural network discrimination model to identify the promoter, poly(A) signal, splice site position of introns and noose structures within genes. They used 256 eukaryotic genes in the training set and 48 genes in the test set and used a multilayer perceptron architecture. They found that as long as the coding length was fixed the artificial neural network would always recognize these gene substructures with 100% accuracy but if the length was variable there was a steep decline in performance. This latter result is disappointing, since in the usual situation of a newly characterized sequence the alignment of that sequence, and hence length between objects, will be unknown.

Sun et al. (1995) have used a back-propagation multilayer perceptron to recognize transfer RNA (tRNA) gene sequences. They used a relatively novel strategy to test for homology between sequences. They take a sequence of DNA as the input data for a network but omit the middle base and train the network to predict what that base will be. The network can be trained on genes from one species, for example *Homo sapiens*, and then tested on a different species. The rate of correct prediction of the middle base will then give an index of the homology of the bases in these regions of DNA for the different species. They used a sliding window of 15 bases as the input layer, a single hidden layer of up to 60 neurons and four output neurons. When using tRNA sequences from mammals the network gave a correct base prediction rate of 73% when trained with mammalian sequences but this fell to 46% when tested on invertebrate tRNA sequences, indicating some, but by no means total, homology in these sequences (there was a 27% correct classification rate for random test sequences, as would be expected with four different bases). The advantages of using this system over straight base homology comparisons is not entirely clear but it could evaluate the pattern of the bases as well as their occurrence in specific locations.

Prediction of protein structure from amino acid sequences

When a segment of DNA has been sequenced and the exons identified within a gene then the chain of amino acid residues for which this DNA will code can be deduced from a simple table. What is much more difficult is the prediction of the structure of the protein that these residues will form. For protein sequences that have significant similarity to sequences with a defined structure then quite accurate predictions of three-dimensional structure can be made but for all other sequences structure prediction is difficult.

Rost (1996) has applied artificial neural network technology to this problem and has developed a sophisticated hybrid system that can predict such features as secondary structure, relative solvent accessibility and transmembrane helices. The part of the system predicting secondary structure and transmembrane helices consists of two consecutive multilayer perceptrons. The input data to the first perceptron is composed of a sequence of 13 amino acid residues (from a sliding window along the sequence) and four other terms – the percentage of each amino acid in the protein, the length of the protein, the distance of the central input residue from the N-terminal end and the distance from the C-terminal end. The network contains a single hidden layer and three output neurons predicting whether the central input residue is in a structural helix, strand or a loop. The network was trained on sequences from proteins with known three-dimensional structures. The second network in the chain has the same structure as the first except that the output prediction from the first network is included as an input. The author explains the rationale behind this by pointing out that training exemplars are chosen at random so adjacent sequences are most unlikely to be presented to the network consecutively. This means that the network does not have the opportunity to learn patterns involving correlations between adjacent sequences such as the known structural fact that helices contain at least three residues. The second network introduced a correlation between adjacent residues, with the effect that predicted secondary structure segments or transmembrane helices have length distributions similar to those observed. The network for predicting relative solvent accessibility was single and had 10 output neurons splitting the prediction into 10 percentage bands (e.g. maximal value in the fourth output neuron indicated a relative solvent accessibility of between 9% and 16%). The author used 'jury' decisions by multiple networks to increase overall accuracy and applied simple filters to the outputs to correct wildly unrealistic predictions (e.g. a helix of fewer than three residues). The accuracy of prediction was $72 \pm 9\%$ for secondary structure, $75 \pm 7\%$ for relative solvent accessibility and $94 \pm 6\%$ for transmembrane helices, which appear quite promising, although it must be remembered that there are a limited number of predictions that can be made (three states for the secondary structure). The author has made the prediction system available to users by email

(http://www.embl-heidelberg.de/predictprotein/predictprotein.html)

and the system had dealt with 30 000 predictions at the time of publication.

Chandonia & Karplus (1996) have also used a multilayer perceptron to predict protein secondary structure. They entered only the amino acid sequence and coded each amino acid by a binary coding in an array of 21 input neurons so the optimal window of 15 amino acid residues required 315 input neurons. They experimented with many different numbers of neurons in the single layer and found eight produced optimal performance. Using this optimized system they produced a 67% accuracy of prediction, which was an improvement on their previous results (63%), which were generated using a smaller training set and fewer hidden neurons. The introduction of sequence profiles to the prediction improved the accuracy to 73%, suggesting that the sequence profiles contain some information that the neural network was not extracting from the raw amino acid input data. A system of predicting the tertiary structure of proteins, by predicting two dihedral angles for each residue, has been developed by Vanhala & Kaski (1993) using a multilayer perceptron. It is difficult to perform formal statistical analysis of the results but the computer-generated pictures of the structure from the neural network predictions are similar to those obtained from crystallographic data. Thompson et al. (1995) have developed a neural network system that predicts the pattern of polypeptides that can be cleaved by human immunodeficiency virus (HIV) 1 protease. The input data was a window of amino acid residues from the protein together with the calculated hydrophobic, α-helix and β-sheet propensities of the protein. The output was a single neuron predicting whether or not the protein would be cleavable. The network achieved an accuracy of 89% on the test set. The authors then used the trained network to investigate the effects of mutations in the protein (producing changes in single amino acid residues) on the cleavability.

Prediction of amino acid sequences from NMR spectra of proteins

In the previous section systems were described that predict protein structure from given amino acid sequences. This section describes a system that acts in reverse; taking a whole protein, examining it by nuclear magnetic resonance (NMR) and predicting the amino acid content from this. The system that Hare & Prestegard (1994) have developed takes an NMR spectra divided into 71 segments (and thus 71 input neurons) and uses this to predict the amino acid residue (one of 17 in their training and test systems). They experimented with different numbers of neurons in a single hidden layer and found four to be optimal; five gave better results on the training set but gave a lower performance on the test set due to a lack of generalization. Using a constraint satisfaction algorithm produced the best results, with 75% correct sequential assignments. The training and test sets contained proteins with 37% sequence homology, which could have led to a bias in the performance, and training on a large database of proteins would be required to produce a more generalized system.

Prediction of chemical mutagenicity

There is a great need to predict the mutagenicity of chemicals from their structural characteristics, since testing for mutagenicity is time-consuming, expensive and cannot be performed at a rate to keep up with the discovery of new chemicals. Brinn et al. (1993) have developed an artificial neural network system that makes prediction of mutagenicity from chemical structure information. The investigators took 607 substances that had been tested for mutagenicity in validated biological systems (488 mutagens, 119 non-mutagens) and deconstructed these into chemical fragments using an established method. Using the 100 most discriminant fragments they trained a multilayer perceptron (with a 100–10–2 architecture) to predict mutagenicity. The network performed with 89% accuracy on the training set and 94% accuracy on the test set (an apparently anomalous increase in performance that is not easily explained). This performance would not be sufficient to classify chemicals as mutagenic or non-mutagenic without biological testing but it does enable the relative risk to be assessed and particular chemicals to have their biological testing prioritized. The authors also used a technique that enabled them to describe the trained weights in the hidden layer in terms of clusters of mutagens and non-mutagens and they found that some of these clusters were structurally homogeneous, providing some demonstration of how the neural network classifier was operating.

Prediction of metastasis from gene expression

Albertazzi et al. (1998) have used neural networks to predict disease progression in breast cancer from the relative expression of the oncogenes h-*mts-1* and *nm23*. They used Kohonen's self-organizing maps and the back-propagation of errors. The input data consisted of levels of expression of h-*mts-1* and *nm23* together with patient age, tumour size, tumour grade, percentage of oestrogen receptor-expressing cells and percentage of progesterone-expressing cells. The study population was relatively small, with 17 cases in the training set and 20 in the test set. The authors state that care was taken to ensure that overtraining did not occur but do not specify the methods that they used to avoid this. Their results appear to show that the presence or absence of metastases in axillary lymph nodes in these patients with breast cancer could be predicted with 100% sensitivity and 80% specificity but they do not explicitly state that these results are for only the test set and it is possible that the results for the training set are included in these figures.

Laboratory information systems

Laboratory medicine generates a large amount of data in both visual (e.g. radiographs, cytology and histology slides) and numerical (e.g. output from parallel chemistry analysers) forms for a large number of patients. Laboratory information systems have to be developed that can assist in the interpretation, storage and retrieval of these data and artificial neural networks can play a role in all three aspects. The theoretical advantages of using neural networks in the interpretation of data in laboratory medicine have been expounded (Eklund & Forsström 1995; Fogel et al. 1995) and many examples are reviewed in the problem-specific sections above. More general references covering generic techniques in image processing and storage are reviewed in the section below.

Image processing

Images in medicine, such as radiographs or histology slides, are interpreted by trained human observers in virtually all applications, with very little contribution from automated measurement systems. The human brain has evolved into a highly efficient processor of visual information that can handle a much higher load of information than any currently available computer systems. In a few environments, such as histological diagnosis of muscle disorders or quantification of metabolic bone disease, objective measurements are made on image analysis systems, but even in these instances the segmentation of the image is usually performed by a human operator in interaction with the computerized system. There is a continuing impetus to develop automated systems that will interpret medical images and so provide objective and reproducible interpretation but the problems in developing such systems are immense and currently the trained human observer provides the most accurate and cost-effective method. Artificial neural networks can play a role in several parts of the automated process including image segmentation (Lin et al. 1996; Schenone et al. 1996; Zhu & Yan 1997), image compression (Dony et al. 1996), feature selection (Sahiner et al. 1996), and higher level interpretation (Nazeran et al. 1995).

Schenone et al. (1996) have used a neural network model, based on a standard competitive self-organization, to produce a completely unsupervised approach to clustering and classification in the process of segmenting images of the brain obtained by MRI. The advantages of this system are two-fold. Firstly, the number of clusters that the network has to partition data is not a parameter for the network but is autonomously discovered during the learning phase. Secondly, the partition of data that comes out of the learning phase takes into account the natural scale of spatial density within the distribution of the data. The authors demonstrate the utility of their system by pictures of processed MR images and graphical representations of voxel classification in the feature space. The classification of voxels to different features appears stable but it is difficult to carry out statistical comparison with other methods. Two independent groups (Lin et al. 1996; Zhu & Yan 1997) have used variants of the Hopfield neural network architecture with unsupervised learning to segment cerebral MRI scans. Lin et al. (1996) have used a fuzzy variant of the Hopfield neural network to segment MRI scans into white matter, grey matter, cerebrospinal fluid, cerebral infarction and background. Their results show correct classification rates varying from 99% for background to 94% for cerebrospinal fluid on normal scans. The classification rate fell to 90% for areas of cerebral infarction but it might be expected that such areas would have properties falling on the boundaries of segmentation of normal tissues. One large advantage of this system is that it interprets multispectral information from the MRI scans, integrating them into a single image. Zhu et al. (Zhu & Yan 1997) have also used a Hopfield neural network to segment the boundaries of cerebral tumours on MRI scans (Figure 2.4). Images presented in that paper show accurate segmentation of the tumours but again comparison with other statistical methods is difficult to perform.

Digitized medical images occupy a huge amount of memory in uncompressed format. With the advent of optical storage devices, such as recordable compact discs, the storage of such images at source is less problematic than it was but it is still a huge problem if these images are to be transmitted to other sites. Any compression method must retain the detail required for diagnosis and must not

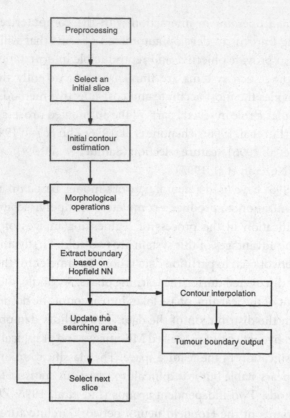

Figure 2.4.   Schematic diagram of the method used by Zhu et al. (Zhu & Yan 1997) define the boundaries of astrocytomas on magnetic resonance imaging scans. NN, neural network.

add spurious information that could be misinterpreted. Dony et al. (1996) have used a neural network-based image compression method to reduce the file size of digital chest radiographs. The method partitions data into a number of discrete regions that form M-dimensional subspaces of the original N-dimensional space. Within each subspace the data are represented by M principal components of the subspace so the technique is a hybrid non-linear principal component/neural network method. Using this method the investigators compressed a number of digital chest radiographs at ratios from 10:1 to 40:1 and by another method (the Karhunen–Loève transform). The images were assessed by seven radiologists and those compressed by the neural network method scored at least as well as the other method, even at lower compression ratios for the other method.

Flow cytometry

Flow cytometry is a widely used technique that can sort cells into different classifications according to their reflectance or absorbance of laser-generated light at a particular wavelength. The technique is often used in ploidy studies including the classification of trophoblastic disease. The usual method of analysis is by analogue circuits in the apparatus but some authors have shown that digital acquisition of the data reveals useful information that is smoothed out by the analogue process. Godavarti et al. (1996) have applied neural network analysis to digital data from flow cytometry with the intention of developing generic techniques of cell classification. They applied both multilayer perceptron and Kohonen-type neural networks to the problem using either features extracted from the pulse waveforms (such as pulse height, pulse width, pulse skewness and discrete Fourier transform) or the raw digital data of the waveform. The networks were trained on 40 waveforms (20 of each dichotomous category) and tested on 1000 waveforms. The most accurate classifications, mean 93.5%, were achieved by a multilayer perceptron with seven input neurons, a single hidden layer of five neurons and two output neurons or by using the unmodified waveform as input data. The performance of the Kohonen network was only slightly inferior, with a mean classification accuracy of 93.2% and all the networks performed better than the k-means algorithm that was used for comparison. Frankel et al. (1996) have also used multilayer perceptrons to analyse flow cytometric data and have developed a system that can operate in real time. They used a neural network classifier to sort human peripheral blood into five categories (CD8 – lymphocytes, CD8 + lymphocytes, monocytes, granulocytes and lymphocytes) training the network (with a 5–8–5 architecture) on 5000 cells and testing it on a further 9443. The network produced accurate classification for each category in the image of 94–100% but this was not compared with conventional statistical methods.

Risk analysis

The introduction of a new laboratory diagnostic test into daily practice is often an economic problem involving many risk factors and it would be useful to model this process before the introduction of the new test. Jabor et al. (1996) have designed such a simulation model that uses neural networks of an unspecified architecture as the CPU. The model is given 10 items of input data and simulations are run on a daily simulation cycle. The output from the model includes total expenses, income, net present value of the project, total number of control samples used, total number of patients evaluated and total number of used kits. The results of the model appear realistic but it would be easier to assess its effectiveness if it were compared with real data from the introduction of a laboratory test.

Summary

This chapter has shown that there are numerous potential applications for artificial neural networks in the analysis of the profusion of data that is produced by laboratory medicine. The fact that many of these applications have not yet been implemented in the live laboratory environment may be due to the problems of interfacing various items of electronic equipment but it also relates to the quality of the current studies and the problems with licensing medical equipment. The population size in the reviewed studies has been stated throughout and it can be seen that many of the studies use small numbers of cases and there is insufficient evidence that the developed method will generalize to an unselected population in a working laboratory. Large numbers of cases are required to show that a system can work in its intended situation. The law on licensing decision support technology varies from country to country but in all cases there must be some proof that use of the decision support system enhances the medical process (Brahams & Wyatt 1989; Hurwitz 1995) and that a neural network system is better than a conventional statistical classifier, such as logistic regression (Hart & Wyatt 1990b; Wyatt & Spiegelhalter 1991; Wyatt 1995; Feinstein 1996). This again requires large numbers of cases and carefully designed trials of the system in the live situation (Heathfield & Wyatt 1993). At present few systems fulfil these requirements.

REFERENCES

Afifi, M. A., Hammad, T. A., Gabr, N. S., El-Shinawi, S. F., Khalifa, R. M. & Azab, M. E. (1995). Application of neural networks to the real-time diagnosis of acute toxoplasmic infection in immunocompetent patients. *Clinical Infectious Diseases* 21, 1411–1416.

Albertazzi, E., Cajone, F., Leone, B. E., Naguib, R. N., Lakshmi, M. S. & Sherbet, G. V. (1998). Expression of metastasis-associated genes h-*mts1* (S100A4) and *nm23* in carcinoma of breast is related to disease progression. *DNA and Cell Biology* 17, 335–342.

Alvager, T., Smith, T. J. & Vijai, F. (1994). The use of artificial neural networks in biomedical technologies: an introduction. *Biomedical Instrumentation and Technology* 28, 315–322.

Astion, M. L. & Wilding, P. (1992). Application of neural networks to the interpretation of laboratory data in cancer diagnosis. *Clinical Chemistry* 38, 34–38.

Baker, J. A., Kornguth, P. J., Lo, J. Y. & Floyd, C. E., Jr (1996). Artificial neural network: improving the quality of breast biopsy recommendations. *Radiology* 198, 131–135.

Baxt, W. G. (1994). Complexity, chaos and human physiology: the justification for non-linear neural computational analysis. *Cancer Letters* 77, 85–93.

Becker, R. L. (1994). Computer-assisted image classification: use of neural networks in anatomic pathology. *Cancer Letters* 77, 111–117.

Boon, M. E. & Kok, L. P. (1993). Neural network processing can provide means to catch errors that slip through human screening of pap smears. *Diagnostic Cytopathology* 9, 411–416.

Boon, M. E., Kok, L. P., Nygaard-Nielsen, M., Holm, K. & Holund, B. (1994). Neural network processing of cervical smears can lead to a decrease in diagnostic variability and an increase in screening efficacy: a study of 63 false-negative smears. *Modern Pathology* 7, 957–961.

Boon, M. E., Beck, S. & Kok, L. P. (1995a). Semiautomatic PAPNET analysis of proliferating (MiB-1-positive) cells in cervical cytology and histology. *Diagnostic Cytopathology* 13, 423–428.

Boon, M. E., Kok, L. P. & Beck, S. (1995b). Histologic validation of neural network-assisted cervical screening: comparison with the conventional procedure. *Cell Vision* 23–27.

Brahams, D. & Wyatt, J. (1989). Decision aids and the law. *Lancet* 2, 632–634.

Brickley, M. R., Cowpe, J. G. & Shepherd, J. P. (1996). Performance of a computer simulated neural network trained to categorise normal, premalignant and malignant oral smears. *Journal of Oral Pathology and Medicine* 25, 424–428.

Brinn, M., Walsh, P. T., Payne, M. P. & Bott, B. (1993). Neural network classification of mutagens using structural fragment data. *Sar and Qsar in Environmental Research* 1, 169–210.

Brouwer, R. K. & MacAuley, C. (1995). Classifying cervical cells using a recurrent neural network by building basins of attraction. *Analytical and Quantitative Cytology and Histology* 17, 197–203.

Burke, H. B. (1994). Artificial neural networks for cancer research: outcome prediction. *Seminars in Surgical Oncology* 10, 73–79.

Burke, H. B., Goodman, P. H., Rosen, D. B., Henson, D. E., Weinstein, J. N., Harrell, F. E., Jr, Marks, J. R., Winchester, D. P. & Bostwick, D. G. (1996). Artificial neural networks improve the accuracy of cancer survival prediction. *Cancer* 79, 857–862.

Cai, Y. & Chen, C. (1995). Artificial neural network method for discriminating coding regions of eukaryotic genes. *Computer Applications in Biosciences* 11, 497–501.

Carpenter, G. A. & Grossberg, S. (1987a). A massively parallel architecture for a self-organizing neural pattern recognition machine. *Computer Vision, Graphics and Image Processing* 37, 54–115.

Carpenter, G. A. & Grossberg, S. (1987b). Discovering order in chaos: stable self-organization of neural recognition codes. *Annals of the New York Academy of Sciences* 504, 33–51.

Carpenter, G. A. & Markuson, N. (1998). ARTMAP-IC and medical diagnosis: instance counting and inconsistent cases. *Neural Networks* 11, 323–336.

Carpenter, G. A. & Tan, A.-H. (1993). Rule extraction, fuzzy ARTMAP, and medical databases. *Proceedings of the World Congress on Neural Networks* 1, 501–506.

Carpenter, G. A., Grossberg, S. & Reynolds, J. H. (1991). ARTMAP: supervised real-time learning and classification of non-stationary data by a self-organizing neural network. *Neural Networks* 4, 565–588.

Carpenter, G. A., Grossberg, S., Markuzon, S., Reynolds, J. H. & Rosen, D. B. (1992). Fuzzy ARTMAP: a neural network architecture for incremental supervised learning of analog multidimensional maps. *IEEE Transactions on Neural Networks* 3, 698–712.

Cenci, M., Nagar, C., Giovagnoli, M. R. & Vecchione, A. (1997). The PAPNET system for quality control of cervical smears: validation and limits. *Anticancer Research* 17, 4731–4734.

Chan, K. H., Johnson, K. A., Becker, J. A., Satlin, A., Mendelson, J., Garada, B. & Holman, B. L.

(1994). A neural network classifier for cerebral perfusion imaging. *Journal of Nuclear Medicine* 35, 771–774.

Chandonia, J. M. & Karplus, M. (1996). The importance of larger data sets for protein secondary structure prediction with neural networks. *Protein Science* 5, 768–774.

Chiou, Y. S. & Lure, Y. M. (1994). Hybrid lung nodule detection (HLND) system. *Cancer Letters* 77, 119–126.

Christy, P. S., Tervonen, O., Scheithauer, B. W. & Forbes, G. S. (1995). Use of a neural network and a multiple regression model to predict histologic grade of astrocytoma from MRI appearances. *Neuroradiology* 37, 89–93.

Chun, J., Atalan, E., Kim, S.-B., Kim, H.-J., Hamid, M. E., Trujillo, M. E., Magee, J. G., Manfio, G. P., Ward, A. C. & Goodfellow, M. (1993). Rapid identification of streptomycetes by artificial neural network analysis of pyrolysis mass spectra. *FEMS Microbiology Letters* 114, 115–120.

Clark, G. M., Hilsenbeck, S. G., Ravdin, P. M., De Laurentiis, M. & Osborne, C. K. (1994). Prognostic factors: rationale and methods of analysis and integration. *Breast Cancer Research and Treatment* 32, 105–112.

Cohen, C. (1996). Image cytometric analysis in pathology. *Human Pathology* 27, 482–493.

Cooper, G. F., Aliferis, C. F., Ambrosino, R., Aronis, J., Buchanan, B. G., Caruana, R., Fine, M. J., Glymour, C., Gordon, G., Hanusa, B. H., Janosky, J. E., Meek, C., Mitchell, T., Richardson, T. & Spirtes, P. (1997). An evaluation of machine-learning methods for predicting pneumonia mortality. *Artificial Intelligence in Medicine* 9, 107–138.

Corrigan, B. W., Mayo, P. R. & Jamali, F. (1997). Application of a neural network for gentamicin concentration prediction in a general hospital population. *Therapeutic Drug Monitoring* 19, 25–28.

Cristea, A. & Zaharia, C. N. (1994). Simulation of a viral epidemic by means of a neural network. *Revue Roumaine de Virologie* 45, 123–133.

Cross, S. S. & Bull, A. D. (1992). Is the informational content of histopathological reports increasing? *Journal of Clinical Pathology* 45, 179–180.

Cross, S. S., Bury, J. P., Stephenson, T. J. & Harrison, R. F. (1997). Image analysis of low magnification images of fine needle aspirates of the breast produces useful discrimination between benign and malignant cases. *Cytopathology* 8, 265–273.

De Laurentiis, M. & Ravdin, P. M. (1994a). A technique for using neural network analysis to perform survival analysis of censored data. *Cancer Letters* 77, 127–138.

De Laurentiis, M. & Ravdin, P. M. (1994b). Survival analysis of censored data: neural network analysis detection of complex interactions between variables. *Breast Cancer Research and Treatment* 32, 113–118.

Denaro, T. J., Herriman, J. M. & Shapira, O. (1997). PAPNET testing system. Technical update. *Acta Cytologica* 41, 65–73.

Dony, R. D., Coblentz, C. L., Nabmias, C. & Haykin, S. (1996). Compression of digital chest radiographs with a mixture of principal components neural network: evaluation of performance. *Radiographics* 16, 1481–1488.

Doornewaard, H., van de Seijp, H., Woudt, J. M., van der Graaf, Y. & van den Tweel, J. G. (1997). Negative cervical smears before CIN 3/carcinoma. Reevaluation with the PAPNET testing system. *Acta Cytologica* **41**, 74–78.

Douglas, T. H. & Moul, J. W. (1998). Applications of neural networks in urologic oncology. *Seminars in Urologic Oncology* **16**, 35–39.

Downs, J., Harrison, R. F. & Cross, S. S. (1995a). A neural network decision-support tool for the diagnosis of breast cancer. In J. Hallam, ed., *Hybrid Problems, Hybrid Solutions. 10th Biennial Conference on Artificial Intelligence and Cognitive Science*. IOS Press, Amsterdam, pp. 51–60.

Downs, J., Harrison, R. F. & Cross, S. S. (1995b). Evaluating a neural network decision-support tool for the diagnosis of breast cancer. In P. Barahona, M. Stefanelli & J. Wyatt, eds., *Artificial Intelligence in Medicine – Lecture Notes in Artificial Intelligence*. Springer-Verlag, Berlin, pp. 239–250.

Downs, J., Harrison, R. F., Kennedy, R. L. & Cross, S. S. (1996). Application of the fuzzy ARTMAP neural network model to medical pattern classification tasks. *Artificial Intelligence in Medicine* **8**, 403–428.

Downs, J., Harrison, R. F. & Cross, S. S. (1998). A decision support tool for the diagnosis of breast cancer based upon fuzzy ARTMAP. *Neural Computing and Applications* **7**, 147–165.

Dwarakanath, S., Ferris, C. D., Pierre, J. W., Asplund, R. O. & Curtis, D. L. (1994). A neural network approach to the early detection of cancer. *Biomedical Sciences Instrumentation* **30**, 239–243.

Dybowski, R. & Gant, V. (1995). Artificial neural networks in pathology and medical laboratories. *Lancet* **346**, 1203–1207.

Dytch, H. E. & Wied, G. L. (1990). Artificial neural networks and their use in quantitative pathology. *Analytical and Quantitative Cytology and Histology* **6**, 379–393.

Einstein, A. J., Barba, J., Unger, P. D. & Gil, J. (1994). Nuclear diffuseness as a measure of texture: definition and application to the computer-assisted diagnosis of parathyroid adenoma and carcinoma. *Journal of Microscopy* **176**, 158–166.

Eklund, P. & Forsström, J. J. (1995). Computational intelligence for laboratory information systems. *Scandinavian Journal of Clinical and Laboratory Investigation – Supplement* **222**, 21–30.

El-Deredy, W. (1997). Pattern recognition approaches in biomedical and clinical magnetic resonance spectroscopy: a review. *NMR in Biomedicine* **10**, 99–124.

Erler, B. S., Hsu, L., Truong, H. M., Petrovic, L. M., Kim, S. S., Huh, M. H., Ferrell, L. D., Thung, S. N., Geller, S. A. & Marchevsky, A. M. (1994). Image analysis and diagnostic classification of hepatocellular carcinoma using neural networks and multivariate discriminant functions. *Laboratory Investigation* **71**, 446–451.

Feinstein, A. R. (1996). Multiple logistic regression. In A. R. Feinstein, ed., *Multivariable Analysis*, 1st edn. Yale University Press, New Haven, CT, pp. 297–330.

Floyd, C. E., Jr, Lo, J. Y., Yun, A. J., Sullivan, D. C. & Kornguth, P. J. (1994). Prediction of breast cancer malignancy using an artificial neural network. *Cancer* **74**, 2944–2948.

Fogel, D. B., Wasson, E. C. & Boughton, E. M. (1995). Evolving neural networks for detecting breast cancer. *Cancer Letters* **96**, 49–53.

Frankel, D. S., Frankel, S. L., Binder, B. J. & Vogt, R. F. (1996). Application of neural networks to flow cytometry data analysis and real-time cell classification. *Cytometry* **23**, 290–302.

Fukuda, H., Inoue, Y., Nakajima, H., Usuki, N., Saiwai, S., Miyamoto, T. & Onoyama, Y. (1995).

Potential usefulness of an artificial neural network for assessing ventricular size. *Radiation Medicine* **13**, 23–26.

Gebbinck, M. S. Verhoeven, J. T., Thijssen, J. M. & Schouten, T. E. (1993). Application of neural networks for the classification of diffuse liver disease by quantitative echography. *Ultrasonic Imaging* **15**, 205–217.

Giger, M. L., Vyborny, C. J. & Schmidt, R. A. (1994). Computerized characterization of mammographic masses: analysis of spiculation. *Cancer Letters* **77**, 201–211.

Godavarti, M., Rodriguez, J. J., Yopp, T. A., Lambert, G. M. & Galbraith, D. W. (1996). Automated particle classification based on digital acquisition and analysis of flow cytometric pulse waveforms. *Cytometry* **24**, 330–339.

Golden, J. B., Torgersen, D. & Tibbetts, C. (1993). Pattern recognition for automated DNA sequencing. I. On-line signal conditioning and feature extraction for basecalling. *Ismb* **1**, 136–144.

Goodacre, R., Howell, S. A., Noble, W. C. & Neal, M. J. (1996a). Sub-species discrimination, using pyrolysis mass spectrometry and self-organising neural networks, of *Propionibacterium acnes* isolated from normal human skin. *Zentralblatt für Bakteriologie* **284**, 501–515.

Goodacre, R., Neal, M. J. & Kell, D. B. (1996b). Quantitative analysis of multivariate data using artificial neural networks: a tutorial review and applications to the deconvolution of pyrolysis mass spectra. *Zentralblatt für Bakteriologie* **284**, 516–539.

Goodacre, R., Timmins, E. M., Rooney, P. J., Rowland, J. J. & Kell, D. B. (1996c). Rapid identification of *Streptococcus* and *Enterococcus* species using diffuse reflectance-absorbance Fourier transform infrared spectroscopy and artificial neural networks. *FEMS Microbiology Letters* **140**, 233–239.

Gross, G. W., Boone, J. M., Greco-Hunt, V. & Greenberg, B. (1990). Neural networks in radiologic diagnosis. II. Interpretation of neonatal chest radiographs. *Investigative Radiology* **25**, 1017–1023.

Gross, G. W., Boone, J. M. & Bishop, D. M. (1995). Pediatric skeletal age: determination with neural networks. *Radiology* **195**, 689–695.

Gurney, J. W. & Swensen, S. J. (1995). Solitary pulmonary nodules: determining the likelihood of malignancy with neural network analysis. *Radiology* **196**, 823–829.

Halford, J. A., Wright, R. G. & Ditchmen, E. J. (1997). Quality assurance in cervical cytology screening. Comparison of rapid rescreening and the PAPNET testing system. *Acta Cytologica* **41**, 79–81.

Hare, B. J. & Prestegard, J. H. (1994). Application of neural networks to automated assignment of NMR spectra of proteins. *Journal of Biomolecular NMR* **4**, 35–46.

Hart, A. & Wyatt, J. (1990a). Evaluating black-boxes as medical decision aids: issues arising from a study of neural networks. *Medical Informatics* **15**, 229–236.

Hart, A. & Wyatt, J. (1990b). Evaluating black-boxes as medical decision aids: issues arising from a study of neural networks. *Medical Informatics* **15**, 229–236.

Heathfield, H. A. & Wyatt, J. (1993). Philosophies for the design and development of clinical decision-support systems. *Methods of Information in Medicine* **32**, 1–8.

Hoda, R. S., Tahirkheli, N. & Koss, L. G. (1997). PAPNET screening of voided urine sediments: a study of 100 cases. *Laboratory Investigations* **76**, 186.

Hurst, R. E., Bonner, R. B., Ashenayi, K., Veltri, R. W. & Hemstreet, G. P. (1997). Neural net-based identification of cells expressing the p300 tumor-related antigen using fluorescence image analysis. *Cytometry* **27**, 36–42.

Hurwitz, B. (1995). Clinical guidelines and the law. *British Medical Journal* **311**, 1517–1518.

Husain, O. A., Butler, E. B., Nayagam, M., Mango, L. & Alonzo, A. (1994). An analysis of the variation of human interpretation: Papnet a mini-challenge. *Analytical Cellular Pathology* **6**, 157–163.

Ikeda, H. (1996). Analysis of diffuse parenchymal liver disease by liver scintigrams: differential diagnosis using neuro and fuzzy. *Osaka City Medical Journal* **42**, 109–124.

Itoh, K. (1994). ID number recognition of X-ray films by a neural network. *Computer Methods and Programs in Biomedicine* **43**, 15–18.

Jabor, A., Vlk, T. & Boril, P. (1996). Introduction of a new laboratory test: an econometric approach with the use of neural network analysis. *Clinica et Chimica Acta* **248**, 99–105.

Jenny, J., Isenegger, I., Boon, M. E. & Husain, O. A. (1997). Consistency of a double PAPNET scan of cervical smears. *Acta Cytologica* **41**, 82–87.

Karakitsos, P., Cochand-Priollet, B., Guillausseau, P. J. & Pouliakis, A. (1996a). Potential of the back propagation neural network in the morphologic examination of thyroid lesions. *Analytical and Quantitative Cytology and Histology* **18**, 494–500.

Karakitsos, P., Stergiou, E. B., Pouliakis, A., Tzivras, M., Archimandritis, A., Liossi, A. I. & Kyrkou, K. (1996b). Potential of the back propagation neural network in the discrimination of benign from malignant gastric cells. *Analytical and Quantitative Cytology and Histology* **18**, 245–250.

Kattan, M. W. & Beck, J. R. (1995). Artificial neural networks for medical classification decisions. *Archives of Pathology and Laboratory Medicine* **119**, 672–677.

Kemp, R. A., MacAulay, C. & Palcic, B. (1997a). Opening the black box: the relationship between neural networks and linear discriminant functions. *Analytical Cellular Pathology* **14**, 19–30.

Kemp, R. A., MacAulay, C., Garner, D. & Palcic, B. (1997b). Detection of malignancy associated changes in cervical cell nuclei using feed-forward neural networks. *Analytical Cellular Pathology* **14**, 31–40.

Kennedy, R. L., Harrison, R. F., Burton, A. M., Fraser, H. S., Hamer, W. G., MacArthur, D., McAllum, R. & Steedman, D. J. (1997). An artificial neural network system for diagnosis of acute myocardial infarction (AMI) in the accident and emergency department: evaluation and comparison with serum myoglobin measurements. *Computer Methods and Programs in Biomedicine* **52**, 93–103.

Keyhani-Rofagha, S., Palma, T. & O'Toole, R. V. (1996). Automated screening for quality control using PAPNET: a study of 638 negative Pap smears. *Diagnostic Cytopathology* **14**, 316–320.

Kippenhan, J. S., Barker, W. W., Pascal, S., Nagel, J. & Duara, R. (1992). Evaluation of a neural-network classifier for PET scans of normal and Alzheimer's disease subjects. *Journal of Nuclear Medicine* **33**, 1459–1467.

Kippenhan, J. S., Barker, W. W., Nagel, J., Grady, C. & Duara, R. (1994). Neural-network classification of normal and Alzheimer's disease subjects using high-resolution and low-resolution PET cameras. *Journal of Nuclear Medicine* **35**, 7–15.

Kok, M. R. & Boon, M. E. (1996). Consequences of neural network technology for cervical screening: increase in diagnostic consistency and positive scores. *Cancer* **78**, 112–117.

Kolles, H., von Wangenheim, A., Vince, G. H., Niedermayer, I. & Feiden, W. (1995). Automated grading of astrocytomas based on histomorphometric analysis of Ki-67 and Feulgen stained paraffin sections. Classification results of neuronal networks and discriminant analysis. *Analytical Cellular Pathology* **8**, 101–116.

Kolles, H., von Wangenheim, A., Rahmel, J., Niedermayer, I. & Feiden, W. (1996). Data-driven approaches to decision making in automated tumor grading. An example of astrocytoma grading. *Analytical and Quantitative Cytology and Histology* **18**, 298–304.

Koss, L. G. (1994). Reducing the error rate in Papanicolaou smears: decreasing false-negatives. *The Female Patient* **19**, 1240–1242.

Koss, L. G., Lin, E., Schreiber, K., Elgert, P. & Mango, L. (1994). Evaluation of the PAPNET cytologic screening system for quality control of cervical smears. *American Journal of Clinical Pathology* **101**, 220–229.

Koss, L. G., Sherman, M. E., Cohen, M. B., Anes, A. R., Darragh, T. M., Lemos, L. B., McClellan, B. J., Rosenthal, D. L., Keyhani-Rofagha, S., Schreiber, K. & Valente, P. T. (1997). Significant reduction in the rate of false-negative cervical smears with neural network-based technology (PAPNET testing system). *Human Pathology* **28**, 1196–1203.

Koss, L. G., Morgenstern, N., Tahir-Kheli, N., Suhrland, M., Schreiber, K. & Greenebaum, E. (1998). Evaluation of esophageal cytology using a neural net-based interactive scanning system (the PAPNET system): its possible role in screening for esophageal and gastric carcinoma. *American Journal of Clinical Pathology* **109**, 549–557.

Lapuerta, P., Azen, S. P. & LaBree, L. (1995). Use of neural networks in predicting the risk of coronary artery disease. *Computers and Biomedical Research* **28**, 38–52.

Liestol, K., Andersen, P. K. & Andersen, U. (1994). Survival analysis and neural nets. *Statistics in Medicine* **13**, 1189–1200.

Lin, J. A., Cheng, K. S. & Mao, C. W. (1996). Multispectral magnetic resonance images segmentation using fuzzy Hopfield neural network. *International Journal of Biomedical Computing* **42**, 205–214.

Lin, J. S., Ligomenides, P. A., Freedman, M. T. & Mun, S. K. (1993). Application of artificial neural networks for reduction of false-positive detections in digital chest radiographs. In *Proceedings of the 16th Annual Symposium on Computer Applications in Medical Care*, McGraw-Hill, New York, pp. 434–438.

Lo, J. Y., Baker, J. A., Kornguth, P. J. & Floyd, C. J. (1995). Computer-aided diagnosis of breast cancer: artificial neural network approach for optimized merging of mammographic features. *Academic Radiology* **2**, 841–850.

Lo, J. Y., Baker, J. A., Kornguth, P. J., Iglehart, J. D. & Floyd, C. E., Jr (1997). Predicting breast cancer invasion with artificial neural networks on the basis of mammographic features. *Radiology* **203**, 159–163.

Lo, S. C., Freedman, M. T., Lin, J. S. & Mun, S. K. (1993). Automatic lung nodule detection using profile matching and back-propagation neural network techniques. *Journal of Digital Imaging* **6**, 48–54.

Maclin, P. S. & Dempsey, J. (1992). Using an artificial neural network to diagnose hepatic masses. *Journal of Medical Systems* **16**, 215–225.

Maclin, P. S. & Dempsey, J. (1994). How to improve a neural network for early detection of hepatic cancer. *Cancer Letters* **77**, 95–101.

Mango, L. J. (1996). Reducing false negatives in clinical practice: the role of neural network technology. *American Journal of Obstetrics and Gynaecology* **175**, 1114–1119.

Mango, L. J. (1997). Clinical validation of interactive cytologic screening. Automating the search, not the interpretation. *Acta Cytologica* **41**, 93–97.

Mango, L. J. & Valente, P. T. (1998). Neural-network-assisted analysis and microscopic rescreening in presumed negative cervical cytologic smears. A comparison. *Acta Cytologica* **42**, 227–232.

Mehdi, B., Stacey, D. & Harauz, G. (1994). A hierarchical neural network assembly for classification of cervical cells in automated screening. *Analytical Cellular Pathology* **7**, 171–180.

Michelow, P. M., Hlongwane, N. F. & Leiman, G. (1997). Simulation of primary cervical cancer screening by the PAPNET system in an unscreened, high-risk community. *Acta Cytologica* **41**, 88–92.

Mitchell, H. & Medley, G. (1998). Detection of laboratory false negative smears by the PAPNET cytologic screening system. *Acta Cytologica* **42**, 265–270.

Molnar, B., Szentirmay, Z., Bodo, M., Sugar, J. & Feher, J. (1993). Application of multivariate, fuzzy set and neural network analysis in quantitative cytological examinations. *Analytical Cellular Pathology* **5**, 161–175.

Moul, J. W. (1995). Proper staging techniques in testicular cancer patients. *Techniques in Urology* **1**, 126–132.

Moul, J. W., Snow, P. B., Fernandez, E. B., Maher, P. D. & Sesterhenn, I. A. (1995). Neural network analysis of quantitative histological factors to predict pathological stage in clinical stage I nonseminomatous testicular cancer [see comments]. *Journal of Urology* **153**, 1674–1677.

Naguib, R. N. & Sherbet, G. W. (1997). Artificial neural networks in cancer research. *Pathobiology* **65**, 129–139.

Naguib, R. N., Adams, A. E., Horne, C. H., Angus, B., Sherbet, G. V. & Lennard, T. W. (1996). The detection of nodal metastasis in breast cancer using neural network techniques. *Physiological Measurement* **17**, 297–303.

Naguib, R. N., Adams, A. E., Horne, C. H., Angus, B., Smith, A. F., Sherbet, G. V. & Lennard, T. W. (1997). Prediction of nodal metastasis and prognosis in breast cancer: a neural model. *Anticancer Research* **17**, 2735–2741.

Narayanan, M. N. & Lucas, S. B. (1993). A genetic algorithm to improve a neural network to predict a patient's response to warfarin. *Methods of Information in Medicine* **32**, 55–58.

Nazeran, H., Rice, F., Moran, W. & Skinner, J. (1995). Biomedical image processing in pathology: a review. *Australasian Physical and Engineering Sciences in Medicine* **18**, 26–38.

Nilsson, T., Bassani, M. R., Larsen, T. O. & Montanarella, L. (1996). Classification of species in the genus *Penicillium* by Curie point pyrolysis/mass spectrometry followed by multivariate analysis and artificial neural networks. *Journal of Mass Spectrometry* **31**, 1422–1428.

O'Leary, T. J., Mikel, U. V. & Becker, R. L. (1992). Computer-assisted image interpretation: use of a neural network to differentiate tubular carcinoma from sclerosing adenosis. *Modern Pathology* 5, 402–405.

Ohno-Machado, L., Walker, M. G. & Musen, M. A. (1995). Hierarchical neural networks for survival analysis. In R. A. Greenes, H. Peterson & D. Protti, eds., *Proceeding of the 8th World Congress on Medical Informatics.* North-Holland, Amsterdam, pp. 828–832.

Ouwerkerk, E., Boon, M. E. & Beck, S. (1994). Computer-assisted primary screening of cervical smears using the PAPNET method: comparison with conventional screening and evaluation of the role of the cytologist. *Cytopathology* 5, 211–218.

Patil, S., Henry, J. W., Rubenfire, M. & Stein, P. D. (1993). Neural network in the clinical diagnosis of acute pulmonary embolism. *Chest* 104, 1685–1689.

Rawlings, C. J. & Fox, J. P. (1994). Artificial intelligence in molecular biology: a review and assessment. *Philosophical Transactions of the Royal Society of London* B344, 353–362; discussion 362–363.

Reinus, W. R., Wilson, A. J., Kalman, B. & Kwasny, S. (1994). Diagnosis of focal bone lesions using neural networks. *Investigative Radiology* 29, 606–611.

Rinast, E., Linder, R. & Weiss, H. D. (1993). Neural network approach for computer-assisted interpretation of ultrasound images of the gallbladder. *European Journal of Radiology* 17, 175–178.

Rosenthal, D. L., Acosta, D. & Peters, R. K. (1996). Computer-assisted rescreening of clinically important false negative cervical smears using the PAPNET testing system. *Acta Cytologica* 40, 120–126.

Rost, B. (1996). PHD: predicting one-dimensional protein structure by profile-based neural networks. *Methods in Enzymology* 266, 525–539.

Sahiner, B., Chan, H. P., Wei, D., Petrick, N., Helvie, M. A., Adler, D. D. & Goodsitt, M. M. (1996). Image feature selection by a genetic algorithm: application to classification of mass and normal breast tissue. *Medical Physics* 23, 1671–1684.

Schechter, C. B. (1996). Cost-effectiveness of rescreening conventionally prepared cervical smears by PAPNET testing. *Acta Cytologica* 40, 1272–1282.

Schenone, A., Firenze, F., Acquarone, F., Gambaro, M., Masulli, F. & Andreucci, L. (1996). Segmentation of multivariate medical images via unsupervised clustering with 'adaptive resolution'. *Computerized Medical Imaging and Graphics* 20, 119–129.

Serón, D., Moreso, F., Gratin, C., Vitria, J., Condom, E., Grinyo, J. M. & Alsina, J. (1996). Automated classification of renal interstitium and tubules by local texture analysis and a neural network. *Analytical and Quantitative Cytology and Histology* 18, 410–419.

Sherman, M. E., Mango, L. J., Kelly, D., Paull, G., Ludin, V., Copeland, C., Solomon, D. & Schiffman, M. H. (1994). PAPNET analysis of reportedly negative smears preceding the diagnosis of a high-grade squamous intraepithelial lesion or carcinoma. *Modern Pathology* 7, 578–581.

Sherman, M. E., Schiffman, M. H., Mango, L. J., Kelly, D., Acosta, D., Cason, Z., Elgert, P., Zaleski, S., Scott, D. R., Kurman, R. J., Stoler, M. & Lorincz, A. T. (1997). Evaluation of PAPNET testing as an ancillary tool to clarify the status of the 'atypical' cervical smear. *Modern Pathology* 10, 564–571.

Shultz, E. K. (1996). Artificial neural networks: laboratory aid or sorcerer's apprentice? *Clinical Chemistry* **42**, 496–497.

Stotzka, R., Manner, R., Bartels, P. H. & Thompson, D. (1995). A hybrid neural and statistical classifier system for histopathologic grading of prostatic lesions. *Analytical and Quantitative Cytology and Histology* **17**, 204–218.

Sturgis, C. D., Isoe, C., McNeal, N. E., Yu, G. H. & DeFrias, D. V. (1998). PAPNET computer-aided rescreening for detection of benign and malignant glandular elements in cervicovaginal smears: a review of 61 cases. *Diagnostic Cytopathology* **18**, 307–311.

Su, M. C. (1994). Use of neural networks as medical diagnosis expert systems. *Computers in Biology and Medicine* **24**, 419–429.

Sun, J., Song, W. Y., Zhu, L. H. & Chen, R. S. (1995). Analysis of tRNA gene sequences by neural network. *Journal of Computational Biology* **2**, 409–416.

Thompson, T. B., Chou, K. C. & Zheng, C. (1995). Neural network prediction of the HIV-1 protease cleavage sites. *Journal of Theoretical Biology* **177**, 369–379.

Tourassi, G. D., Floyd, C. E., Sostman, H. D. & Coleman, R. E. (1993). Acute pulmonary embolism: artificial neural network approach to diagnosis. *Radiology* **189**, 555–558.

Tourassi, G. D., Floyd, C. E., Sostman, H. D. & Coleman, R. E. (1995). Artificial neural network for diagnosis of acute pulmonary embolism: effect of case and observer selection. *Radiology* **194**, 889–893.

Tourassi, G. D., Floyd, C. E. & Coleman, R. E. (1996). Improved noninvasive diagnosis of acute pulmonary embolism with optimally selected clinical and chest radiographic findings. *Academic Radiology* **3**, 1012–1018.

Truong, H., Morimoto, R., Walts, A. E., Erler, B. & Marchevsky, A. (1995). Neural networks as an aid in the diagnosis of lymphocyte-rich effusions. *Analytical and Quantitative Cytology and Histology* **17**, 48–54.

Usenius, J. P., Tuohimetsa, S., Vainio, P., Ala-Korpela, M., Hiltunen, Y. & Kauppinen, R. A. (1996). Automated classification of human brain tumours by neural network analysis using in vivo ^{1}H magnetic resonance spectroscopic metabolite phenotypes. *Neuroreport* **7**, 1597–1600.

Vanhala, J. & Kaski, K. (1993). Protein structure prediction system based on artificial neural networks. *Ismb* **1**, 402–410.

Wallace, B. H., Lott, J. A., Griffiths, J. & Kirkpatrick, R. B. (1996). Isoforms of alkaline phosphatase determined by isoelectric focusing in patients with chronic liver disorders. *European Journal of Clinical Chemistry and Clinical Biochemistry* **34**, 711–720.

Warner, A., Bencosme, A., Polycarpou, M. M., Healy, D., Verme, C., Conway, J. Y. & Vemuri, A. T. (1996). Multiparameter models for the prediction of sepsis outcome. *Annals of Clinical and Laboratory Science* **26**, 471–479.

Weid, G. L., Dytch, H., Bibbo, M., Bartels, P. H. & Thompson, D. (1990). Artificial intelligence-guided analysis of cytologic data. *Analytical and Quantitative Cytology and Histology* **12**, 417–428.

Wells, C. A., Ellis, I. O., Zakhour, H. D. & Wilson, A. R. (1994). Guidelines for cytology procedures and reporting on fine needle aspirates of the breast. *Cytopathology* **5**, 316–334.

Wilding, P., Morgan, M. A., Grygotis, A. E., Shoffner, M. A. & Rosato, E. F. (1994). Application of backpropagation neural networks to diagnosis of breast and ovarian cancer. *Cancer Letters* **77**, 145–153.

Winkel, P. (1994). Artificial intelligence within the chemical laboratory. *Annales de Biologie Clinique* **52**, 277–282.

Wolberg, W. H. & Mangasarian, O. L. (1993). Computer-designed expert systems for breast cytology diagnosis. *Analytical and Quantitative Cytology and Histology* **15**, 67–74.

Wu, C. H. (1996). Gene classification artificial neural system. *Methods in Enzymology* **266**, 71–88.

Wu, C. H. (1997). Artificial neural networks for molecular sequence analysis. *Computers and Chemistry* **21**, 237–256.

Wu, C., Berry, M., Fung, Y. S. & McLarty, J. (1993). Neural networks for molecular sequence classification. *Ismb* **1**, 429–437.

Wu, Y., Giger, M. L., Doi, K., Vyborny, C. J., Schmidt, R. A. & Metz, C. E. (1993). Artificial neural networks in mammography: application to decision making in the diagnosis of breast cancer. *Radiology* **187**, 81–87.

Wu, Y. C., Doi, K. & Giger, M. L. (1995a). Detection of lung nodules in digital chest radiographs using artificial neural networks: a pilot study. *Journal of Digital Imaging* **8**, 88–94.

Wu, Y. C., Freedman, M. T., Hasegawa, A., Zuurbier, R. A., Lo, S. C. & Mun, S. K. (1995b). Classification of microcalcifications in radiographs of pathologic specimens for the diagnosis of breast cancer. *Academic Radiology* **2**, 199–204.

Wyatt, J. (1995). Nervous about artificial neural networks. *Lancet* **346**, 1175–1177.

Wyatt, J. & Spiegelhalter, D. (1991). Field trials of medical decision-aids: Potential problems and solutions. In P. Claydon, ed., *Proceedings of the 15th Symposium on Computer Applications in Medical Care*. Washington. McGraw Hill Inc., New York, pp. 3–7.

Zhang, W., Doi, K., Giger, M. L., Wu, Y., Nishikawa, R. M. & Schmidt, R. A. (1994). Computerized detection of clustered microcalcifications in digital mammograms using a shift-invariant artificial neural network. *Medical Physics* **21**, 517–524.

Zhu, Y. & Yan, H. (1997). Computerized tumor boundary detection using a Hopfield neural network. *IEEE Transactions in Medical Imaging* **16**, 55–67.

3

Using artificial neural networks to screen cervical smears: how new technology enhances health care

Mathilde E. Boon and Lambrecht P. Kok

Screening for carcinoma of the cervix

In this chapter, we present our experience of 9 years of using neural network technology to screen for cervical carcinoma. In 1928 Papanicolaou presented in Battle Creek, Michigan, his chance observation that cervical cancer cells can be found in a vaginal smear. He realized that the method could be used to recognize cervical carcinoma and treat it in its early stages thereby preventing death from cancer in these women. In addition, he found that the preinvasive stages of cervical carcinoma could be detected in the smear. Removal of the abnormal tissue at this stage before spread would in essence therefore provide 'curative' treatment. Mass screening of asymptomatic women to detect cervical carcinoma at a curable stage began in the USA in 1945. Abnormal cells were to be detected in cervical smears by trained cytotechnologists, cytologists, or pathologists by means of light microscopy, a technique still used in the vast majority of modern laboratories.

Human screening is far from ideal as cancer cells can easily be overlooked, resulting in a 'false negative' diagnosis. The risk of consequent litigation has become a major concern within the cytology community in the USA (Frable 1994; DeMay 1996) and Australia (Mitchell 1995). Significant laboratory incidents with adverse medicolegal consequences have also been reported in the UK (Cogan 2000). One of the approaches taken to facilitate the detection of abnormal cells in cervical smears has been the application of neural network technology.

Population screening for cervical cancer implies screening women who consider themselves to be healthy. Without an invitation by the screening organization, there would be no reason at all for women to perceive the need for a cervical smear. Screening is therefore a difficult balancing act. This is because women who need treatment have to undergo further gynaecological examination, whilst women without important cervical abnormalities must be kept out of hospital. Because of the (relatively) low prevalence of true abnormality, the system must be capable of high specificity, in order to minimize both unnecessary repeat investigation and anxiety. At the same time, sensitivity must be high enough to produce an acceptable false negative rate. One is necessarily a trade-off for the other.

With conventional screening by light microscopy it is virtually impossible to increase sensitivity without simultaneously decreasing specificity. If the rate of histological diagnosis of cancer is higher than the cytological one, we speak of cytological underdiagnosis, with cytological overdiagnosis representing a higher pick-up rate with cytology rather than histology. Note that not only overdiagnosis but also regression and progression are directly related to degree of abnormality: mild dysplasias regress more often and display less progression than carcinomas in situ.

Definitions of cytologic and histologic entities

The aim of screening is to detect the preinvasive and early invasive stage of cervical carcinoma such that deeply invasive carcinoma cannot develop. In this chapter, the following terms for the various stages of preinvasive lesions are used. ASCUS stands for atypical squamous cells of unknown significance. The pre-invasive lesions are, in increasing severity, mild dysplasia, moderate dysplasia, severe dysplasia, and carcinoma in situ. With the exception of ASCUS (a purely cytological concept; in the UK the term 'borderline smear' is used), these terms are used throughout the text for both cytology and histology, as is the term 'invasive carcinoma'. In this context it is important to mention that certainly not all preinvasive lesions progress into invasive carcinoma: many regress in time.

Screening cervical smears using neural network technology: the PAPNET system

Neural network-based systems for cervical screening have been available since the early 1990s. For practising pathologists the literature on neural networks seems complex and difficult to understand: the systems made available to us at the time were, however, apparently easy to understand in their operation, and were presented as a finished product ready for laboratory implementation. The original neural network-based systems were, however, to remain separate from the laboratory, with slides being sent away for remote analysis.

This chapter concerns our experience with the PAPNET system, developed by Neuromedical Systems, Inc. (Suffern, New York). We wished to use this neural network-based technology to:

1. analyse conventionally prepared smears, without changing standard clinical practice,

2. automate only the search for diagnostic images, not the diagnostic decision itself,
3. reduce the amount of non-diagnostic visual information, and
4. exploit fully the ability of the screeners to recognize diagnostic information as presented by the system.

Neural network-based systems have been shown not only to be as capable as human beings as image recognition tools, but in some cases possibly superior, in that they are capable of flagging abnormalities in smears established as false negative (Kok & Boon, 1996b). It should be noted that this was a study, and it is well known that screeners working in an unsupervised 'real life' situation perform quite differently (Van Ballegooijen et al. 1998). Whether neural network-based screening (NNS) should be adopted depends on its applicability in a routine setting which in turn depends on how it interacts with the staff of the diagnostic screening laboratory.

The hardware employed by PAPNET consists of two units: the scanning station and the review station. They are fully separate instruments that can be located far apart. The scanner includes a robotic arm for loading and unloading slides, an automated microscope plus colour camera, a high-speed image processor, and an 80486 computer for operator interface and system control. Three objectives (50 ×, 200 ×, and 400 × magnification) are used in different stages of scanning. The first (low-power) scan maps slide cellularity and optimises focusing. The second (medium-power) scan enables an algorithmic image processor using colour processing and mathematical morphology to locate the set of potentially abnormal cells and clusters. One neural network then processes the individual cells and a second neural network processes the clusters. Both neural networks use a feedforward architecture, trained by back-propagation. The two neural networks used during the processing of each smear produce similarity scores for each object. These scores depend on how closely the object resembles those in the training libraries (containing a large number of positive and negative cells, and clusters, respectively). During scanning, the 64 highest scoring objects for each neural network are chosen as the most diagnostic. A final rescan collects high-resolution colour images of the 64 objects selected by each of the two neural networks. These 128 cellular fields include diagnostic cells, epithelial fragments, and backgrounds, which are stored on a digital tape (DAT) or a CD-ROM. The object's coordinates, identifying its location on the slide, are also recorded on this medium. The 128 images contain diagnostic information, which is reviewed by the cytologist.

The diagnostic station is located in the cytology laboratory. It includes a desktop computer with mouse and keyboard, a tape drive for reading the digital tapes (or CD-ROM), and a large high-resolution monitor for displaying colour

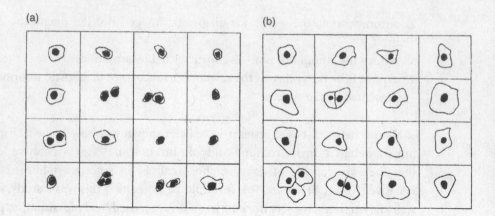

Figure 3.1.   Visual depiction of cells detected by the neural network system in two cases.

images. Our laboratory protocol consists of a summary screen of each case displaying the 16 most diagnostic tiles selected from the original NNS-selected 128 video images or 'tiles'. The light microscope is calibrated such that the coordinates of the tiles match the x/y coordinates in the smear, in order that the cytologist can easily find the cells selected and displayed by the system on the original slide. Figure 3.1 demonstrates the nature of the objects the networks detect.

The figure demonstrates camera lucida drawings, obtained from the printouts of cells detected and highlighted by PAPNET as needing review. Figure 3.1a shows cells detected by the system in a case originally diagnosed as ASCUS. This case subsequently had a histological diagnosis of CIN III. Note that the system has detected cells with a high nuclear/cytoplasmic ratio, consistent with the eventual histological diagnosis. Figure 3.1b shows cells highlighted by the system in a case originally diagnosed as ASCUS. This case was subsequently found to be normal at follow up. Note that the nuclear/cytoplasmic ratio is low.

In order to exploit the NNS, the cytologist must be trained to interpret the video images and to make informative summary screens. This is because it is necessary to develop an appreciation of the novel way in which diagnostic data are represented by the system. In this case, cytologists are trained with known examples (cases with known follow-up and/or histologic validation) in order that they may appreciate the diagnostic potential of the video images provided by the system, and to exploit the information of the summary screen.

The screener's detection role can be divided into three steps:

Step 1: amongst the more than 300 000 normal cells the (potentially) abnormal cells are recognized (the screening step).

Step 2: the degree of abnormality of these selected cells is established.

Step 3: on the basis of the sum of the selected cells and on other diagnostic information ('soft signs' visible in the background of the smear), the smear diagnosis is described in histological terms.

Step 1 is performed by the neural networks. In this case, the networks' ability to extract the most abnormal cellular appearances from the slide consistently and reliably is of vital importance. We investigated this by scanning twice 1200 smears from Zurich, Switzerland, including 516 smears obtained from patients with positive histological findings (Jenny et al. 1997). We saw that in both scans, the diagnostic cells were selected by PAPNET (Jenny et al. 1997). In the very few cases erroneously signed out as negative by the pathologist examining the network-selected tiles, we found that the negative diagnosis had been released as a result of the cytologist's faulty interpretation of the tiles containing abnormal cells. Thus, in these cases, step 2 of the screening process was incorrectly carried out. From 1992 to 2000, we have screened over 500 000 cases with the NNS. We *did* find a few false negatives (smears erroneously signed out as negative) in this large series. Once again, in all these cases it was not the neural network that failed to select the abnormal cells (step 1 of the screening process). Instead, the human diagnostician failed to realize that the selected cells were from a significant cervical lesion, and failed to construct an informative summary screen of these cells to come to the correct diagnosis (steps 2 and 3).

With increasing use, the screener learns to rely more on the videotiles and the power of the summary screen, and needs less light microscopy. When we started neural network-based screening in our laboratory in 1992, we used a protocol based on the premise that the technology was not proven. In cases in which the videoscreen *might* not display the diagnostic information, we turned to the light microscope. In short, we were not certain about the abilities of the neural network. As a result, over 70% of the smears needed additional light microscopy (Ouwerkerk-Noordam et al. 1994). Screening by light microscopy, however, revealed no new diagnoses so we changed our protocol, spending more time looking closely at the videotiles and less on light microscopy.

The decision for additional light microscopy depends on the videoscreen and the macroscopic appearance of the smear. Bloody smears need extra attention, since the cancer cells can be hidden in the blood and are difficult to see on the videoscreen.

In summary, more recently we have profited not from designing better neural network-based systems, but from adapting our screening methods to make full use of the strategic advantage that neural network-based technology offers us.

The parties involved

There are several parties involved in screening for cervical cancer, and each one has a different view of what neural network technology has to offer for screening cervical smears.

Firstly, the epidemiologist plays a part in shaping the screening policy. For the epidemiologist, it is important that the cytologic diagnosis will predict the histological one accurately. In the ideal world, cytological diagnosis is always equal to the histological diagnosis. In the real world, this is often *not* the case. Because the diagnostician using NNS can collect the individual malignant cells (which in reality are scattered over the microscope slide) on the computer screen, he/she can 'glue' these together into a 'histological section' and accordingly it is easier to predict what the histologic diagnosis of the lesion will be. The improved match between cytology and histology which NNS deliver has accordingly been demonstrated (Boon et al. 1995). This fact alone should prompt the epidemiologist to favour NNS.

Secondly, there is then the healthy woman who is invited for a smear to be taken. Her main concern is that no cancer cells are missed. Any pathologist who has tried to explain to a woman why the cancer cells in her smear were left undetected is confronted with her strong opinion that this only happened because the screener failed to do a good job while screening her smear. Litigation against the laboratory might ensue, as has been seen both in the USA (Frable 1994) and in Europe (Cogan 2000). False negatives *do*, however, occur, even in the best laboratories. These concerns prompted us to keep smears of women who were subsequently proven to have invasive carcinoma which were originally incorrectly reported by us. These 'false negative' smears often contain few, small cancer cells, frequently obscured by blood. These cells would therefore be very difficult to detect by conventional means. We submitted these smears to neural network-based analysis: PAPNET detected the cancer cells in all 10 cases (Boon & Kok 1993). These findings were reconfirmed in a study using 63 false negative smears from a population screening program in Denmark (Boon et al. 1994). PAPNET proved to be superior in finding abnormal cells of the reserve cell lineage, diagnostically the most important subgroup (Kok et al. 1998). In Jenny et al.'s (1997) study of a large clinical material it was shown that the false negative rate of 5.7% in conventional screening was reduced to 0.4%.

Thirdly, there is also the clinician who takes the smear, who expects consistency of laboratory results, which in turn depends on consistent diagnostic performance on the part of the cytologists. The degree to which individual cytologists vary in their diagnostic performance is reduced when neural networks are used in the screening process (Kok & Boon 1996b), which can be anticipated because the abnormal cells are selected by the same neural network. To evaluate the consistency of diagnostic performance in our own laboratory for both neural network- and conventionally based screening, we followed up seven of our screeners in the 3 years 1992, 1993 and 1994. Diagnostic consistency was enhanced by PAPNET, especially for the more severe lesions, which are also clinically the most important ones (Kok & Boon 1996b).

Fourthly, there are the screeners themselves. For the screener it is important that the fear of missing a diagnostic cell decreases, making the job of screening less stressful (Boon et al. 1994, 1995). One should also realize that screening means looking at moving cells, which is very tiring. With NNS, the cells are shown on the computer screen and are static, allowing for physically less demanding observation.

Lastly, there is the pathologist, who must not only have insight but also a firm control on the screening procedure performed by his/her coworkers, the screeners. The pathologist must be able to audit a screening colleague's performance and actions – something that is difficult with conventional microscopy. However, with NNS, the summary screens of the screened cases can be stored and these can be checked by the pathologist. We have learned to evaluate summary screens to gain insight into whether the screener scrutinizes the important cells in the smear, and whether informative summary screens are made of the cases. Hard copies of summary screens of pathological cases can be used during the screening process as 'gold standards' for upcoming cases. The hard copies can serve as visual examples and for streamlining the diagnostic process. Recently, it has become possible to view summary screens at all work stations in the laboratory, because the images can be retrieved from storage units (virtually instantaneously) via the computer local area network.

Of all these parties, the screener is most aware of the dangers of human screening. In this context it is important to mention that not one of our 11 screeners is willing to go back to conventional screening after having got experience with NNS. This is at least partly because any system which 'enriches' for abnormality must by definition be found to be more inviting to the scrutineer. Our laboratory has no problem in attracting young people into screening cervical smears (in a tense labour market) because they all like working with computers. The new technology not only enhanced health care for our patients, but also improved the quality of the jobs in our laboratory.

Summary

The careful, evidence-based stepwise development of screening with neural network technology in our laboratory in the past 9 years has had a significant impact on our screening performance.

The woman has become more certain that the laboratory does not miss cancer cells in her smear because these are brought to the attention of the screener evaluating her smear.

The clinician can be more confident that the cytological diagnosis coming back from the laboratory is correct.

The screener, effectively presented with diagnostic images, has learned to exploit this type of visual information. His/her job has become more satisfactory.

The pathologist can now monitor and control the screening process in an effective manner.

The gynaecologist is less often confronted with unnecessary referrals, because the diagnosis has become more precise (Kok & Boon 1996a).

REFERENCES

Boon, M. E. & Kok, L. P. (1993). Neural network processing can provide means to catch errors that slip through human screening of Pap smears. *Diagnostic Cytopathology* 9, 411–416.

Boon, M. E., Kok, L. P., Nygaard-Nielsen, M., Holm, K. & Holund, B. (1994). Neural network processing of cervical smears can lead to a decrease in diagnostic variability and an increase in screening efficacy: a study of 63 false-negative smears. *Modern Pathology* 7, 957–961.

Boon, M. E., Kok, L. P., & Beck, S. (1995). Histologic validation of neural network-assisted cervical screening: comparison with the conventional procedure. *Cell Vision* 2, 23–27.

Cogan, T. J. (2000). Litigation and the Canadian Pap Test: perspectives from a single-payer system. *Diagnostic Cytopathology* 22, 207–210.

DeMay, R. M. (1996). To err is human – to sue, American. *Diagnostic Cytopathology* 15, 3–6.

Frable, W. J. (1994). Litigation cells: definition and observations on a cell type in cervical vaginal smears not adressed by the Bethesda system. *Diagnostic Cytopathology* 11, 213–215.

Jenny, J., Isenegger, I., Boon, M. E. & Husain, O. A. N. (1997). Consistency of a double PAPNET scan of cervical smears. *Acta Cytologia* 41, 82–7.

Kok, M. R. & Boon, M. E. (1996a). Effects of applying neural networks in cervical screening: lower overtreatment rates and less overdiagnosis for patients with mild/moderate dysplasia smears. *Journal of Cell Pathology* 3, 109–114.

Kok, M. R. & Boon, M. E. (1996b). Consequences of neural network technology for cervical screening: increase in diagnostic consistency and positive scores. *Cancer* 78, 112–117.

Kok, M. R., Habers, M. A., Schreiner-Kok, P. G. & Boon, M. E. (1998). New paradigm for ASCUS diagnosis using neural networks. *Diagnostic Cytopathology* 19, 361–366.

Mitchell, H. (1995). Cancer screening: protecting the public's health. *Diagnostic Cytopathology* **12**, 199–200.

Ouwerkerk-Noordam, E., Boon, M. E. & Beck, S. (1994). Computer-assisted primary screening of cervical smears using the PAPNET method: comparison with conventional screening and evaluation of the role of the cytologist. *Cytopathology* **5**, 211–218.

Papanicolaou, G.N. (1928). New cancer diagnosis. In *Proceedings of the Third Race Betterment Conference*, Battle Creek, MI. Race Betterment Foundation, 528–534.

Van Ballegooijen, M., Beck, S., Boon, M. E., Boer, R. & Habbema, J. D. F. (1998). Rescreen effect in conventional and PAPNET screening: observed in a study using material enriched with positive smears. *Acta Cytologia* **42**, 1133–1138.

4

Neural network analysis of sleep disorders

Lionel Tarassenko, Mayela Zamora and James Pardey

Introduction

It is well known that quality of life is critically dependent on quality of sleep. Consequently, the evaluation of sleep disorders is one of the fastest growing sectors of US and European health care. Patients suffering from sleep disorders or excessive daytime sleepiness are referred to *sleep laboratories.* In these laboratories, sleep is monitored continuously for a whole night using the electroencephalogram (EEG) recorded from the scalp, the electro-oculogram (EOG), the chin electromyogram (EMG) and other physiological signals. There is a need for an automated analysis system to identify anomalies in the sleep patterns (primarily from the EEG) and help to decide on possible therapeutic measures. The standard method for analysing the EEG during sleep is a *rule-based system* (Rechtschaffen & Kales 1968) developed 30 years ago, which assigns consecutive 30-second segments uniquely to one of six categories (wakefulness, dreaming sleep or rapid eye movement (REM) sleep, and four stages of progressively deeper sleep, stages 1 to 4). The rules, however, are notoriously difficult to apply and inter-observer correlation can be as low as 51% in the classification of intermediate stages (Kelley et al. 1985). The lack of agreement amongst trained human experts has made the automation of the rule-based 'sleep scoring' process a very difficult task.

A problem such as this presents an ideal application domain for neural networks. We have developed an approach for the analysis of the sleep EEG that combines both unsupervised and supervised learning. In the initial unsupervised learning phase, we attempt to learn as much as possible about the distribution of the parameterized EEG signal in input space. The results obtained with unsupervised learning are then used in a *subsequent* supervised learning phase that is governed by the results obtained in the initial phase. We have previously reported on this approach in some detail (Roberts & Tarassenko 1992, 1995; Pardey et al. 1996a,b) and so this chapter presents only a broad overview and gives our latest results from its application to one of the commonest disorders, obstructive sleep apnoea (OSA).

Materials and methods

The database that we used in our original studies was assembled from nine whole-night sleep records (total sleep time = 71 hours), acquired from healthy adults with no history of sleep disorders. Three human experts, all trained in the same clinical department, used the standard rules to 'score' each sleep record from visual inspection of the central EEG, EOG and chin EMG, the last two being used to decide when the subject is in dreaming sleep. As the classification of consecutive 30-second EEG segments over several hours is required, it takes between 2 and 5 hours for an expert to score a typical sleep record. Those 30-second epochs from each EEG record to which all three experts independently assigned the same sleep stage were archived.

In the neural network analysis system, the EEG signal is sampled at a rate of 128 Hz with 8-bit accuracy, following an anti-aliasing filter. The digitized signal is low-pass filtered with a linear-phase (finite impulse response) digital filter with a pass-band cut-off frequency of 30 Hz and then parameterized as described below.

Input representation

Since conventional neural networks are *static* pattern classifiers, the EEG signal must be segmented into 'frames' during which the statistical properties are assumed to be stationary. The EEG is usually considered to be quasi-stationary over intervals of the order of 1 second, as this is the characteristic time of key transient features such as sleep spindles. The important information in the EEG is in the frequency domain. In our earlier work (Roberts & Tarassenko 1992), we used a 10-coefficient Kalman filter as an autoregressive (AR) model of the EEG signal. Filter coefficients were calculated *for each input sample* and then averaged over 1 second to give a 10-dimensional input vector for every 1-second segment. The problem with this approach is the high computational overhead incurred in computing these coefficients: the time required to analyse a whole night's sleep was not acceptable for a commercial system. As a result, we switched to a less computationally intensive representation that required the AR coefficients to be computed only once for each 1-second frame.

Frequency-domain representation

AR modelling is best known as an alternative to the discrete Fourier transform (DFT), which is traditionally used for the spectral analysis of sampled signals. With 1-second segments and a sampling rate of 128 Hz, there would be 64 DFT or fast Fourier transform (FFT) coefficients to characterize the amplitude spectrum of each segment. A low-dimensional representation is essential for a trained neural network to be able to generalize on previously unseen patterns (Tarassenko 1998). A coarse, low-dimensional representation of the amplitude spectrum could be generated by grouping successive FFT coefficients together; for example, averaging each block of eight coefficients to obtain a single value over that frequency band would give a reduction from 64 to 8 input dimensions. However, this succeeds only in blurring the details of the EEG spectrum to such an extent that the discriminatory information is mostly lost. What is required is an accurate characterization of the dominant frequencies in the EEG so that changes in these over time can be tracked as a function of sleep state. Such a characterization is provided by an all-pole AR model that allows the spectral *peaks* to be tracked even with a low-order model (Pardey et al. 1996a).

The theoretical basis for AR modelling of the EEG has been explored in detail elsewhere (Pardey et al. 1996a). The key concept is the assumption that the sequence $\{s_k\}$ of values from the sampled EEG signal is the *output* of a linear system driven by white noise. If successive samples from the output sequence $s_j, j = 0, 1, \ldots, (N-1)$ are available, we can estimate a sample s_k by the linearly weighted summation of the previous p sample values:

$$\hat{s}_k = -\sum_{i=1}^{p} a_i s_{k-i},$$

where p is the model order. At time $t = kT$, where T is the sampling interval (equal to 1/128 second, i.e. 7.8 milliseconds in our work), we can calculate the error e_k between the actual value and the predicted one;

$$e_k = s_k - \hat{s}_k = s_k + \sum_{i=1}^{p} a_i s_{k-i}.$$

The parameters a_i of the model (the AR coefficients) are estimated by minimizing the expectation of the squared error E over the N samples in the sequence:

$$E = \frac{1}{N}\sum_{k=1}^{N} e_k^2 = \frac{1}{N}\sum_{k=1}^{N}\left(s_k + \sum_{i=1}^{p} a_i s_{k-i}\right)^2.$$

The minimization is performed by setting $\partial E/\partial a_i$ to zero, which yields p linear equations known as the Yule–Walker equations from which the p AR coefficients can be determined by inverting a $p \times p$ matrix. Since this matrix is a Toeplitz matrix (the elements along any diagonal are identical), a more efficient solution is to use a recursive procedure known as the Levinson–Durbin algorithm.

An intermediate set of values, known as the *partial correlation* or *reflection coefficients*, are also produced as part of this recursive procedure. The κ_i reflection coefficients encode the same information as the AR coefficients but they have an important advantage in that it can be ensured that they satisfy the following condition

$$|\kappa_i| \leq 1.$$

This means that the distribution of values is bounded for each reflection coefficient and hence no scaling needs to be applied before they are used as inputs to a neural network. For these reasons, all of our recent sleep EEG analysis work has used reflection coefficients as input features in preference to AR coefficients (Holt et al. 1998; Tarassenko et al. 1998).

Unsupervised learning – 2-D visualization

There are a number of clustering algorithms (for example, k-means clustering; Tarassenko 1998) that could be used to investigate the structure of the 10-dimensional (10-D) parameterization of the EEG data (the 10 reflection coefficients generated for each 1-second frame). In our early work, we used mainly Kohonen's feature map (Kohonen 1982, 1990), which can be viewed as a form of k-means clustering with a neighbourhood that allows the preservation of *topology* in the structuring of the 2-D representation. The units (also known as centres) in a Kohonen map are ordered on a grid such that nearest neighbours in the grid correspond to prototypical input vectors that are also close in the original high-dimensional input space (10-D in our case). The number of centres is usually fixed a priori (most often, we chose 100 centres distributed on a 10×10 square grid). In more recent work (Holt et al. 1998), we have used instead the generative topographic mapping (GTM) algorithm (Bishop et al. 1998) for 2-D visualization of EEG data. The GTM algorithm is a generative model that defines a mapping from the visualization or latent space *onto* the n-dimensional space of the input vectors. For the purposes of data visualization, the mapping is then inverted using Bayes' theorem.

Visualization algorithms invariably assume that the different types of input vector occur in roughly equal numbers in the training set (i.e. that they have approximately equal prior probabilities). This is manifestly not true in the case of the sleep EEG, as periods of wakefulness will normally be few and far between. Thus the input vectors generated when the subject is awake are hardly represented at all in the training set. It is therefore important to construct a training database in which this imbalance is corrected, otherwise an underrepresented class of feature vectors will hardly have any centres assigned to it and will occupy only a small area of the 2-D visualization map.

A balanced training database was therefore constructed, consisting of 24 000 vectors of 10-D reflection coefficients, i.e. 4000 vectors for each of the six stages of the standard rule-based system, as assessed independently by the three expert scorers. When this dataset is visualized in 2-D, three non-overlapping clusters are clearly visible on the map. These can readily be identified (from the consensus-scored labels) as corresponding to wakefulness, dreaming or light sleep (REM/stage 1, which cannot be separated without either EOG or chin EMG information) and deep sleep (stage 4). Most importantly, the intermediate stages (stages 2 and 3 of the rule-based system) are *not* mapped onto separate clusters. The evolution of the sleep–wake continuum throughout the night can thus be described in its entirety as a combination of three time-varying processes.

Supervised learning

The conclusions drawn from the unsupervised learning phase suggest the construction of a supervised neural network mapping from the input reflection coefficients to three output classes corresponding to wakefulness (W), REM/light sleep (R) and stage 4 (deep sleep) (S). In our early work (Tarassenko & Roberts 1994; Roberts & Tarassenko 1995), the neural network was a radial basis function (RBF) network, but the BioSleep system (see below) uses a standard multilayer perceptron (MLP) with one layer of hidden units. This network is trained using gradient descent to minimize the squared output error, the error back-propagation algorithm (Tarassenko 1998) being used to calculate the weight updates in each layer of the network. (Typically, a learning rate of 0.01 and a momentum term of 0.5 may be used, but these values are not critical.)

The hidden layer activities of the MLP, h_j, are calculated from the weighted summation of the input reflection coefficients, x_i, passed through a saturating non-linearity known as a sigmoid, f_σ (Tarassenko 1998):

$$h_j = f_\sigma \left(\sum_{i=1}^{10} w_{ij} x_i + w_{0j} \right),$$

where h_j is the output of the j-th hidden unit, w_{ij} is the weight connecting the i-th input to it and w_{0j} is a bias weight.

The output classification vector y is generated in the second layer of the MLP from the weighted summation of the hidden-layer activities, also passed through a sigmoid:

$$y_k = f_\sigma \left(\sum_{j=1}^{J} w_{jk} h_j + w_{0k} \right),$$

where y_k is the k-th component of the classification vector, w_{jk} is the weight connecting the j-th hidden unit to it and w_{0k} is a bias weight. The target value for y_k

is 1 if the input vector x belongs to class k and 0 otherwise (1-out-of-k coding). Thus, for all patterns in the training database for the supervised learning phase, we have the following target vectors: $y = \{1, 0, 0\}$ for the W class, $y = \{0, 1, 0\}$ for the R class and $y = \{0, 0, 1\}$ for the S class.

As the number of inputs in the MLP is set by the number of reflection coefficients (usually 10 in our work), the network architecture is effectively determined by the choice of number of hidden units. For a given network architecture, the weights are initialized with small random values and the patterns in the training set are repeatedly presented in random order to the network. The weight update equations are applied after the presentation of each pattern. The training process is controlled by monitoring the classification error on an independent set of labelled patterns called the *validation* set. When this error stops decreasing or even starts to rise, training should stop. The stopping criterion is therefore the point at which the minimum classification error on the validation set is reached (a method known as 'early stopping' Tarassenko 1998).

Training runs are repeated with the number of hidden units gradually increased from a small initial value. As more hidden units are added, the minimum classification error obtained on the validation set decreases: the complexity of the neural network model more closely matches the complexity of the required input–output mapping. The optimal number of hidden units is that number for which the lowest classification error is achieved on the validation set. (If the number of hidden units is increased beyond this, performance does not improve and soon begins to deteriorate as the complexity of the neural network model is increased beyond that which is required for the problem.) Once the optimal network architecture has been determined, the performance can be evaluated on a third dataset, the *test* set, which should always consist of independent data *not* used in the training procedure, either to determine the weights (training set) or decide when to stop training (validation set). In biomedical signal processing, an independent data set is one that consists of signals recorded from subjects *not* in the training or validation sets.

When the intermediate stages of sleep (stages 2 or 3 in the conventional rule-based system) occur in test data, they are indicated at the output of the trained classifier by y_k values which lie *between* 0 and 1 ($\Sigma_k y_k$ always being equal to 1.0). Thus we use the *interpolation properties* of neural networks to quantify the depth of sleep. This description of the sleep–wake continuum in terms of three values that can vary *continuously* between 1 and 0 turns out to be much more precise than the *discrete* six-state classification of the rule-based system. The three outputs y_W, y_R and y_S correspond to the (posterior) probabilities of the subject being awake, in REM/light sleep or in deep sleep. Since these probabilities always sum to 1.0, they are not independent and the preferred option for tracking the sleep–wake continuum has been to display the difference between y_W and y_S on a second-by-second basis (1.0 corresponding to wakefulness, 0.0 to light sleep and − 1.0 to deep sleep).

Development of QUESTAR/BioSleep

Between 1993 and 1995, we collaborated with the Medical Systems Division of Oxford Instruments to develop a commercial version of our neural network system, known as QUESTAR (QUantification of EEG and Sleep Technologies Analysis and Review). In the QUESTAR system, the neural network software developed at the University of Oxford on a Unix workstation was ported onto a Windows-based environment running on a desktop computer.

For QUESTAR to be adopted as a new system for sleep analysis, there were two essential steps that had to be taken; firstly, the neural analysis had to be related to the method in regular clinical use, in this case the traditional rule-based sleep scoring. This was done in an extensive submission to the Food and Drug Administration (FDA), in which the correlation of the neural network outputs with the six discrete stages of the rule-based system was demonstrated. FDA approval was granted in 1996, one of the first neural network systems to obtain this certification. Secondly, extensive clinical studies needed to be carried out in order to demonstrate the value of the novel analysis. The system has already proved its clinical usefulness in studies carried out on patients with a variety of sleep disorders (Stradling et al. 1996; Davies et al. 1999) and with major learning disabilities (Espie et al. 1998). The latest version of the commercial system is known as BioSleep (available from Oxford BioSignals Ltd) and is an upgraded version of QUESTAR. In the rest of this chapter, we report on our work on the analysis of obstructive sleep apnoea (OSA).

Obstructive sleep apnoea

About 2% of the population is affected by daytime sleepiness, mainly caused by sleep breathing disorders. Most patients (85%) are middle-aged men, about half of them weighing at least 30% more than their ideal body weight. Sleep breathing disorders fragment the sleep continuum with hundreds of *micro-arousals*, but the patient is rarely aware of this. During sleep, some patients experience apnoeic events, when the upper airway, usually crowded by obesity, enlarged glands, or other kinds of obstruction, collapses as the muscles lose their tone. Then, as is shown in Figure 4.1, the patient increases his respiratory efforts gradually, until the intrathoracic pressure drops to a subatmospheric value. Either the repeated attempts to breathe or the rise in carbon dioxide level and the drop in oxygen level,

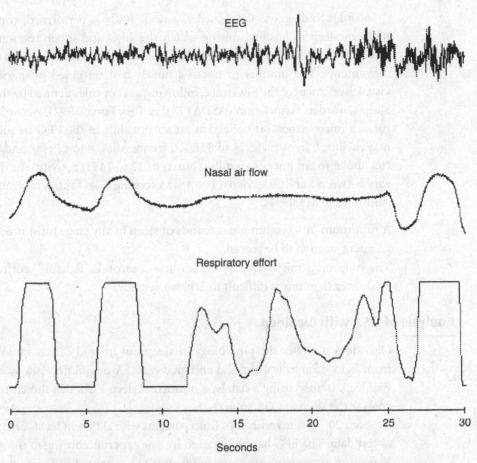

Figure 4.1.   Central EEG signal, nasal air flow and respiratory effort during a 15-second apnoeic event.

eventually awake the cortex respiratory mechanism, and the returning muscle tone unblocks the upper airways and restores ventilation. This kind of arousal is short in time, the subject rarely noticing it, and is known in the literature as a micro-arousal. A patient with a chronic history of OSA may experience more than one micro-arousal per minute, and up to 400 micro-arousals per night (Stradling 1993). The quality of sleep deteriorates as a result of the large number of micro-arousal disturbances.

About 10% of the male population suffers from this sleep disorder. The problem usually arises in middle age, when the muscles become less rigid, and a decrease in subject daily activity increases their weight. The main consequence is progressive sleepiness during daytime, starting with some loss of vigilance when performing repetitive tasks, and ending with a severe condition in which the subject falls asleep during the day.

In order to diagnose the disorder, a sleep study is performed, consisting of a night of sleep in hospital during which the EEG and other respiratory related signals are monitored continuously. A video recording is also made to follow body movements. The number of micro-arousals is determined primarily from the visual assessment of the EEG trace, following a set of rules defined by the American Sleep Disorders Association (ASDA) (Atlas Task Force 1992). According to these rules, a micro-arousal is defined as an abrupt shift in the EEG frequency, which may include θ frequencies (4 to 8 Hz), α frequencies (8 to 12 Hz), and/or frequencies above 16 Hz, but not spindles (bursts of 12 to 14 Hz activity). Its duration can vary between 3 and 20 seconds. The ASDA scoring rules for micro-arousals may be summarized as follows:

A minimum of 10 continuous seconds of sleep in any stage must precede an EEG micro-arousal to be scored.

The minimum micro-arousal duration is 3 seconds. Reliable scoring of events shorter than this is difficult to achieve visually.

Analysis of OSA with BioSleep

OSA does not alter the physiology of sleep but instead causes rapid transitions from light sleep to wakefulness and vice versa. A neural network system such as BioSleep, trained using a database of normal sleep EEG, can therefore be used to analyse the sleep of OSA subjects.

Seven 20-minute recordings from patients with different levels of OSA are used as test data. The EEG has been scored by one expert according to the ASDA rules. Reflection coefficients are extracted from the segmented EEG signal as described above, before being passed to the trained MLP. The output of the MLP, $y_W - y_S$ is thresholded in order to identify the micro-arousals. Any micro-arousal detected by the MLP within 10 seconds of the expert label is considered to be a match (true positive). Transients shorter than 3 seconds are discarded.

Figure 4.2 shows a 2-minute section of EEG from one of the OSA patients, the corresponding scores from the expert and the MLP output $y_W - y_S$. The latter is highly oscillatory around the time of an arousal, a phenomenon that has no physiological explanation. The oscillations are caused by instabilities in the values of the reflection coefficients as the assumption of stationarity begins to break down at the time of an arousal. A 5-point median filter is therefore applied to the MLP output and this has the effect of removing short pulses of 1 to 2 second duration. The filtered output and the resulting detection of an arousal after thresholding are also shown in Figure 4.2. The latter indicates that the identification of an arousal by the MLP is highly correlated with the expert's scoring, as confirmed by Figure 4.3, which shows the whole 20-minute record.

Values of sensitivity (Se) and positive predictive accuracy (PPA) can also be

Table 4.1. Sensitivity (Se) and positive predictive accuracy (PPA) for each of the seven patients in the OSA database

Patient	1	2	3	4	5	6	7
Se	0.94	1.00	0.92	0.71	0.97	1.00	1.00
PPA	0.94	0.96	0.92	0.96	0.90	0.88	1.00

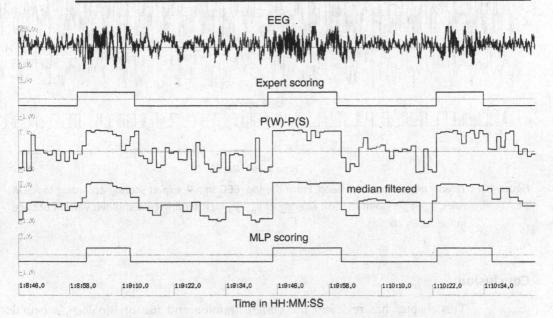

Figure 4.2. Two minutes of OSA sleep. From the top: EEG signal, expert scoring according to ASDA rules, $y_w - y_s$, 5-point median filtering of $y_w - y_s$, MLP scoring (thresholded version of trace immediately above).

calculated in order to quantify the MLP's performance for each of the seven patients. Sensitivity and positive predictive accuracy are defined as follows;

$$Se = \frac{TP}{TP + FN},$$

$$PPA = \frac{TP}{TP + FP},$$

where TP is the number of true positives, FP is the number of false positives and FN is the number of false negatives. The results are given in Table 4.1 for the whole database. These numbers (except perhaps for the sensitivity for patient 4) confirm the very high correlation between the neural network analysis and the expert's scoring.

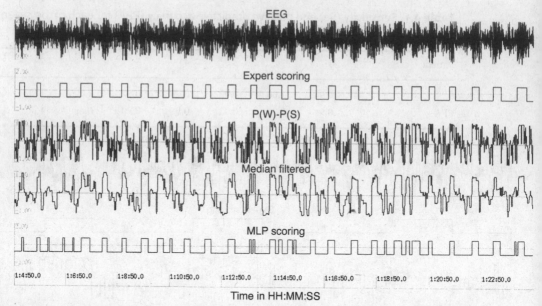

Figure 4.3.   Twenty minutes of OSA sleep. From the top: EEG signal, expert scoring according to ASDA rules, $y_W - y_S$, 5-point median filtering of $y_W - y_S$, MLP scoring (thresholded version of trace immediately above).

Conclusion

This chapter has reviewed the design, training and use of BioSleep, a neural network system for the analysis of sleep disorders. The sleep EEG is segmented into consecutive 1-second frames, or epochs, and its frequency content during each of these intervals is characterized by a set of autoregressive reflection coefficients. As a result of visualizing the distribution of these in a balanced database recorded from nine healthy subjects, it is clear that there are three main clusters of reflection coefficients, corresponding to wakefulness, REM/light sleep and deep sleep. A neural network is therefore trained to construct a mapping from the 10 input reflection coefficients to the three output classes, using examples that are typical of each class. The ability of a neural network to interpolate on test data allows the sleep–wake continuum to be tracked on a second-by-second basis. When the trained network is tested on EEG recordings made from patients suffering from OSA, it is clearly able to detect micro-arousals accurately with excellent sensitivity and specificity, an important result because it has not been possible, up until now, to automate the scoring of this type of disturbed sleep.

REFERENCES

Atlas Task Force of the American Sleep Disorders Association (1992). EEG arousals: Scoring rules and examples. *Sleep* 15(2), 174–184.

Bishop, C. M., Svensen, M. & Williams, C. K. I. (1998). GTM: the generative topographic mapping. *Neural Computation* 10, 215–234.

Davies, R. J. O., Bennet, L. S., Barbour, C., Tarassenko, L. & Stradling, J. R. (1999). Second by second patterns in cortical electroencephalograph and sub-cortical (systolic blood pressure) arousal during Cheyne–Stokes breathing. *European Respiratory Journal* 14, 940–945.

Espie, C. A., Paul, A., McFie, J., Amos, P., Hamilton, D., McColl, J. H., Tarassenko, L. & Pardey, J. (1998). Sleep studies of adults with severe or profound mental retardation and epilepsy. *American Journal of Mental Retardation* 103, 47–59.

Holt, M. R. G., Tooley, M., Forrest, F., Prys-Roberts, C. & Tarassenko, L. (1998). Use of parametric modelling and statistical pattern recognition in the detection of awareness during general anaesthesia. *IEE Proceedings in Science, Measurement and Technology* 145, 307–316.

Kelley, J. T., Reilly, E. L., Overall, J. E. & Reed, K. (1985). Reliability of rapid clinical staging of all night sleep EEG. *Clinical Electroencephalography* 16, 16–20.

Kohonen, T. (1982). Self-organized formation of topologically correct feature maps. *Biological Cybernetics* 43, 59–69.

Kohonen, T. (1990). The self-organizing map. *IEEE Proceedings* 78, 1464–1480.

Pardey, J., Roberts, S. & Tarassenko, L. (1996a). A review of parametric modelling techniques for EEG analysis. *Medical Engineering and Physics* 18, 2–11.

Pardey, J., Roberts, S., Tarassenko, L. & Stradling, J. (1996b). A new approach to the analysis of the human sleep/wakefulness continuum. *Journal of Sleep Research* 5(4), 201–210.

Rechtschaffen, A. & Kales, A., eds. (1968). *A Manual of Standardized Terminology, Techniques and Scoring System for Sleep Stages of Human Subjects*. Brain Research Institute, UCLA, Los Angeles.

Roberts, S. J. & Tarassenko, L. (1992). The analysis of the sleep EEG using a multi-layer network with spatial organisation. *IEE Proceedings F*, 139, 420–425.

Roberts, S. J. & Tarassenko, L. (1995). Automated sleep EEG analysis using an RBF network. In A. F. Murray, ed., *Applications of Neural Networks*. Kluwer Academic Publishers, Dordrecht, pp. 305–322.

Stradling, J.R. (1993). *Handbook of Sleep-Related Breathing Disorders*. Oxford University Press, Oxford and New York.

Stradling, J. R., Partlett, J., Davies, R. J. O., Siegwart, D. & Tarassenko, L. (1996). Effect of short term graded withdrawal of nasal continuous positive airway pressure on systemic blood pressure in patients with obstructive sleep apnoea. *Blood Pressure* 5, 234–240.

Tarassenko, L. (1998). *A Guide to Neural Computing Applications*. Edward Arnold, London.

Tarassenko, L. & Roberts, S. J. (1994). Supervised and unsupervised learning in radial basis function classifiers. *IEE Proceedings in Vision, Image and Signal Processing* 141, 210–216.

Tarassenko, L., Khan, Y. U. & Holt, M. R. G. (1998). Identification of inter-ictal spikes in the EEG, using neural network analysis. *IEE Proceedings in Science, Measurement and Technology* 145, 270–278.

5

Artificial neural networks for neonatal intensive care

Emma A. Braithwaite, Jimmy Dripps, Andrew J. Lyon and Alan Murray

Introduction

Neonatal units care for sick newborn babies. Although problems can arise in infants of all gestational ages, the premature infant with immature lung development contributes a significant workload to these units. These babies often require respiratory support, and throughout their clinical course need careful monitoring to detect changes in their respiratory status. In many cases important changes are detected only once there has been a significant deterioration in respiratory status. Earlier detection of these changes will allow intervention to prevent serious deterioration and will improve the outcome for the baby.

The use of artificial neural networks in medicine is increasing, predominantly in the areas of image processing (Farnsworth et al. 1996; Hintz-Madsen et al. 1996) and pattern recognition (Reddy et al. 1992; Reggia 1993). This chapter describes a prototype system developed at Edinburgh to investigate the use of neural networks for the early diagnosis of common physiological conditions found in neonatal infants by using multiple time-series traces that are already stored as part of the current monitoring system.

Results show that, although it may be possible to use neural networks in this domain, substantial work is needed into both the current monitoring processes and the techniques to be used before a system can be developed that will be usable.

Neonatal intensive care

The neonatal unit in Edinburgh uses a computerized monitoring system to collect, display and log physiological data from the dedicated monitors surrounding any incubator (see Figure 5.1). The system, called *Mary* (named after the first nurse to use it), is also networked to enable clinical staff to access patient history and to enable data collected to be used as part of the teaching process. *Mary* is also capable of storing clinical information by 'time-stamping' clinical treatment

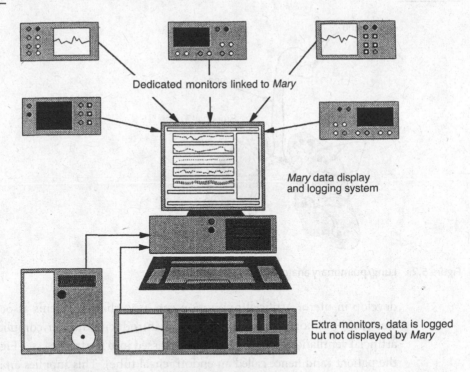

Dedicated monitors linked to *Mary*

Mary data display
and logging system

Extra monitors, data is logged
but not displayed by *Mary*

Figure 5.1.   A schematic of the single cot *Mary* data-logging system.

entries, and these can then be recalled when previous physiological data are examined. This system relies on clinicians to enter details of treatment programmes as they are completed. Data from other non-standard monitors or measuring devices can also be stored by *Mary* but not in the same time-indexed manner.

Problems faced in intensive care

An intensive care unit (ICU) is often seen as a working environment where clinicians are constantly fighting to save the lives of people who are seriously ill and require round the clock attention. This portrayal is not entirely accurate. Although the majority of patients in an ICU require greater attention than other patients within a hospital, the patient is not in a state of permanent crisis and often has sustained periods of stability. During these periods, problems can develop undetected and it is only when a crisis point is reached that a diagnosis is made or clinicians are alerted to the condition. The development of respiratory problems is an example of this.

Many patients in ICUs need respiratory support with ventilators. This is especially true in the preterm neonate as the respiratory system is one of the last to

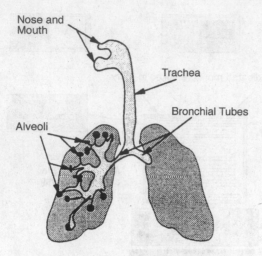

Figure 5.2.   Lung/pulmonary anatomy, including trachea.

develop in utero. Artificial respiration can exacerbate problems associated with weakened pulmonary function as well as introducing further complications. In artificial ventilation, a tube is commonly passed into the trachea (see Figure 5.2) of the patient (and hence called an endotracheal tube). This supplies an air/oxygen mixture under pressure to the lungs of the patient when he or she is unable to provide either the musculatory movement that would enable them to complete the respiratory process or the correct levels of gaseous exchange in the lungs. In neonates, the trachea is approximately 1 cm in diameter and the endotracheal tube even smaller and it can block easily with mucus. If the tube becomes blocked the patient can be starved of oxygen and in severe cases brain damage can result. Also when a tube is blocked the treatment involves removing and replacing the tube (reintubation) and this can damage the trachea. High pressure ventilation itself damages the lungs and can lead to an air leak outside the lung (pneumothorax). These are associated with a collapse of the lung and severe deterioration in the clinical state of the baby. Although the fabric of the lung can heal, the scarring can permanently reduce pulmonary function and the neonate may require further therapy. If a system can be designed to detect the development of these common problems, a substantial improvement in patient care and future prognosis could be made. The methods described in this chapter were designed to perform this task and were an initial investigation into the use of a neural network for this type of application.

Another problem faced by clinicians is that every patient is unique. This is particularly true in the neonatal ICU (NICU), as each patient has developed differently and what may be normal behaviour for one patient may cause concern if exhibited by another.

One approach

As multilayer perceptron (MLP) neural networks have previously been used in medical applications (Jansen 1990; Artis et al. 1992), fault detection (Ayanoglu 1992; Smyth & Mellstrom 1994) and condition monitoring (Hatzipantelis et al. 1995; Ramdén 1995) it was decided that initial investigations into the use of neural networks for this application would include their use. It was also decided that the maximum amount of expert knowledge on the development of the problems under investigation would also be included in the preprocessing phase of the system.

Expert knowledge and preprocessing

The build-up of secretions resulting in the blockage of an endotracheal tube can take several hours (A. Lyon & N. McIntosh, personal communication) therefore the system must contain some temporal information of the previous behaviour of the patient. Expert knowledge also tells us that, despite the development of certain respiratory problems remaining undiagnosed, clinicians can often, with hindsight, identify the onset of a particular problem. In respiratory difficulties the precursors to a condition are often present in the blood gas concentrations. Carbon dioxide (CO_2) and oxygen (O_2) play an important part in determining the current pulmonary function of an individual and therefore should be included in any system designed to aid the diagnosis of respiratory problems (Guyton 1956). Clinicians at Edinburgh also wondered whether the inclusion of a further measure, that of the fraction of inspired oxygen concentration (FiO_2), would have an effect on the ability of the system to determine the onset of respiratory difficulties. This last hypothesis was made because, during ventilation, the O_2 value of the baby is controlled by altering the FiO_2. This means that the O_2 value can be artificially maintained and that if FiO_2 is ignored the underlying process may be disguised.

For this application, expert knowledge of the development of the conditions was essential to the design of the initial stages of the system. Firstly, the signals of interest were isolated from the data archived by *Mary* and treated identically (i.e. each selected signal was processed using the same methods). In each case minute-average data are used. These are generated by averaging the standard 1-second data from *Mary* every minute and are available from clinical archives. Second-average data are also available but it was thought that it would be unnecessary to use these as the conditions under investigation develop over hours rather than minutes. Each of these signals were low-pass filtered to extract the long-term trend information and to remove artefact. Artefact was often due to the monitoring probe being moved to another location on the body. This lasted a few minutes.

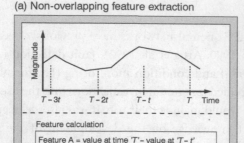
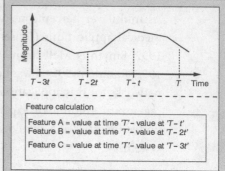

Figure 5.3.   Feature extraction processes.

The filtered signals were then passed to the feature extraction stage of preprocessing. Here, information corresponding to the development of respiratory problems was maximized by including temporal information regarding the previous behaviour of each of the physiological signals. Figure 5.3a and b shows graphical representations of the feature extraction processes. Two processes were tested to determine whether the method of inclusion of the temporal information had an impact on the ability of the system to determine the development of respiratory problems. In both cases clinical data of previous patients have been used to identify regions that should be typical of both a developing problem and an area where no concern was expressed. This was achieved by examining the clinical treatment records stored by *Mary*, and where a blocked tube or pneumothorax was entered or where the patient had been reintubated (endotracheal tube replaced) the area preceding the entry was assumed to be indicative of the problem. Conversely, where no clinical comment was made for a period of at least 3 hours, the central hour was assumed to be indicative of normal patient behaviour for that particular patient. Where a problem had developed, the time of diagnosis was taken to be T and features were extracted back from that. In the case of the non-concern examples, T was taken to be 120 minutes into the 3 hour period. The overall period over which features were extracted was 30 minutes prior to diagnosis. The subdivision of time t was defined to be 10 minutes (during the project, investigation of other time periods was also made but the results will not be presented here; Braithwaite 1998). Therefore two feature extraction processes could be tested:

Three non-overlapping features
Three nested (overlapping) features

Possible inputs	Outputs
Oxygen	Perceived problem
Carbon dioxide	
Fraction of oxygen	No problem

Figure 5.4.   Possible inputs and defined outputs.

The two approaches were designed to determine whether the system would require long-term trend (nested) or a series of shorter-term trends (non-overlapping). Once features were extracted from the three signals (CO_2, O_2 and FiO_2) the resultant vector was passed on to the classification stage of the process (see Figure 5.4).

Multilayer perceptron

The classifier chosen for this application was a simple MLP classifier trained using conjugant gradient descent. The size of the input layer was determined by which physiological signals were being used and therefore consisted of either six or nine neurons. The output layer was two dimensional, the two neurons representing either concern or no concern with regards to a developing respiratory problem. The size of the hidden layer was determined by successive tests, and results from the optimum network found will be presented. Training, validation and test vectors were formed from the sets of feature vectors generated. In total, approximately 6000 feature vectors were produced and these were not biased to either concern or no-concern. For each network, 50% of the total available data set was used for training (again unbiased) as the remainder divided between validation and test. Each network architecture was tested 10 times in order to produce an average network performance. In each case the data set was randomly partitioned into its respective parts and the progress of training was checked using the validation set.

The output of the MLP was therefore designed to produce an indicator that the particular patient was developing respiratory difficulties. A comparison was also made with results obtained from a general linear discriminant classifier.

Final system

The final system used was designed to test a number of hypotheses:

Can a neural network (MLP) be used to detect the onset of certain respiratory problems?

Does the use of the fraction of inspired oxygen have an effect on the ability of the system?

Does the method by which temporal information is included affect the performance of the system?

Figure 5.5 shows a graphical representation of the final system.

Results and discussion

Results obtained from the study can be separated into three categories:

Neural network for neonatal intensive care
Impact of including fraction of inspired oxygen
Differences between two feature extraction processes

Neural network for neonatal intensive care

To ascertain the effectiveness of the MLP as a classifier of multiple physiological
time series, results obtained from the classifier were compared with those obtained
from a general linear discriminant classifier. Results of this comparison are shown
in Table 5.1, where the percentage classification rate of a linear classifier is
compared with that of the optimal MLP architecture.

Comparison of feature extraction techniques

As it can be seen, the MLP classifier consistently outperforms the linear classifier
in terms of its accuracy or classification rate on the test set. Using this knowledge,
further tests could be carried out to determine which feature extraction process
should be used and which signals are of most relevance to the diagnostic process.
Table 5.1 also indicates that the overlapping feature extraction approach yields
greater accuracy. This does not, however, completely compare the two approaches. Table 5.2 shows some performance characteristics of the classifier when
the two different feature extraction processes are used. As it is shown, the
approach of overlapping feature extraction yields better accuracy (classification
rate), sensitivity (detection of problem rate) and lower specificity (correct identification of no-concern areas) and selectivity (a measure of the false alarm rate
(Tarassenko et al. 1997)). Therefore the conclusion can be drawn that, from a
clinical point of view, if this time interval is used overlapping features should be
chosen as they yield a higher classifier accuracy and sensitivity rate.

It should be noted that during the development phase of a system being
designed for a medical application, the selectivity measure is important as it gives
an indication of how many false alarms the system will eventually produce. This is
extremely important when the final clinical system requires low levels of false
alarm. However, in the clinical environment, sensitivity is of extreme importance

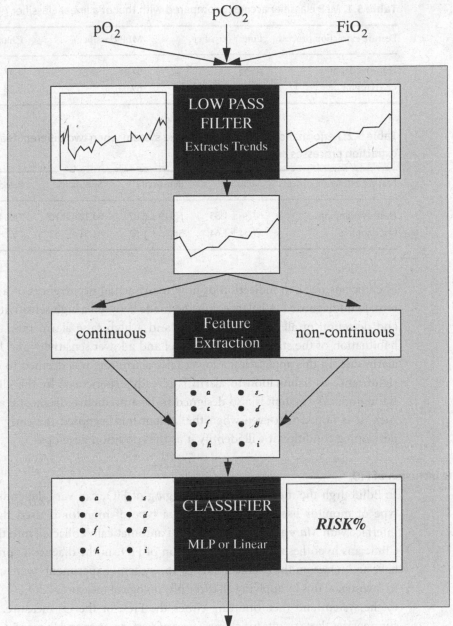

Figure 5.5.   Final system.

Table 5.1. MLP classifier accuracy compared with that of a linear classifier (%)

Feature extraction process	Linear classifier	MLP classifier	Change
Non-overlapping	65.65	67.86	3.37
Overlapping	64.76	69.04	4.28

Table 5.2. Performance characteristics of the system when two different feature extraction processes are used (%)

Feature extraction process	Accuracy	Sensitivity	Specificity	Selectivity
Non-overlapping	67.86 ± 1.85	53.49 ± 6.07	83.12 ± 8.16	76.04 ± 3.85
Overlapping	69.04 ± 1.64	56.86 ± 1.52	81.31 ± 2.62	75.28 ± 2.74

as clinicians need an indication of how many actual occurrences of a condition remain undiagnosed. A balance must be made between a high sensitivity measure and detection of all possible problems and a high false alarm rate, and hence habituation of the staff to the alarm level and a lower sensitivity and lower false alarm rate. In this application a lower false alarm rate was deemed to be of high significance as habituation to alarm is already experienced by the clinicians at Edinburgh. The system is also designed to be a predictive diagnostic aid and, as such, it is hoped that even when the system misdiagnosed the early signs of a developing condition it will identify it as the condition develops.

The inclusion of FiO$_2$

In Edinburgh the measurement and logging of FiO$_2$ can vary depending on the type of monitor used. In certain cases a type of monitor is used that cannot interface with *Mary* and hence FiO$_2$ is not automatically collected into the system. Clinicians hypothesized that the inclusion of FiO$_2$ in the diagnostic process may have an impact on the overall ability of the system. Experiments were carried out to investigate this by applying all three physiological measures (CO$_2$, O$_2$ and FiO$_2$) to the system and then omitting either the FiO$_2$ or the O$_2$ measure. Table 5.3 summarizes these results for all measures of performance and Figure 5.6a–d shows graphically the results of these experiments.

As both Table 5.3 and Figure 5.6 show, there is an improvement in all the performance measures when FiO$_2$ is included in the classification process. The improvement can also be seen, but to a lesser extent, when the fraction of inspired oxygen is substituted for the blood gas oxygen measure. These results suggest that the measure of the fraction of inspired oxygen in the air/oxygen mixture should be

Table 5.3. Performance measures (%) when different physiological signals are used

Physiological measures	Accuracy	Sensitivity	Specificity	Selectivity
CO_2, O_2 and FiO_2	69.04 ± 1.64	56.86 ± 1.52	81.31 ± 2.62	75.28 ± 2.74
CO_2 and O_2	63.66 ± 1.52	49.31 ± 4.65	78.61 ± 4.05	69.86 ± 3.49
CO_2 and FiO_2	66.11 ± 1.79	49.18 ± 5.34	83.71 ± 4.68	75.2 ± 2.98

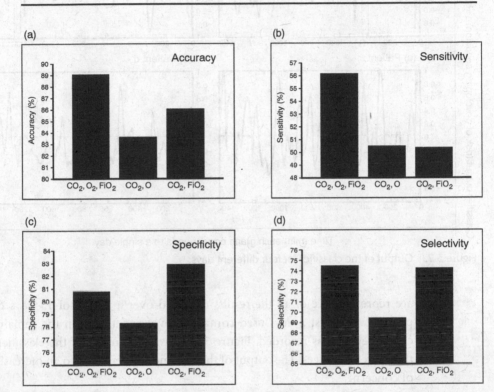

Figure 5.6.   Physiological signal relevance (using performance measures).

used in the diagnosis of developing respiratory problems to increase the likelihood of diagnosis before further invasive therapy is required.

Testing on real-time data

Although these results are encouraging and tentative conclusions can be drawn, the classifier has not yet been tested for the purpose for which it was designed: the early diagnosis of respiratory problems. The method chosen to evaluate this aspect of the classifier was to train the classifier on the preselected regions of interest and then test it on a series of complete days of physiological data. For the purposes of illustration, 4 days of physiological data will be used. However, the results shown

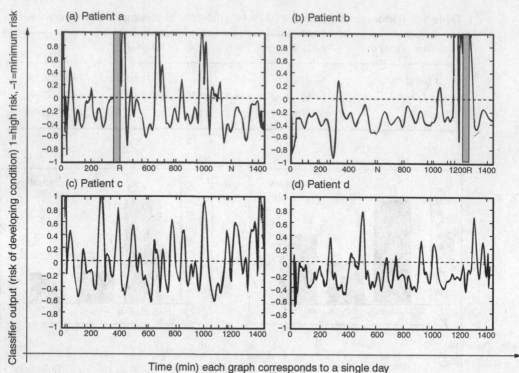

Figure 5.7. Output of the classifier for four different days.

are representative of all the results obtained over a period of 15 days from 15 patients. The first 2 days used contain known events and in the remainder no clinical event was recorded. Figure 5.7 shows the output of the classifier under these circumstances. The output of the classifier corresponds to an increasing level of concern.

As it can be seen in the first two patients (patients a and b) where the patient has been reintubated (denoted by R on the x-axis of Figure 5.7), the classifier output exhibits a significant peak. The peak also appears at least 30 minutes before the diagnosis (denoted by the grey shaded area in the figure). However, in the case of patient a other equally large peaks appear in the output, indicating that the system detected problems with the patient that clinicians had not identified at the time of entry into the record. On examination of the record there were entries made around the times of these peaks that may partially explain the classifier output. In the first instance the patient underwent 'all-care', which can include a suctioning of the endotracheal tube. This means that the condition may have been developing and was stopped before clinicians diagnosed any problems. In the case of the second peak the patient experienced a heel stab, which is a stressful procedure and may have had an adverse affect on some of the physiological control processes. In

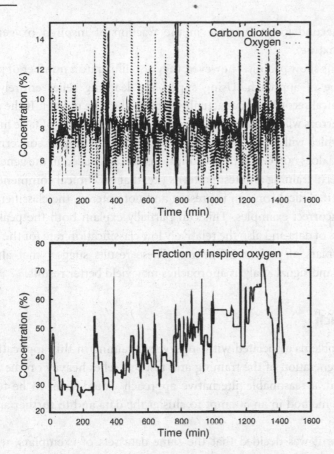

Figure 5.8.   Physiological data for patient c. (Note the long-term increase in FiO$_2$.)

the patients where no concern was entered onto the clinical record (patients c and d) it would be expected that little or no activity would occur; however, as it can be seen this is not the case. In particular in patient c multiple peaks occur that indicate a high level of concern. Examining the patient record yields no clues as to the reason for the peaks; however, returning to the physiological data (see Figure 5.8) it can be seen that, throughout the day, clinicians increased the levels of oxygen in the air/oxygen mixture, i.e. they had some concern about the respiratory function of the patient but no clinical comment was made to this effect. This illustrates the need for complete clinical records and close collaboration between clinical staff and designer. It also illustrates that, by using expert knowledge as the core of the feature extraction and preprocessing stages of the system, it is possible to determine why the classifier may have behaved in certain ways. The graph generated by patient d also shows significant peaks; however, these are lower than in the case of patient c and in the first case correspond to all care being carried out and in the second to an increase in the fraction of inspired oxygen in the air/oxygen mixture.

These results show promise; however, they also illustrate a number of problems with this type of approach. Using supervised learning relies entirely on the historical clinical record of what actually happened to the patient. If the record is incomplete, errors will occur. This is especially true in the case of false high levels of concern, which will occur when the physiological data suggest concern and the clinical record does not. Given the assumptions that were used in the generation of the 'no-concern' training and test patterns (i.e. that no clinical comment implied no concern), if clinical concern is present and not entered, the classifier is being trained on incorrect examples. This can partially explain both the peaks in the complete days of data and also the relatively low classification rate for the classifier on the exemplars of patient behaviour. These results suggest that alternative classification and signal analysis approaches may yield better results.

An alternative approach

Given the problems associated with supervised training in this application area, i.e. that the generation of the training and test sets relies heavily on the available clinical record, a reasonable alternative approach would seem to be to use an unsupervised method in an attempt to cluster the data and to further analyse its structure.

In this case it was decided that the same data sets of exemplars, with their associated problems, would be used and preprocessing and feature extraction would be carried out as before. This time, however, the feature vectors would be applied to a Kohonen network (Pao 1989) to determine whether there was any intrinsic structure in the data set that may correspond to clinical problems. A Kohonen network was chosen for these trials as a commercial neural network simulation package was used and Kohonen networks were the only unsupervised technique available. Again the size of the network was varied but this time the criteria for choosing the network size were based on which network seemed to exhibit the most clustering. Figures 5.9 and 5.12 show examples of the activation frequencies of all the nodes in a network after clustering has occurred and different data sets were applied. Figure 5.9 shows the activation frequency of the map's nodes when the entire data set that it clustered has been applied. It can be seen that there are significant clusters in the data set. To determine whether these clusters represent particular examples of patient behaviour, three further data sets were applied to the network once all weights were fixed (i.e. once the network had performed its mapping of the input space). The three data sets were the data that had previously been used to described normal patient behaviour (Figure 5.10), the

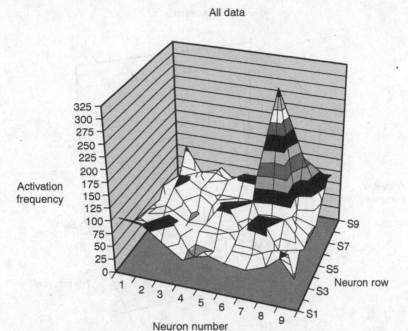

Figure 5.9.   Activation frequencies of a Kohonen network.

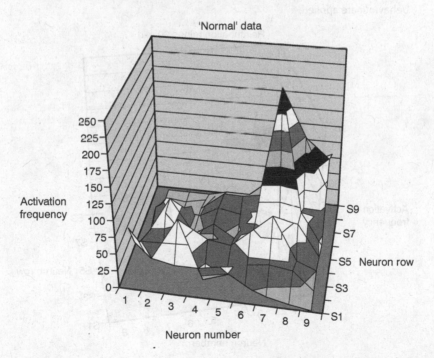

Figure 5.10. Activation frequencies of a Kohonen network when data corresponding to normal patient behaviour are applied.

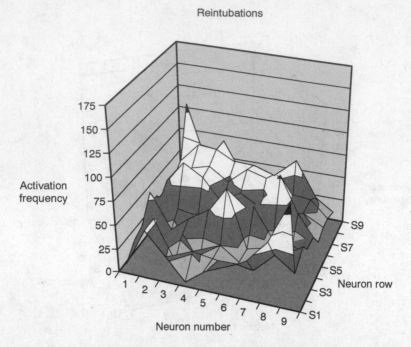

Figure 5.11. Activation frequencies of a Kohonen network when data corresponding to abnormal patient behaviour are applied.

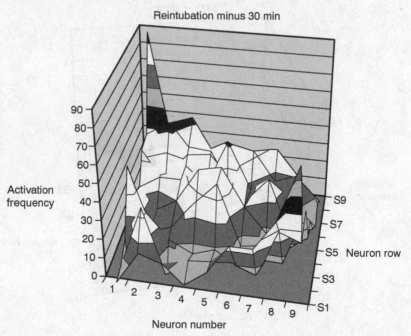

Figure 5.12. Activation frequencies of a Kohonen network when data corresponding to abnormal patient behaviour 30 minutes prior to diagnosis are applied.

data that had previously been used to describe abnormal patient behaviour (Figure 5.11), and a subset of the latter containing examples of patient behaviour 30 minutes prior to diagnosis (Figure 5.12). Examining the frequency activation of the Kohonen network under these circumstances shows that certain regions of the network seem to correspond to one type of input data, and that the clusters associated with abnormal patient behaviour become more pronounced as the catalogued time of diagnosis approaches.

These results suggest that an unsupervised approach to training a neural network may be used for this type of application but problems remain. In order to evaluate and analyse the clusters that have formed it is necessary to use clinical records (this is true even if complete days of data are used) and therefore assumptions must be made about the data and clinical record. Given the current monitoring techniques in place at Edinburgh it will only ever be possible to analyse the periods in the physiological records of a patient where a clinical entry has been made to the effect that the patient suffered some form of respiratory disorder.

Further work

As the work presented here shows, a significant amount of further investigation must be carried out before the developed system can operate to the degree of accuracy that the clinicians require. However, the work also points out several areas meriting further investigation. Given the problems associated with the supervised learning approaches of generating good example data sets, it is suggested that either an unsupervised approach should be adopted or that careful consideration should be given to the method of collection of clinical data.

Assuming that the collection method remains the same, an unsupervised approach must surely be used and attention given to the preprocessing and feature extraction stages of the system. During the filtering stage of the system it may be that information is lost which is necessary to the diagnosis of these types of respiratory problems. Again, close collaboration with clinicians and examining patient records may point towards a new preprocessing system. Expanding the number of signals under investigation, for example respiratory rate, may also have an effect on the outcome. The feature extraction process should also be refined. In other time-series, fault diagnosis application ARX modelling has been used to parameterize the time-series (Smyth 1994a) and this approach may prove to be more effective. However, if this type of approach is used, the historical information of previous patient behaviour, which clinicians know to be so important, will be lost and alternative methods of incorporating it must be found, such as hidden Markov model/artificial neural network hybrids, as previously used in speech processing (Boite et al. 1994; Reichl & Ruske 1995) and other fault diagnosis

(Smyth 1994b), and classification problems (Kundu & Ghen 1995) or in novelty detection.

Conclusions

This chapter has detailed work that has been carried in Edinburgh for the early diagnosis of common respiratory problems occurring in neonatal intensive care units. The approaches used combine expert knowledge, historical information of the patient behaviour, and a simple MLP classifier to produce an indicator of the development of a respiratory problem. Results show promise but also illustrate many of the problems associated with the medical domain. The data on which analysis is carried out are not ideal and compromises and assumptions must be made at every stage of the development process. Expert knowledge should be included to improve the acceptability of the final system to the end user, and this may in fact be at the expense of performance as more conditions being detected may be achieved by permitting a high level of false alarm.

To summarize, results from the work described suggest that a neural network can be used as part of an early diagnosis system for neonatal intensive care. However, significant work is required before any system could be in place in an NICU and relied upon by clinicians and diagnosticians.

Acknowledgements

This work was sponsored by the Scottish Office Home and Health Department (grant no. K/MRS/50/C2664).

REFERENCES

Artis, S., Mark, R. & Moody, G. (1992). Detection of atrial fibrillation using artificial neural networks. *Computers in Cardiology (1991)*, IEEE, Los Alamitos, CA, pp. 173–176.

Ayanoglu, E. (1992). Robust and fast failure detection and prediction for fault tolerant communication links. *Electronics Letters* 28, 940–941.

Boite, J., Bourlard, H., D'Hoore, B., Accaino, S. & Vantieghern, J. (1994). Task independent and dependent training: performance comparison of HMM and hybrid HMM/MLP applications. In *International Conference on Acoustics, Speech and Signal Processing*, vol. 1. IEEE, San Diego, CA, pp. I.617–I.620.

Braithwaite, E. A. (1998). Neural networks for medical condition prediction: an investigation of neonatal respiratory disorder. PhD thesis, University of Edinburgh.

Farnsworth, A., Chambers, F. & Goldschmidt, C. (1996). Evaluation of the PAPNET system in a general pathology service. *Medical Journal of Australia* 165, 429–431.

Guyton, A. (1956). Respiratory insufficiency – pathophysiology, diagnosis, oxygen therapy. In

Textbook in Medical Physiology, 8th edn., pp. 454–462. W. B. Saunders, New York.

Hatzipantelis, E., Murray, A. & Penman, J. (1995). Comparing hidden Markov models with artificial neural network architectures for condition monitoring applications. In *Artificial Neural Networks*, 4th International Conference on Artificial Neural Networks, pp. 369–374.

Hintz-Madsen, M., Hansen, L., Larsen, J., Olesen, E. & Drzewiecki, K. (1996). Detection of malignant melanoma using neural classifiers. In *Proceedings of the International Conference on Engineering Applications of Neural Networks (EANN)*, pp. 395–398.

Jansen, B. (1990). Artificial neural nets for K-complex detection. *IEE – Engineering in Medicine and Biology* 9(9), 50–52.

Kundu, A. & Ghen, G. (1995). An integrated hybrid neural network and hidden Markov model classifier for sonar signal classification. In *International Conference on Acoustics, Speech and Signal Processing*, vol. 5. IEEE, San Diego, CA, pp. IV/3587–3509.

Pao, Y.-H. (1989). *Adaptive Pattern Recognition and Neural Networks*, 1st edn. Addison-Wesley Publishing Company, Inc., Reading, MA.

Ramdén, T. (1995). On condition monitoring of fluid power pumps and systems. Master's thesis, Linköping University, Sweden. Licentiate thesis.

Reddy, M., Edenbrandt, L., Svensson, J., Haisty, W. & Pahlm, O. (1992). Neural network versus electrocardiographer and conventional computer criteria in diagnosing anterior infarction from the ECG. In *Proceedings of a Conference on Computers in Cardiology*, IEEE, San Diego, CA, 667–670.

Reggia, J. A. (1993). Neural computation in medicine. *Artificial Intelligence in Medicine* 5, 143–157.

Reichl, W. & Ruske, G. (1995). A hybrid RBF–HMM system for continuous speech recognition. In *International Conference on Acoustics, Speech and Signal Processing*, vol. 5. IEEE, pp. IV/3335–3338.

Smyth, P. (1994a). Hidden Markov models for fault detection in dynamic systems. *Pattern Recognition* 27, 149–164.

Smyth, P. (1994b). Markov monitoring with unknown states. *IEEE Journal on Selected Areas in Communications* 12, 1600–1612.

Smyth, P. & Mellstrom, J. (1994). Fault diagnosis of antenna pointing systems using hybrid neural networks and signal processing techniques. In *Advances in Neural Information Processing Systems*, vol. 4, pp. 667–674. Morgan Kaufmann, San Mateo, CA.

Tarassenko, L., Nairac, A. & Townsend, N. (1997). Novelty detection. In *Neural Computing – The Key Questions*, NCAF, Bath.

6

Artificial neural networks in urology: applications, feature extraction and user implementations

Craig S. Niederberger and Richard M. Golden

Introduction

Urology is a diverse surgical specialty that includes disorders of the urinary and male reproductive systems. As such, it includes diagnosis and treatment of cancers, urinary stones, male infertility, impotence, urinary diseases in children, neurological and anatomical disorders resulting in an inability to properly empty the bladder, trauma to the urinary and male reproductive systems, and other diseases. This diversity contributes to the challenging nature of diagnosing and treating urological disorders, and to the difficulty in modelling urological data sets.

In this chapter, we review urological diagnostic and prognostic modelling problems that we found intractable to discriminant function analysis in which neural computational modelling was superior in performance. Because of its simplicity and explicit nature, we chose discriminant function analysis (DFA) as a traditional, linear statistical approach with which we compared neural computational modelling (Duda & Hart 1973). This analysis does not prove that neural computational modelling is superior to all forms of classical data modelling; rather, we found neural computational modelling to be a useful and robust technique for a variety of diverse urological data sets.

In this chapter we also review two aspects of neural computational modelling that, while not necessarily central to modelling per se, are of substantial interest to physicians entrenched in the clinical realm. The first is feature extraction. Physicians encountering our trained and tested neurological models invariably asked which feature or features were significant to the model. 'Was it important if the patient had stone fragments on X-ray to the network that predicted stones on future exam?' Did giving patient chemotherapy affect the outcome of the network that predicted kidney cancer metastases?' We applied Wilk's generalized likelihood ratio test (Wilk's GLRT) as a feature extraction method for neural computation, and discuss the technique in this chapter.

The second aspect of neural computational modelling essential to physicians that we discuss here is availability of the trained model to practising physicians. Physicians may read with interest in journals reports of trained models, but without a readily, widely available, and easily implemented model, the tool will be little more than a curious toy. We used commonly available resources in conjunction with the World Wide Web to develop interfaces in which users could run trained networks on either a centralized server or a distributed client. We end this chapter with a discussion of these strategies and their implementation.

Neural computational model building for the urological data sets

Because little a priori knowledge was available about the urological modelling problems, we designed neural computational models with a generic approach. We built a programming environment to rapidly prototype neural computational models, naming the environment 'neUROn' (neural computational environment for urological numericals). NeUROn was initially designed as a general purpose neural programming environment in C rather than a single program, and was recently ported to C++. Neural network architecture features are coded in preprocessor directives, and are specified by a single header file. By defining preprocessor variables, programmers can generate during compilation machine code highly tailored to a specific medical application. The reduction of computing cost in this approach is desirable, as neural network training may require billions of iterations through a training data set before a solution is achieved.

Although neUROn contains several training engines as encoded objects, our approach was to model first with canonical back-propagation, with the exception that the cross-entropy error function was used at the output node rather than least mean squared error (Werbos 1974; Golden 1996). This error function is described in the next section. We built networks with one hidden node layer and bias nodes on all layers. Ten hidden nodes were initially encoded in the neural architecture, and hidden nodes were reduced (pruned) until overlearning ceased. Cessation of overlearning was noted when training and test set classification error versus training iteration curves were non-divergent. The networks with the hidden node number so determined were trained to completion, which was defined either as an error function value that was less than the numerical precision of the C compiler (10^{-12}) or if the error increased over a given window width of iterations through the training set. The strict local minimum thus found was tested by arbitrarily changing individual weights by small random numbers, and demonstrating that the weights returned on retraining to the weight vector found on initial training to completion.

Feature extraction using Wilk's GLRT

Although neUROn is typically described as a back-propagation neural network, neUROn may also be expressed as a non-linear regression model (Golden 1996). Let matrix v denote the pattern of connections from the m hidden units to the output unit, let scalar b denote the bias for the output unit, let matrix q_j denote the connections from the input layer to the j-th hidden unit $(j=1\dots m)$, and let z denote the biases for the hidden units. The elements of all four of these parameter vectors may be arranged in a single d-dimensional parameter vector w.

Consider a statistical environment defined by a sequence of n independent and identically distributed random vectors (the notation $\tilde{o}$ is used to indicate that o is a random variable),

$$\{(\tilde{s}_1, \tilde{o}_1), \dots, (\tilde{s}_n, \tilde{o}_n)\},$$

with common probability mass function $p([s, o])$. Assume that

$$p([s, o]) = p(s)p(o \mid s, w);$$

where $p(s)$ is the probability mass that stimulus input vector s will be presented to neUROn (which is not functionally dependent upon the connection strength parameter vector w), and the conditional probability mass function $p(o \mid s, w)$ maps a given stimulus input vector s and connection strength parameter vector w into the probability that outcome o will occur. It is assumed that o can take on exactly one of two values 0 or 1, so that $o \in \{0, 1\}$.

Let $\mathscr{S}$ be a sigmoidal function defined such that for any real number x: $\mathscr{S}(x) = 1/(1 + \exp(-x))$. The formula for $p(o=1 \mid s, w)$ (which is the activation level r of the output unit of neUROn) is given by the expression:

$$r = p(o=1 \mid s, w) = \mathscr{S}\left(\sum_{j=1}^{m} v_j h_j + b\right), \tag{6.1}$$

where the activation level of the j-th hidden unit $(j=1\dots m)$ is given by the formula:

$$h_j = \mathscr{S}(q_j^T s + z_j),$$

where z_j is the j-th element of z. Note that since $o \in \{0, 1\}$, we have $p(o \mid s, w) = or + (1-o)(1-r)$.

Learning in neURO proceeds by using a gradient descent algorithm that seeks a strict local minimum of the negative log-likelihood function. A strict local minimum of the error function E is sought, where E is defined such that, for any given connection strength parameter vector w,

$$E(w) = -(1/n) \sum_{i=1}^{n} \log[p(o^i \mid s^i, w)],$$

where (o^i, s^i) is the i-th record in the set of n data records used to 'train' (or equivalently estimate the parameters of) neUROn. Golden (1996) has noted that, on completion of network training, Wilk's generalized likelihood ratio test (GLRT) may be used to determine which input nodes in the back-propagation network have connection strengths to the rest of the network that are effectively equal to zero. This capability is of particular interest to medical researchers who desire to 'open the black box', and dissect the importance of specific clinical parameters.

Use of Wilk's GLRT begins with training of a network on a particular data set, and recording the network error $E_{full}(w^{full})$ for the *full model*. One or more input node(s) representing a feature are then removed from the full model by setting u of the weights that connect the selected input nodes to the rest of the network equal to zero. The network is then retrained on the same data set and the network error $E_{red}(w_{red})$ is recorded. The procedure requires that both error estimates are associated with strict local minima of their respective error surfaces and the same strict local minimum of the 'true' error function. The procedure also requires that the full model, which contains all of the input nodes, generates probabilities that are a 'good fit' to the observed statistical data. The question to test is whether the increase in error is statistically significant (i.e. whether the u weights in the original network were really equal to zero).

Using Wilk's GLRT, the null hypothesis that the two networks are equally effective (aside from sampling error) in classification can be rejected if

$$-2n[E_{full}(w^{full}) - E_{red}(w^{red})] > \chi_\alpha^2, \tag{6.2}$$

where χ_α^2 is a constant with the property that a chi-squared random variable with u degrees of freedom exceeds χ_α^2 with probability α.

To summarize, the procedure to use Wilk's GLRT for feature extraction is as follows:

1. The full network is trained to a strict local error minimum. The trained network is then examined to determine whether the model is a 'good fit' (it would be useless to perform feature extraction if the model was no better than the flip of a coin). The modeller also demonstrates that the model was trained to a strict local error minimum, for example by arbitrarily altering individual trained weights and observing the network on further training to return to the same local error minimum.
2. The cross-entropy error function is calculated at the strict local error minimum

for the full model,

$$E_{\text{full}}(w^{\text{full}}) = -\sum_{k=1}^{n}\sum_{i=1}^{d}[o_i^k \log(r_i^k) + (1-o_i^k)\log(1-r_i^k)], \tag{6.3}$$

where n is the number of records in the data set, d is the number of output nodes, o is an output node's value derived by the network, and r is the 'real' value of that output in the data set. It is important to note that in this use of Wilk's GLRT, output values must be constrained to $\{0,1\}$.

3. The number of network connections C_{full} is calculated for the full model. For example, for a fully interconnected network with one hidden node layer and biases on the input and hidden layers, the number of connections C is

$$C = (N_i + 1)N_h + (N_h + 1)N_o, \tag{6.4}$$

where N_i is the number of input nodes, N_h is the number of hidden nodes, and N_o is the number of output nodes.

4. A feature-deficient network is trained by holding all of the input nodes corresponding to that feature in the data set to 0, and retraining the network to a strict local error minimum. The strict local error minimum is demonstrated as in the first step of the procedure, with the additional requirement that the strict local error minima of the full model and feature deficient model correspond to the same strict local minimum of the 'true' error function. The modeller observes the error curve while training for rapid changes indicating a possible 'leap' into another, different error minimum.

5. The cross-entropy error function for the feature deficient network $E_{\text{red}}(w^{\text{red}})$ is calculated as in Eq. 6.3.

6. The number of network connections C_{red} for the feature deficient network is calculated as in Eq. 6.4.

7. A chi-squared value is calculated,

$$\chi_\alpha^2 = -2n[E_{\text{full}}(w^{\text{full}}) - E_{\text{red}}(w^{\text{red}})], \tag{6.5}$$

where n is the number of records in the data set, and the cross-entropy errors for the full and feature deficient data sets are calculated as described above.

8. The number of degrees of freedom (df) for the test is calculated by

$$\text{df} = C_{\text{full}} - C_{\text{red}}, \tag{6.6}$$

where C_{full} is the number of network connections for the full model, and C_{red} is the number of network connections for the feature deficient model.

9. The probability p_α that the modeller can reject the null hypothesis that the full network and feature deficient networks are the same is then determined for the

chi-squared value χ^2_α with degrees of freedom df either by examination of a table of chi-squared values, or using the incomplete gamma function.

A neural network to model testis biopsy outcomes

As an example of neural computational modelling of a difficult urological diagnostic problem, and of use of Wilk's GLRT for feature extraction, we modelled outcomes of patients undergoing testis biopsies. A commonly encountered infertile male is one who has no or very few sperm in his semen. These patients are referred to as 'azoospermic' or 'near azoospermic'. When evaluating such a patient, the urologist must identify him as one who has no sperm in the semen as a result of failure to make sperm in the testis, or of blockage of the tiny ductal system that carries the sperm from the testis to the outside world. This diagnosis is typically made by surgically removing a small piece of testis, and examining it under the microscope. If sperm cells are present in the testis in various stages of development and in normal numbers, then the patient has presumptive ductal obstruction, and is scheduled for surgery so that a search may begin to identify and correct the obstruction. If no mature sperm cells are present in the testis specimen, the patient is counselled that fathering biological children is not yet possible. Clearly the two outcomes have vastly different implications, and it is desirable to predict as early on as possible in the diagnostic evaluation of the patient into which category he belongs.

Urologists have long noticed certain associations of various features of a patient with the outcome of testis biopsy. Taking a clue from their counterparts in animal husbandry, urologists have observed that the smaller the testis size, the less likely the patient is to have sperm made in the testis. However, this association is far from perfect, as while some men may normally have larger ears than others without any effect on hearing, some men may have smaller testes than others without any effect on fertility. Urologists have also observed that a specific hormone level in the blood, follicle-stimulating hormone (FSH), is inversely correlated with the likelihood of finding sperm in a testis biopsy. Presumably, as sperm cells are depleted in the testis, their influence wanes on the secretion of an inhibitory factor, inhibin, by their neighbouring cells, the Sertoli cells. As blood inhibin levels fall, blood FSH levels rise. However, this too is an imperfect association. Certainly, the patients with very high levels of FSH, the probability of finding sperm in the testis is low, although this rule is occasionally broken. For normal or near normal levels of FSH, however, inspection of this single feature tells us very little about the probability of finding sperm on testis biopsy.

In a sense then, urologists have adopted a somewhat imperfect 'expert system', or algorithmic approach, to the problem of modelling testis biopsy outcomes. If the FSH level was elevated past a threshold value, usually twice the laboratory upper limit of normal, then the patient was counselled to use donor sperm or to adopt. If the FSH level was not elevated, then the patient underwent testis biopsy to determine whether mature sperm was present in the testis. We sought to substitute a more robust and accurate model for this simple algorithmic approach that relied on one single clinical parameter, the FSH level.

We chose neural computation as a non-linear computational method for modelling testis biopsy outcomes in a pilot study of 36 patients. Five features were encoded into eight input nodes. The first two input nodes corresponded to the FSH value, with the first input node representing whether or not $(0, 1)$ that data value was available for that patient, and the second input node was the normalized value for FSH, with

$$FSH = \frac{FSH_{value} - FSH_{low}}{FSH_{high} - FSH_{low}},$$

where FSH_{low} was the lower limit and FSH_{high} was the upper limit of normal for the laboratory determination of FSH_{value}. In this way, FSH values from different laboratories could be used in the built model. In a similar manner, two input nodes were encoded for blood luteinizing hormone (LH) and two for blood testosterone levels. As seminal fructose (semen sugar) and testis size measurements were available for all patients, one input node was encoded for each. One output variable was encoded, with 0 representing no mature sperm, and 1 representing mature sperm seen on testis biopsy. The data set was randomly divided into a training set of 24 records and a test set of 12 records. Sequential random sets of training and test sets were generated until the frequency of records with outputs 1 and 0 was the same in both training and test sets. This procedure generated test set data with the property that the estimated overall expected likelihood of observing a mature sperm was the same as the corresponding training data set, and was designed to bias the generation of the test set data so that more representative test data sets would be generated (under the assumption that the training data set was fairly representative of the population distribution).

Canonical back-propagation as described by Werbos (1974) was used as the training algorithm, with the exception that the cross-entropy error function was substituted for a least mean squared error at the output node (Golden 1996). Our general strategy for neural computational model building has been to begin with a fully interconnected network with one hidden layer and biases on both input and hidden node layers, and to reduce hidden nodes until overlearning is observed to cease. Overlearning usually occurs when a network has so many resources (i.e. parameters) that it can 'memorize' the training data and is not forced to extract useful discriminatory features from the training data set. Overlearning is detected by plotting classification errors in the test set at intervals during training. If the test set error initially decreases, then increases as the training set error continues to decrease, overlearning is evident. We began with 10 hidden nodes in the hidden layer, and reduced one at a time until overlearning ceased, at which point two hidden nodes remained in the hidden layer. The network was then trained to completion. The final cross-entropy error recorded at completion of training was 3.07e-16. At completion of training, the classification accuracy was 100% in the training set, and 91% in the test set. In comparison, the classification accuracies of linear and quadratic discriminant function analysis were both 21% in the training set, and 25% in the test set.

Feature extraction was then performed using Wilk's GLRT. *Beginning with the weights and biases of the trained model,* the network was retrained with each input feature removed by setting its respective input node activation levels to 0. For example, the activation levels of the two nodes representing FSH were held to 0 and the network was retrained, with a final cross-entropy error recorded to be 3.81e-15. Thus, in Eq. 6.5, with $n = 24$ records in the training set,

$$\chi^2_\alpha = -2n[E_{full}(w^{full}) - E_{red}(w^{red})],$$
$$\chi^2_\alpha = -2(24)[3.07 \times 10^{-16} - 3.81 \times 10^{-15}],$$
$$\chi^2_\alpha = 1.68 \times 10^{-13}.$$

It is essential to note that both the full and feature-depleted models were trained to a critical point, as partial training invalidates Wilk's GLRT. We empirically defined a critical point as either a change in output node error over one training iteration to be less than the numerical precision of the compiler, or an increase in output node error after a discrete number of training iterations (error window). The former definition is obvious, as training will conclude when the executable code is no longer able to process the difference in output node error. The latter definition is more ambiguous and is obtained empirically. The error window cannot be so small as to cease training during a small increase in error prior to a large decline. However, if the error is fluctuating over a small value for a large number of iterations, it can be surmised that the error gradient in weight space is oscillating in the vicinity of a local error minimum, and training is complete. This error window is different for every training set, and was determined by empirical observation of plots of cross-entropy error versus training iterations to be 8000 for this example.

In order to calculate the degrees of freedom for Wilk's GLRT, the number of network interconnects for the full and feature deficient models are calculated. The full model consisted of a fully connected network with eight input nodes, two hidden nodes, one output node, and biases on the input and hidden layers. Thus,

Table 6.1. Wilk's generalized likelihood ratio test p values for feature deficient networks trained to model testis biopsy outcomes

Feature extracted	χ^2_α	df	p
FSH	1.68e-13	4	≈ 1
LH	1.65e-13	4	≈ 1
Testosterone	1.67e-13	4	≈ 1
Fructose	1.66e-13	2	≈ 1
Testis size	2.80	2	0.247

FSH, follicle-stimulating hormone; LH, luteinizing hormone.

from Eq. 6.4,

$$C_{full} = (N_i + 1)N_h + (N_h + 1)N_o,$$
$$C_{full} = (8 + 1)2 + (2 + 1)1 = 21.$$

The reduced model consisted of six input nodes (two input nodes encoded the FSH feature, one node for the presence or absence of the feature, and one node for the FSH value), two hidden nodes, one output node, and biases on the input and hidden layers. Thus, from Eq. 6.4,

$$C_{red} = (N_i + 1)N_h + (N_h + 1)N_o,$$
$$C_{red} = (6 + 1)2 + (2 + 1)1 = 17.$$

From Eq. 6.6,

$$df = C_{full} - C_{red},$$
$$df = 21 - 17 = 4.$$

Inspection of a table of chi-squared values showed that, for $\chi^2_\alpha = 1.68e-13$ with 4 degrees of freedom, $p \approx 1$. The null hypothesis that the feature-deficient model was the same as the full network cannot be rejected. This result is not surprising, as simple inspection of the final errors of the full and reduced networks appeared very similar. Use of Wilk's GLRT allows the conclusion that FSH, *as a single parameter*, does not affect the model's performance.

Results of extracting FSH and other single features are shown in Table 6.1. For no single feature extracted was $p < 0.05$. The only single feature extracted with an obvious difference in final trained error was testis size. However, the test did not reveal a significant difference for testis size. This failure to find a significant difference is probably due to the small number (24) of records in the training data set. Combinations of features were then extracted, first two at a time, then three at a time. When FSH and testosterone and testis size were extracted together, χ^2_α was

18.53, and with 10 degrees of freedom, $p = 0.047$. Thus, for our chosen level of significance ($p < 0.05$), a feature-deficient model lacking FSH and testosterone and testis size performed significantly worse than the full model. We can thus deduce from the model that these are the three most significant clinical features in predicting the relevant outcome; that is, whether or not mature sperm will be found on testis biopsy.

A neural network to model outcomes of patients with renal cancer

Outcomes of patients with renal carcinoma are among the most difficult to model in medicine (de Kernion 1986; Williams 1987; Montie 1994). For most cancers, the prognosis of a patient is fundamentally altered when the tumour migrates to a distant site, a process known as metastasis. It is generally useless to surgically remove a metastasis in an attempt to cure cancer, as invariably more metastases follow. Unlike in other cancers, however, in renal cancer, the removal in certain patients leads to long-term survival (Jett et al. 1983). Renal cancer thus behaves in a very 'illogical' way.

Physicians have long devised descriptive categories in an attempt to correlate prognostic outcomes with a categorical state. These categories are referred to as 'stages' of cancer, and the application of a stage to a patient is referred to as 'staging'. Stages are chosen so that, if left unchecked, the cancer would evolve from one stage to another in an orderly fashion. The staging exercise in cancer is the basis on which therapeutic choices are made in an algorithmic approach. As an example, a renal tumour that is smaller than 2.5 cm in diameter and limited to the kidney, and that has not migrated to the lymph nodes or other distant organs, is termed 'stage T1' in the 'TNM' classification system. Surgical removal of such a tumour results in 60–82% of patients alive at 5 years. A renal tumour that has pushed its way outside of the kidney's capsule and into the surrounding fat is termed 'stage T3a', and surgical removal of this type of tumour leads to a 5-year survival rate of 47–80% (de Kernion 1986). Two additional problems are thus evident in the staging of renal cancer and render this an 'illogical' cancer. The first is the substantial degree of overlap in the outcomes of patients undergoing surgical therapy for different stages. One would expect high survival for lower stages, and lower survival for more advanced stages. This is not necessarily the case for renal cancer. In addition, renal cancer may remain quiescent for many years and suddenly erupt with distant metastases, 'skipping' stages (de Kernion 1986; Williams 1987; Montie 1994).

We therefore sought to computationally model outcomes of patients with renal cancer in an attempt to more accurately predict progression of this odd disease (Qin et al. 1994; Niederberger et al. 1997). We chose to model two outcomes: the

Table 6.2. Feature encoding for renal cancer data sets

Number input nodes	Variable	Type
4	Ethnicity	Categorical
1	Gender	Binary
1	Diagnosis date available (Yes, No)	Binary
1	Age = Date of diagnosis − Date of birth	Numerical
1	T stage available (Yes, No)	Binary
1	T stage	Numerical
1	N stage available (Yes, No)	Binary
1	N stage	Numerical
1	M stage available (Yes, No)	Binary
1	M stage	Numerical
1	Nephrectomy (Yes, No)	Binary
1	Nephrectomy date available (Yes, No)	Binary
1	Date of surgery − Date of birth	Numerical
1	Lung metastases information available (Yes, No)	Binary
1	Lung metastases (Yes, No)	Binary
1	Bone metastases information available (Yes, No)	Binary
1	Bone metastases (Yes, No)	Binary
10	Histologic subtype	Categorical
1	Tumour size (centimetres)	Numerical
7	Treatment choice	Categorical

occurrence of metastases and patient mortality, for example whether or not a patient was alive or dead at a specific time point. Encoded input variables are shown in Table 6.2. Categorical variables such as ethnicity were encoded into multiple binary variables; for example African-American was encoded as (1,0,0,0), Caucasian (0,1,0,0), Hispanic (0,0,1,0), and Asian (0,0,0,1). Although this method of encoding categorical variables is not as efficient as assigning binary values to each category, for example African-American would be encoded as (0,0), Caucasian (0,1), Hispanic (1,0), and Asian (1,1), the one-node-per-category strategy is more amenable to subsequent analysis with Wilk's GLRT. Two data sets were obtained, one with 341 records of patients with known mortality (alive or dead), and one with 232 patients in which metastases were known. The data set of 341 patients with known mortality was randomized into a training set of 257 and a test set of 84 patients in the same manner as described in the previous section describing modelling of testis biopsy outcomes. The data set containing 232 entries of patients with known metastatic status was randomized into 174 patients in the training set and 58 in the test set. In the case of the mortality data set, the

Table 6.3. Classification accuracies of methods modelling new metastases in the renal cancer data set

Data set	LDFA (%)	QDFA (%)	Neural network (%)
Training	68.4	69.0	92.5
Test	67.2	69.0	84.5

Table 6.4. Classification accuracies of methods modelling new mortality in the renal cancer data set

Data set	LDFA (%)	QDFA (%)	Neural network (%)
Training	40.1	39.3	90.3
Test	40.5	39.3	71.4

LDFA, linear discriminant function analysis; QDFA, quadratic discriminant function analysis.

outcome node was encoded as (1,0) for alive or dead at the measured time point. For the metastases data set, the outcome was encoded as (1,0) for new or no metastases at the measured time point.

Fully interconnected networks with one hidden layer and biases on the input and hidden layers were constructed for both data sets as described in the testis biopsy model. Canonical back-propagation was used as the training method, except for the use of the cross-entropy error function for the output node. Hidden nodes were sequentially removed from the hidden node layer until cessation of overlearning was noted. For both data sets, the resulting networks had six hidden nodes in the hidden layer. These networks were then trained to completion, in a fashion similar to the testis biopsy experiments. The data sets were previously modelled with linear and quadratic discriminant function analysis. Performance of these models is shown in Table 6.3. Performance of discriminant function analyses and the neural network training to model mortality is shown in Table 6.4. In both models, neural computation yielded higher classification accuracies in the test set than discriminant function analysis. However, the neural network modelling patient mortality fared worse than that modelling the development of metastases. This is not surprising, as modelling survival involves non-disease specific factors such as the degree of health of the patient's cardiovascular system prior to development of the tumour, factors that we could not specify or access for every patient.

Because the neural network modelling the development of metastases performed reasonably well, it was interesting to ask what patient features were

Table 6.5. Wilk's GLRT feature extraction results for the renal cancer metastasis model

Feature extracted	p
Ethnicity	1.000
Gender	0.009[a]
Age	< 0.001[a]
T stage	0.004[a]
N stage	0.007[a]
M stage	0.428
Nephrectomy	1.000
Surgery date	1.000
Lung metastases	0.807
Bone metastases	1.000
Histologic subtype	< 0.001[a]
Tumour size	0.739
Treatment choice	1.000

[a] $p < 0.05$.

significant to the model. For example, did the model rely on tumour size? Did the type of therapy, surgery or chemotherapy, determine the model's outcome? Was the presence of metastases in the past necessary to the model of future metastases? To answer these questions, we performed feature extraction with Wilk's GLRT as described in the previous section detailing feature extraction in modelling testis biopsy outcomes. The result of Wilk's GLRT for the metastatic model is shown in Table 6.5. Inspection of Table 6.5 reveals that patient gender, age, T stage, N stage and histologic subtype of the tumour all significantly degraded network perform-ance when these features were extracted from the full network. The findings of T and N stages as significant features to the model substantiate the TNM system as one that has at least some place in the staging of renal cancer. What are perhaps as interesting as those features that were significant to the model are those features that were not. Surprisingly, the presence of a past metastasis was not a feature essential to the model's performance in predicting a new metastasis. This observa-tion is in agreement with the odd behaviour of renal cancer in that surgical removal of a metastasis may lead to long-term survival. It is also interesting that the choice of treatment was not one of the features significant to the model. Surgeons that remove renal tumours and medical oncologists that use chemother-apy would probably desire to have choice of therapy significantly affect a model of new metastases to argue for the selection of one type of therapy versus another. Yet, in this model, other features were more significant than type of therapy. This example of the use of Wilk's GLRT thus serves as one in which analysis of a model built without the inherent clinical biases of physicians aids clinicians in making new inferences about a disease.

A neural network to model extracorporeal shock wave lithotripsy outcomes

One urological disease that has recently undergone a revolution in therapy is urinary lithiasis, or the formation of stones in the urinary tract (Lange 1986; Chaussy & Fuchs 1987). Urinary stones form when various inorganic and organic substances in the urine exceed their solubility product. This process depends on the urinary pH, as well as various substances that inhibit or promote stone formation. A wide variety of risk factors have been identified that lead to new or recurrent urinary stones, and these include environmental, nutritional, metabolic, anatomic, infectious and other factors. When urinary stones do form, they often obstruct the urinary system, leading to great pain and possible damage to the kidneys from back pressure.

The traditional therapy for urinary stones was surgical removal. Since the early 1980s, a technological advance, extracorporeal shock wave lithotripsy (ESWL), obviated surgery for over 90% of patients with large urinary stones. Shock waves are generated from a submersed spark-plug with opposing electrodes. The underwater spark vaporizes adjacent water molecules, causing a primary shock wave and a secondary shock wave from collapse of gas bubbles formed during the spark discharge. These shock waves are focused by a rotationally symmetrical semi-ellipsoid bath, and the focused shock waves so generated fragment the stone. Thus a non-invasive therapy replaced surgery for a majority of patients.

However, the new therapy was not without its new problems. ESWL often left behind small, non-obstructing fragments, whereas surgery generally removed the entire stone. The urologist was left with the dilemma of how to manage these residual stone fragments. Sometimes these fragments would grow into another obstructing stone. At other times, these stones would remain small and clinically insignificant. At times, even when no fragments were left after ESWL, stones would recur. We sought to build a computational model that would predict, given a patient profile, stone recurrence after ESWL. The clinically relevant outcome was chosen; that is, if no stone fragments were present after ESWL, the model would predict whether new stones would form, or, if stone fragments were present after ESWL, the model would predict whether these fragments would grow.

Data were encoded with the general strategy in the previous section describing modelling of renal cancer data. Sixteen input variables were encoded into 37 input

Table 6.6. Performance of methods modelling stone recurrence in the ESWL data set

Method	Train Class Acc (%)	Test Class Acc (%)	Sens (%)	Spec (%)	PPV (%)	NPV (%)	ROC area
NNET	100	90.9	90.5	91.7	95.0	85.0	0.964
LDFA	32.3	36.4	0	100	NaN	39.4	0.524
QDFA	32.3	36.4	0	100	NaN	39.4	0.524

Sens, sensitivity; Spec, specificity; PPV, positive predictive value; NPV, negative predictive value; ROC area, receiver operator characteristic curve area; NaN indicates division by zero; Acc, accuracy.

nodes. These included (1) patient age, (2) gender, (3) ethnicity, (4) stone chemistry, (5) location, (6) configuration, (7) metabolic disease, (8) infectious disease, (9) time since last follow-up, (10) presence of fragments after ESWL, (11) other procedures, (12) medical therapy, (13) anatomical abnormality, (14) presence of catheter, (15) history of previous stone and (16) concurrent stones. One output node was encoded as 0 if no stones were seen on follow-up, or if fragments were present, they did not grow. The output node was 1 if stones were present on follow-up, or if fragments were present, they grew. The full data set consisted of 98 records randomized into a training set of 65 and a test set of 38 records using the strategy described in the previous section describing modelling of testis biopsy outcomes (Michaels et al. 1998).

Fully interconnected networks with one hidden layer and biases on the input and hidden layers were constructed for both data sets as described in the testis biopsy and renal cancer models. Canonical back-propagation was used as the training method, with the exception of the use of the cross-entropy error function for the output node. Hidden nodes were sequentially removed from the hidden node layer until overlearning was noted to cease. The resulting network had five hidden nodes in the hidden layer. The network was then trained to completion, in a fashion similar to that of the testis biopsy and renal cancer experiments. The data sets were previously modelled with linear and quadratic discriminant function analysis. Performance of these models is shown in Table 6.6.

As in the previous examples for models of testis biopsy and renal cancer outcomes, feature extraction was performed with Wilk's GLRT. All features extracted resulted in p values ≈ 1. This result indicates a high degree of redundancy of informational content of the input feature set. What was perhaps most surprising was the superior performance in every parameter measured of the neural computational method compared with discriminant function analysis.

A perusal of receiver operator characteristic (ROC) curve area alone is revealing, with 1.0 representing a perfect model, and 0.5 a completely imperfect model, the neural network resulted in an ROC curve area of 0.964, whereas both discriminant function analysis methods resulted in an ROC curve area of 0.524. It was thus desirable to make the trained neural model available for practising physicians treating patients after ESWL, so that they could use the prognostic information afforded by this tool. Our strategy for making available to remote physicians this and other networks is discussed in the following section.

Remote user implementations of trained neural models

Without the ability to use trained neural computational models, physicians are unlikely to treat these models as little more than intriguing diversions. It is desirable to make these models widely available and easy to use. The internet offers computational resources that achieve both goals.

Two general strategies are available to modellers using the Internet to increase availability of their models. Although the details of the implementations will undoubtedly change, and change rapidly, the two general strategies will remain as options. In the first strategy, the modeller builds a model and interface on a server computer, and the remote user accesses the model, using the server computer's processes to run the neural network on remote data. We will refer to this as the 'Central Server' strategy. The advantage of this strategy is that the remote, or client, computer needs very few resources of its own to access the model. The disadvantage is that the server assumes all of the processing burden of all clients accessing it. In the second strategy, the server simply serves model code to the client. We will refer to this as the 'Distributed' strategy. The advantage of this strategy is that the only burden placed on the server is that of sending code. The disadvantage is that the client computer must possess the resources to interpret the code. Fortunately, with the current state of widely available World Wide Web browsers supporting the JavaScript language, this disadvantage is lessened substantially.

The following serves as an example of the 'Central Server' strategy. The user is assumed to have a World Wide Web browser that is capable of the forms standard protocol. This example uses the Common Gateway Interface (CGI) as the interface between browser and server. The example implementation is from a Unix V system with an installed http daemon. The HTML scripts were placed in the directory /export/http/htdocs, and the common gateway interface files, Perl program, and executable model code were placed in the directory /export/http/cgi-bin. These locations are not necessary for the implementation, but will serve to orient the reader to the following code.

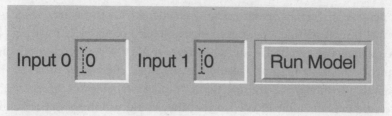

Figure 6.1.   HTML form for a neural network interface.

Three different codes were written. The first was HTML code that the browser will initially interpret. The HTML code then calls Perl code which handles running of the neural model, as well as generating HTML code that reports the result back to the end user. The neural model is executable code that was programmed to take the input features as arguments and to return a text message that includes the result of the model. For brevity, a neural network was trained to model the exclusive–or problem, which is $(0,0) = 0$, $(0,1) = 1$, $(1,0) = 1$, $(1,1) = 0$.

The following HTML code, xor_example.html, was placed in the /export/http/ htdocs directory:

```
<FORM ACTION="/cgi-bin/xor.pl" METHOD="POST">
Input 0 <INPUT TYPE="text" NAME="input_0" VALUE="0" SIZE=3>
Input 1 <INPUT TYPE="text" NAME="input_1" VALUE="0" SIZE=3>
<INPUT TYPE="submit" VALUE="Run Model">
</FORM>
```

The first line of the HTML code identifies a form that will hand data to a Perl script, xor.pl. This Perl script is placed in the /export/http/cgi-bin directory. The next two lines define the form. The variables are labelled as Input 0 and Input 1, and defined for passage to the Perl script as input_0 and input_1. The variables are given the arbitrary default value 0, which may then be changed by the user. The fourth line of the HTML code completes the form, and labels the button that is assigned to the Perl routine. The appearance of this HTML code as viewed by a forms-compliant browser is shown in Figure 6.1.

The Perl script referenced by xor_example.html, xor.pl, was placed in the /export/http/cgi-bin directory:

```
#!/usr/bin/perl
require "cgi-lib.pl";

&ReadParse();
print &PrintHeader();

$input_0=$in{'input_0'};
$input_1=$in{'input_1'};

print './xor_model $input_0 $input_1';

1;  #return true
```

The first of the Perl code identifies the code as a Perl program. The next three lines reference the Common Gateway Interface library, which must be present on the server, and contain the routines for the form and passage of arguments. The fifth and sixth lines get the input variables from the form. The seventh line runs the executable code, xor_model, which takes as its arguments the values of the input variables, and returns a message with the result of the trained neural network. If xor_model were run directly on the server, the following would result:

$ xor_model 0 0
My guess is 1.546861e-07 which is LESS than the threshold

Thus, when the user 'presses the button' on the HTML form, the following is returned,

My guess is 1.546861e-07 which is LESS than the threshold

We built a number of interfaces to neural networks trained to model urological data sets using this Central Server strategy. One was even used by a remote physician who pitted his clinical judgement against the neural model, and reported his findings at a meeting where we encountered them for the first time (Gardner et al. 1996). This then was an implementation in which the remote physician needed no personal assistance from us to use the model. For model-builders who are concerned about training physicians to use the model, this is a clear advantage. However, as we built more models, the load on our server became more substantial every time a remote physician would access one using this Central Server strategy. We thus turned to developing user interfaces and trained models using a Distributed strategy.

Following is a JavaScript program that also implements an exclusive-or neural network. The network is entirely encoded within JavaScript, including the architecture and trained weights and biases. The server need only pass the JavaScript code to the client, and this is generally performed using a JavaScript-compliant browser. Thus the computational load of actually executing the code is shifted to the client computer.

```
1:   <html>
2:   <head>
3:   <title>XOR</title>
4:   <script language="JavaScript">
5:   <!-- hide script
6:
7:   function MakeArray (v) {// generic array constructor
8:   for (var i=0; i <=MakeArray.arguments.length; i++) {
9:   this[i]=MakeArray.arguments[i];
10:  }
```

```
11:  }
12:
13:  INPUT=new MakeArray();
14:  HIDDEN=new MakeArray();
15:  NUMBER_INPUT=2;
16:  NUMBER_HIDDEN=3;
17:  INPUT_LBOUND=−0.9;
18:  INPUT_HBOUND=0.9;
19:
20:  function Sigmoid(sum) {// sigmoidal transfer function
21:  neg_sum=−1.0 * sum;
22:  return 1.0 / (1.0 + Math.exp(neg_sum));
23:  }
24:
25:  // Argument list should be non-radio button values only
26:  function Predict(I0) {
27:
28:  // Replace INPUT[x] below if it is a radio button with its function
29:  INPUT[0]=I0.value;
30:  getI1();
31:
32:  minimax=new MakeArray();
33:  minimax[0]=new MakeArray(1.000000e+01,1.000000e+01,0.000000e+00);
34:  minimax[1]=new MakeArray(2.000000e+01,2.000000e+01,1.000000e+00);
35:
36:  hidden_weights=new MakeArray();
37:  hidden_weights[0]=new MakeArray(−5.631417e+00,5.631364e+00);
38:  hidden_weights[1]=new MakeArray(−4.747887e+00,4.747892e+00);
39:  hidden_weights[2]=new MakeArray(−4.719451e+00,4.719454e+00);
40:
41:  hidden_bias=new MakeArray(−4.985623e+00,4.172563e+00,4.146893e+00);
42:
43:  output_weights=new MakeArray(1.935789e+01,−9.816044e+00,−9.656253e+00);
44:
45:  output_bias=9.498419e+00;
46:
47:  // Scale input vector
48:  for (var i=0; i < NUMBER_INPUT; i++)
49:  INPUT[i] = (((INPUT[i] − minimax[0][i])
50:  / (minimax[1][i] − minimax[0][i]))
51:  * (INPUT_HBOUND − INPUT_LBOUND)) + INPUT_LBOUND;
52:
53:  // Propagate to hidden layer
54:  for (var h=0; h < NUMBER_HIDDEN; h++) {
```

```
55:   var sum=0;
56:   for (var i=0; i < NUMBER_INPUT; i++)
57:   sum += INPUT[i] * hidden_weights[h][i];
58:   sum += hidden_bias[h];
59:   HIDDEN[h]=Sigmoid(sum);
60:   }
61:
62:   // Propagate to output
63:   var sum=0;
64:   for (var h=0; h < NUMBER_HIDDEN; h++)
65:   sum += HIDDEN[h] * output_weights[h];
66:   sum += output_bias;
67:   var OUTPUT=Sigmoid(sum);
68:
69:   if (OUTPUT < 0.5)
70:   document.writeln("Predict: less than threshold <br>");
71:   if (OUTPUT >=0.5)
72:   document.writeln("Predict: greater than threshold <br>");
73:
74:   }
75:
76:   // Put in radio buttons below
77:   INPUT[1]=10;// initialize I1
78:   function getI1 () {
79:   if (document.forms[0].I1[0].checked) INPUT[1]=10;
80:   if (document.forms[0].I1[1].checked) INPUT[1]=20;
81:   }
82:
83:   <!-- end of script -->
84:   </script>
85:   </head>
86:
87:   <body>
88:   <form method="post">
89:   The exclusive-or problem. In this example, 10 is boolean 0, 20 is boolean
90:   1. Here is given a numeric field type example as well as a radio button
91:   type example. Since this program is written in JavaScript, Netscape 2.0 or
92:   greater <b>must </b> be used.<br>
93:   I[0]: <input type="number" name="I0" value=10> <br>
94:   I[1]: <input type="radio" name="I1" onClick="getI1 ()" value=0 checked> 10
95:   <input type="radio" name="I1" onClick="getI1 ()" value=1> 20 <br>
96:   <input type="button" value="predict" onClick="Predict(this.form.I0);">
97:   </body>
98:   </html>
```

Lines 7–11 set up a two-dimensional array structure in JavaScript that will be used throughout the program. Lines 13 and 14 initialize the input and hidden arrays. Lines 15–18 define the number of input and hidden nodes, and the bounds for the input values. Lines 20–23 define the sigmoidal transfer function. Lines 26–74 are the main function, which will return the result of the trained model. Lines 29 and 30 obtain the input variable values from the form at the end of the code; in this example, the first input variable is accessed as a text box in the form, whereas the second input variable is a radio button. Lines 32–34 define the minimum and maximum values for the input and output nodes, so that input nodes may be scaled to the boundaries defined in lines 17 and 18. Lines 36–39 populate the hidden weight array with the trained hidden weights. Line 41 populates the hidden bias array, line 43 the output weight array and line 45 the output bias array with the trained hidden biases, output weights and hidden weights, respectively. Lines 47–51 scale the input variables with the limits defined in lines 17, 18 and 32–34. Lines 53–59 propagate to the hidden layer using the sigmoidal feedforward transfer function, and lines 62–67 propagate to the output node. Lines 69–72 write the result to a page readable by the JavaScript-compliant browser. Lines 76–81 serve as an example definition for a radio button. Lines 88–96 define the user interface form.

The upper region of a JavaScript implementation of the neural network trained to model ESWL outcomes is shown in Figure 6.2. Advantages of the JavaScript implementation include decreased server load; the server is required only to serve the code to the client computer. The client computer executes the JavaScript code, usually using JavaScript-compliant World Wide Web browsers, which, at this time, are widely available. An additional advantage is the use of Graphical User Interface (GUI) tools such as radio buttons with JavaScript. Physicians are more likely to use models if they are easily available and easy to use.

Conclusions

In this chapter, we give three examples of clinically relevant urologic modelling problems that were intractable to discriminant function analysis, yet modelled well with neural computation. However, the challenge to the clinician, engineer or scientist does not end with the building of a successful model. Clinicians may glean useful information from examination of the built model by feature extraction. We describe one method of feature extraction, Wilk's GLRT, and give examples and clinical interpretations. We hope that the reader will find this form of feature extraction useful and insightful. Finally, these models, no matter how well they perform, would be largely useless without an effort to make them widely available and easy to use. Fortunately, at the time of this writing, the internet has

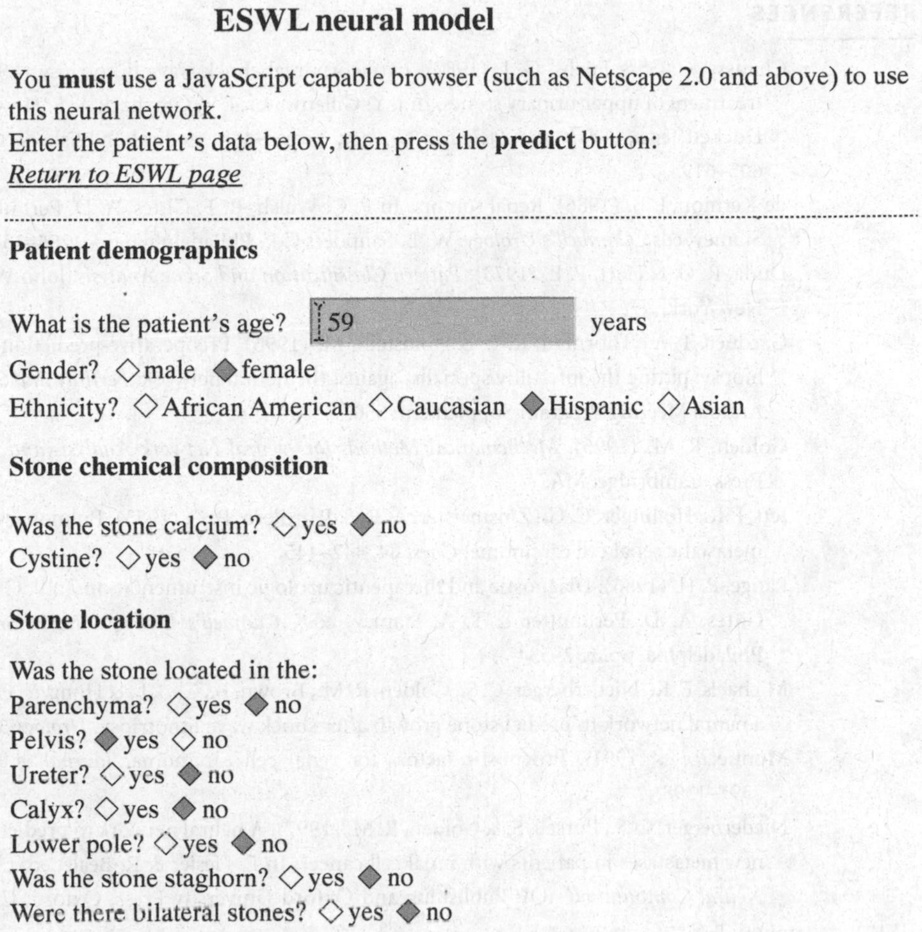

ESWL neural model

You **must** use a JavaScript capable browser (such as Netscape 2.0 and above) to use this neural network.
Enter the patient's data below, then press the **predict** button:
Return to ESWL page

Patient demographics

What is the patient's age? ⎸59   years
Gender? ◇ male ◆ female
Ethnicity? ◇ African American ◇ Caucasian ◆ Hispanic ◇ Asian

Stone chemical composition

Was the stone calcium? ◇ yes ◆ no
Cystine? ◇ yes ◆ no

Stone location

Was the stone located in the:
Parenchyma? ◇ yes ◆ no
Pelvis? ◆ yes ◇ no
Ureter? ◇ yes ◆ no
Calyx? ◇ yes ◆ no
Lower pole? ◇ yes ◆ no
Was the stone staghorn? ◇ yes ◆ no
Were there bilateral stones? ◇ yes ◆ no

Figure 6.2.   JavaScript implementation of trained ESWL neural model.

developed to the point where clinicians will generally find a connection nearby, and resources have developed so that 'point and click' graphical user interfaces make user-friendly distributed computing a reality. We give examples of World Wide Web implementations using a Central Server and a Distributed strategy, and encourage model-builders to use these examples and strategies to make their own trained models widely available and easy to use for physicians.

Acknowledgement

The authors would like to thank Dolores Lamb, Larry Lipshultz, Lawrence Ross, Eli Michaels, Vinod Kutty, Yuan Qin, Joe Jovero, Young Hong, Sue Ting and Luke Cho for their substantial contributions to the projects described in this chapter, and Karen Lewak for her assistance in editing the manuscript.

REFERENCES

Chaussy, C. G. & Fuchs, G. J. (1987). Extracorporeal shock wave lithotripsy (ESWL) for the treatment of upper urinary stones. In J. Y. Gillenwater, J. T. Grayhack, S. S. Howards & J. W. Duckett, eds., *Adult and Pediatric Urology*. Year Book Medical Publishers, Chicago, pp. 605–619.

de Kernion, J. B. (1986). Renal tumors. In P. C. Walsh, R. F. Gittes, A. D. Perlmutter & T. A. Stamey, eds., *Cambell's Urology*. W. B. Saunders Co., Philadelphia, pp. 1294–1342.

Duda, R. O. & Hart, P. E. (1973). *Pattern Classification and Scene Analysis*. John Wiley & Sons, New York.

Gardner, T. A., Thornhill, K. E. & Goldstein, M. (1996). Preoperative prediction of testicular biopsy: pitting the infertility specialist against the neural network. *Fertility and Sterility*, 1996 Annual Meeting Program Supplement: S50.

Golden, R. M. (1996). *Mathematical Methods for Neural Network Analysis and Design*. MIT Press, Cambridge, MA.

Jett, J. R., Hollinger, C. G., Zinsmeister, A. R. & Pairolero, P. C. (1983). Pulmonary resection of metastatic renal cell carcinoma. *Chest* **84**, 442–445.

Lange, P. H. (1986). Diagnostic and therapeutic urologic instrumentation. In P. C. Walsh, R. F. Gittes, A. D. Perlmutter & T. A. Stamey, eds., *Cambell's Urology*. W. B. Saunders Co., Philadelphia, pp. 532–534.

Michaels, E. K., Niederberger, C. S., Golden, R. M., Brown, B., Cho, L. & Hong, Y. (1998). Use of a neural network to predict stone growth after shock wave lithotripsy. *Urology* **51**, 335–338.

Montie, J. E. (1994). Prognostic factors for renal cell carcinoma. *Journal of Urology* **152**, 1397–1398.

Niederberger, C. S., Pursell, S. & Golden, R. M. (1997). A neural network to predict lifespan and new metastases in patients with renal cell cancer. In E. Fiesler & R. Beale, eds., *Handbook of Neural Computation*. IOP Publishing and Oxford University Press, Oxford, Chapter G5.4, pp. 1–6.

Qin, Y., Lamb, D. J., Golden, R. M. & Niederberger, C. (1994). A neural network predicts mortality and new metastases in patients with renal cell cancer. In M. Witten, ed., *Proceedings of the First World Congress on Computational Medicine, Public Health and Biotechnology – Building a Man in the Machine*, Part III, *Series in Mathematical Biology and Medicine*, vol. 5. World Scientific, River Edge, NJ, pp. 1325–1334.

Werbos, P. (1974). Beyond regression: new tools for prediction and analysis in the behavioral sciences. PhD thesis, Harvard University.

Williams, R. D. (1987). Renal, perirenal, and ureteral neoplasms. In J. Y. Gillenwater, J. T. Grayhack, S. S. Howards & J. W. Duckett, eds., *Adult and Pediatric Urology*. Year Book Medical Publishers, Chicago, pp. 513–554.

7

Artificial neural networks as a tool for whole organism fingerprinting in bacterial taxonomy

Royston Goodacre

Introduction

There is a continuing need for the rapid and accurate identification of micro-organisms, particularly in the clinical laboratory. Recent advances in analytical instruments have allowed the characterization of microbes from their phenotypic make-up, but these techniques tend to produce vast amounts of multivariate data that can be extremely hard to interpret. There is therefore a need to exploit modern statistical and related (chemometric) methods to facilitate automatic microbial identification. A particularly powerful set of methods is based on the use of artificial neural networks (ANNs). Over the last few years the availability of powerful desktop computers in conjunction with the development of several user-friendly packages that can simulate such ANNs has led to these 'intelligent systems' increasingly been adopted by the microbial taxonomist for pattern recognition. The nature, properties and exploitation of ANNs for the classification and the identification of microorganisms by whole-organism fingerprinting is reviewed.

In just about every area of microbiology the more rapid, but still accurate, characterization of microorganisms is a desirable objective. In medicine, shortening the time taken to identify a pathogenic bacterium, yeast or fungus will accelerate targeted prescription and should lead to improvements in epidemiological studies. In industry, speedy characterization will allow for better-quality control procedures on both raw materials and finished products, and allow accurate microbial screening for isolates producing novel pharmacophores, thus saving time and money. In pure science the ability to characterize numbers of microorganisms quickly will be beneficial, for example in ecological studies involving bacteria from aquatic or soil habitats (Amann et al. 1995).

To achieve accurate classifications of bacterial groups at the subspecies level, it is considered that the number of characters (variables) that should be studied for each operational taxonomic unit (OTU) should lie between 100 and 200 (Sokal & Sneath 1963; Austin & Preist 1986); indeed, it has been shown statistically (Sokal &

Sneath 1963) that the optimum number seems to be between 100 and 150. Classical bacteriology has traditionally relied upon colonial and microscopic morphology, although over the last 20 years or so these have been supplemented by analysing a large number of biochemical characteristics. With the recent advances in analytical chemistry instruments, various automated easy-to-use spectroscopic methods that carry out 'whole-organism fingerprinting' (Magee 1993) are now entering the microbial laboratory; of these physicochemical techniques pyrolysis mass spectrometry (PyMS) (Magee 1993; Goodacre 1994), Fourier transform infrared spectroscopy (FT-IR) (Helm et al. 1991), ultraviolet (UV) resonance Raman spectroscopy (Nelson et al. 1992) and flow cytometry (Boddy & Morris 1993a; Davey & Kell 1996) are the most popular. Other rapid methods have also been developed to assay only part of the cell, and the more commonly employed include protein and lipid profiling (Howard & Whitcombe 1995); whilst DNA homologies have been expressed in terms of DNA and 16 S ribosomal RNA (rRNA) sequences (Howard & Whitcombe 1995), and more rapid characterization of the organism's genotype effected by the random amplified polymorphic DNA method (RAPD) (Williams et al. 1990) and amplified fragment length polymorphisms (AFLP) (Janssen et al. 1996).

Each of the above analytical methods has the potential to create large amounts of multivariate data characteristic of the OTUs under study. Multivariate data of this nature consist of the results of many different characters or variables (Martens & Næs 1989); each of which may be regarded as constituting a different dimension, such that if there are n variables (characters) each object may be said to reside at a unique position in an abstract entity referred to as n-dimensional hyperspace. This hyperspace is necessarily difficult to visualize, and the underlying theme of multivariate analysis (MVA) is thus *simplification* (Chatfield & Collins 1980) or dimensionality reduction, which usually means that we want to summarize a large body of data by means of *relatively* few parameters, preferably the two or three that lend themselves to straightforward graphical display, with minimal loss of information.

Conventionally, within microbial systematics, the reduction of the multivariate data is carried out using principal components analysis (PCA; Jolliffe 1986) or discriminant function analysis (DFA; Chatfield & Collins 1980; Manly 1994), which typically produce two- or three-dimensional ordination plots; alternatively hierarchical cluster analysis (HCA) can be employed to produce dendrograms, cherished by most taxonomists (for the usual taxonomic procedure used please refer to Figure 7.1). However, the relevant multivariate algorithms used by these methods seek 'clusters' in the data (Everitt 1993), thereby allowing the investigator to group objects together on the basis of their perceived closeness (Figure 7.2), and fall into the category of 'unsupervised learning', since their chief purpose is merely

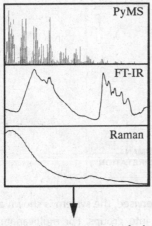

Spectra are high dimensional:

- 150 masses from PyMS

- 882 wavenumbers from FT-IR

- 2283 wavenumbers from Raman

Principal Components Analysis

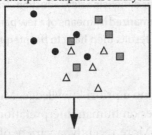

PCA transforms the original set of variables to a new set of uncorrelated variables called PCs. PCA is a data reduction process and the first few PCs will typically account for >95% variance

Discriminant Function Analysis

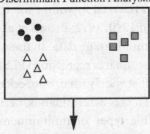

DFA has a priori information based on spectral replicates and uses this to minimize within-group variance and maximize between-group variance

Hierarchical Cluster Analysis

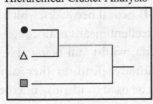

A similarity matrix can be constructed from the DFA space. HCA can then use this to produce a dendrogram, using average linkage clustering

Figure 7.1. Flowchart of the usual taxonomic procedure used to perform cluster analyses on high-dimensional spectra. PyMS, pyrolysis mass spectrometry; FT-IR, Fourier transform infrared spectroscopy; PCA, principal components analysis; PC, principal components; DFA, discriminant function analysis; HCA, hierarchical cluster analysis.

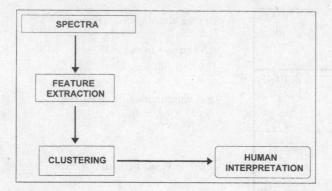

Figure 7.2.   Unsupervised learning: when learning is unsupervised, the system is shown a set of inputs (spectra) and then left to cluster the spectra into groups. For multivariate analysis this optimization procedure is usually *simplification* or dimensionality reduction. This means that a large body of data (the spectral inputs) are summarized by means of a few parameters, with minimal loss of information. After clustering the results then have to be interpreted.

to *distinguish* objects or populations using no a priori knowledge. Moreover, this approach is often subjective because it relies on human interpretation of complicated ordination plots and dendrograms. More recently, a variety of related but much more powerful methods, most often referred to within the framework of chemometrics (Massart et al. 1988; Brereton 1990, 1992; Brown et al. 1994), have been applied to the 'supervised' analysis of multivariate data. In these methods, of which multiple linear regression, partial least squares regression (PLS) and principal components regression (PCR) are the most widely used, one seeks to relate the multivariate inputs to the concentrations of target determinands, i.e. to generate a quantitative analysis, essentially via suitable types of multidimensional curve fitting or regression analysis (Martens & Næs 1989).

A related approach is the use of (artificial) neural networks, which are increasingly being exploited because they are an excellent means of uncovering complex, non-linear relationships in multivariate data, whilst still being able to map the linearities. In addition to mapping quantitative features they can also effect qualitative pattern recognition and thereby be used to identify microorganisms.

Introduction to artificial neural networks

The following texts and books are recommended as excellent introductory texts to artificial neural networks (Rumelhart et al. 1986; Wasserman 1989; Simpson 1990; Hertz et al. 1991; Richard & Lippmann 1991; Zupan & Gasteiger 1993; Haykin 1994; Ripley 1994, 1996; Werbos 1994; Baxt 1995; Bishop 1995; Dybowski & Gant

1995; Goodacre et al. 1996b). The following is a brief introduction to the reasoning behind and the implementation of ANNs.

ANNs are biologically inspired; they are composed of processing units that act in a manner that is analogous to the basic function of the biological neuron. In essence, the functionality of the biological neuron consists in receiving signals, or stimuli, from other cells at their synapses, processing this information, and deciding (usually on a threshold basis) whether or not to produce a response that is passed on to other cells. In ANNs these neurons are replaced by very simple 'computational units' that can take a numerical input and transform it (usually via summation) into an output. These processing units are then organized in a way that models the organization of the biological neural network, the brain.

Despite the rather superficial resemblance between the artificial and biological neural network, ANNs do exhibit a surprising number of characteristics similar to those of the brain. For example, they learn from experience, generalize from previous examples to new ones, abstract essential characteristics from inputs containing irrelevant data, and make errors (although this usually because of badly chosen training data; Zupan & Gasteiger 1993; Kell & Sonnleitner 1995); all these traits are considered more characteristic of human thought than of serial processing by computers. What these 'intelligent' systems can offer the microbial taxonomist is the capability of performing pattern recognition on very complex uninterpretable (at least to the naked eye) multivariate data.

For a given analytical system used there are some patterns (e.g. the multivariate data) that have known desired responses or values (e.g. the identity of a group of bacteria). These two types of data form pairs called inputs and targets. The goal of supervised learning is to find a *model* or *mapping* that will correctly associate the inputs with the targets (Figure 7.3).

The relevant principle of supervised learning in ANNs is that the ANNs take numerical inputs (the training data) and transform them into 'desired' (known, predetermined) outputs. The input and output nodes may be connected to the 'external world' and to other nodes within the network (for a diagrammatic representation see Figure 7.4). The way in which each node transforms its input depends on the so-called 'connection weights' (or 'connection strengths') and 'bias' inputs of the node, which are modifiable. The output of each node to another node or the external world then depends on both its weight strength and bias and on the weighted sum of all its inputs, which are then transformed by a (normally non-linear) weighting function referred to as its activation or squashing function. The great power of neural networks stems from the fact that it is possible to 'train' them. One can acquire sets of multivariate data from standard bacteria of known identities and train ANNs using these identities as the desired outputs. Training is effected by continually presenting the networks with the 'known'

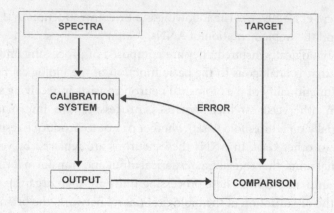

Figure 7.3.   Supervised learning: when we know the desired responses (targets) associated with each of the inputs (spectra) then the system may be supervised. The goal of supervised learning is to find a model that will correctly associate the inputs with the targets; this is usually achieved by minimizing the error between the target and the model's response (output).

inputs and outputs and modifying the connection weights between the individual nodes and the biases, typically according to some kind of back-propagation algorithm (Rumelhart et al. 1986; Werbos 1994; Chauvin & Rumelhart 1995), until the output nodes of the network match the desired outputs to a stated degree of accuracy. For any given network, set of weight values, and set of training patterns there exists an overall root mean squared (RMS) error value. If one dimension in a multidimensional space is put aside for each weight, and one more for the RMS error, one can construct an error surface. The back-propagation algorithm performs gradient descent on this error surface by modifying each weight in proportion to the gradient of the surface at its location. Two parameters, *learning rate* and *momentum*, control this process. Learning rate scales the size of the step down the error surface taken by each iteration, and momentum acts as a low-pass filter, smoothing out progress over small bumps in the error surface. After training, the ANNs may then be exposed to unknown inputs (i.e. spectra) when they will immediately provide the globally optimal best fit to the outputs.

It is known (Martens & Næs 1989; Wasserman 1989; Goodacre & Kell 1993; Goodacre et al. 1994b; Bishop 1995; Kell & Sonnleitner 1995) that supervised learning methods such as neural networks (and partial least squares) can overfit data. An overtrained neural network has usually learnt perfectly the stimulus patterns it has seen but cannot give accurate predictions for unseen stimuli, i.e. it is no longer able to generalize. For supervised learning methods accurately to learn and predict the identities of bacteria the model must obviously be calibrated to the correct point. This is usually accomplished by partitioning the data into three sets:

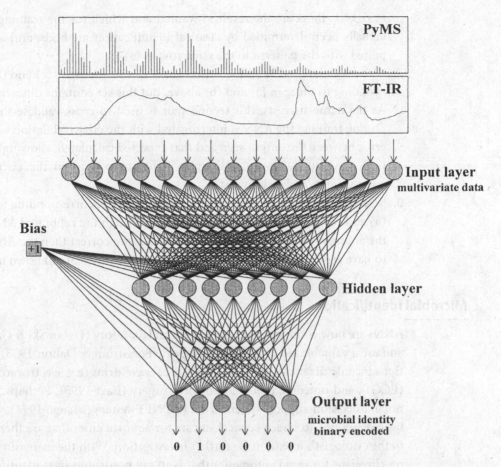

Figure 7.4.　A multilayer perceptron neural network consisting of an input layer connected to a single node in the output layer by one hidden layer. In the architecture shown, adjacent layers of the network are fully interconnected, although other architectures are possible. Nodes in the hidden and output layers consist of processing elements that sum the input applied to it and scale the signal using a sigmoidal logistic squashing function. PyMS, pyrolysis mass spectrometry; FT-IR, Fourier transform infrared spectroscopy.

1. 'Training data', which is used to calibrate the model consist of (a) a matrix of s rows and n columns in which s is the number of objects and n the number of variables (for FT-IR these characters may be the absorbance at particular wavelengths, the normalized ion intensities at a particular m/z for PyMS, or light scattered or fluorescence for flow cytometry), and (b) a second matrix, again consisting of s rows and the same number of columns as there are classes to be identified. For microbial identification these are binary encoded such that if there are four classes there would be four variables such that class A would be represented by 1,0,0,0, class B by 0,1,0,0, class C by 0,0,1,0, and class D encoded

as 0,0,0,1; these are the result(s) wanted and which for the training set have actually been determined by classical identification methods, and are always paired with the patterns in the same row in (a).

2. 'Cross-validation data', which also consist of two matrices, (c) and (d), corresponding to those in (a) and (b) above, but this set contains different objects. As the name suggests, this second pair is used to cross-validate the system. During training the ANN is interrogated with the cross-validation set and the error between the output seen and that expected calculated, allowing a calibration curve to be drawn; training will be stopped when the error on the cross-validation data is lowest.

3. 'Test data', which again also consist of two matrices corresponding to those in (a) and (b) above. These data are 'passed' through the calibrated ANN to test the accuracy of the system. If these responses are correct then the ANN is said to have generalized and may then be used to identify real unknown microbes.

Microbial identification

ANNs are now common place in the clinical laboratory (Dybowski & Gant 1995) and are a valuable aid for decision support (Forsström & Dalton 1995); applications include diagnosis, imaging, analysis of waveforms (e.g. electrocardiography (ECG)), and outcome prediction before surgery (Baxt 1995). Perhaps, the most notable decision-support system is the PAPNET system (Mango 1994), which has been developed to screen cervical smears for abnormalities that are then brought to the cytologist's attention for further investigation. With the increasing demand on clinicians for rapid automatic (that is to say non-subjective) identification of bacteria, ANNs are increasingly being explored in a wide range of taxonomic applications. Simulations of neural networks are computationally intense and it is likely that the availability of more powerful desktop computers over the last 7 years has given life to these exciting intelligent methods. The following summarizes the most significant application areas within whole-organism fingerprinting.

Flow cytometry

Flow cytometry (FCM) permits the rapid acquisition of light-scattering and fluorescence characteristics of individual cells within a (mixed) population (Figure 7.5); data acquisition is very rapid and 10^3–10^4 cells or more can be characterized per second (Davey & Kell 1996). The ANN analysis of flow cytometry data was first applied to the analysis of phytoplankton (Frankel et al. 1989), and this approach was later used by Smits and his colleagues to effect the automatic identification of groups of cyanobacteria (e.g., algae) (Balfoort et al. 1992; Smits et al. 1992). In the latter study (Smits et al. 1992), ANNs were trained with the data

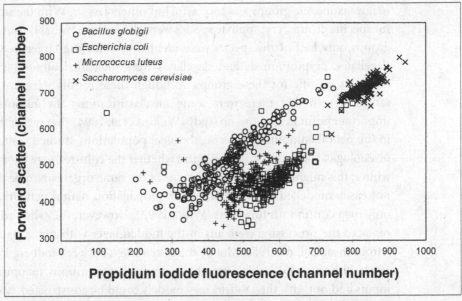

Figure 7.5.   Raw data from the flow cytometry of *Bacillus globigii*, *Escherichia coli*, *Micrococcus luteus*, and *Saccharomyces cerevisiae* cells. The forward scatter and propidium iodide fluorescence parameters are plotted.

from axenic cultures of eight algal species. These data were: forward and perpendicular light scattering, which are related to cell size and structure, respectively; time of flight, which is related to cell length; and three fluorescence parameters that gave information on phycoerythrin, chlorophyll and phycocyanin. After the 6–12–8 ANNs were trained with data from monocultures, they were interrogated with data from mixtures of laboratory cultures and could distinguish cyanobacteria from other algae with 99% accuracy. The identification of the eight algal species was less accurate, and was generally > 90%; given that the authors had a systematic error of 5–10% in the preparation of the mixtures these results were very encouraging.

A more elegant approach to the identification of marine phytoplankton has been recently demonstrated by Boddy et al. (1994). Flow cytometry data (time of flight, horizontal and vertical forward light scatter, 90° light scatter, and 'red' and 'orange' autofluorescence) were collected for laboratory cultures of 40 phytoplankton species from Dinophyceae, Bacillariophyceae, Prymnesiophyceae, Cryptophyceae and other flagellates. Two back-propagation neural networks were assessed: the first was a hierarchy of small networks, the first identifying to which major taxonomic group a cell belonged, and then another ANN for that taxonomic group to identify the species; this was then compared with a single large network identifying all 40 phytoplankton species. Discrimination of some of the major taxonomic groups was successful but others less so. With the smaller ANNs for specific groups, cryptophyte species were all identified reliably, but in the other groups only half of the species were identified. With the larger network, dino-flagellates, cryptomonads and flagellates were identified almost as well as by networks specific for these groups. Although these results were not completely satisfactory in that there were some misclassifications the authors made the important point in a follow-up study (Wilkins et al. 1994) that rather than a failing in the neural computation per se, the algal populations studied contained major physiological differences depending on whether the cultures were from summer or winter; this might cause two populations of the same organism to be disjoint, and not easily modelled by a standard back-propagation neural network, which can only map continuous functions (White 1992). However, they showed that if they replaced the processing elements in the hidden layer with radial basis functions (Broomhead & Lowe 1988; Moody & Darken 1989; Park & Sandberg 1991; Haykin 1994; Bishop 1995), which are able to map discontinuous mappings between inputs and outputs, then satisfactory models could be constructed. More recently Wilkins et al. (1996) have tested a number of other popular neural network algorithms for the identification of phytoplankton from flow cytometry data.

Back-propagation neural networks have also been evaluated for identifying fungal species from flow cytometric measurements of spores (Morris et al. 1992). Only three flow cytometry parameters were used to train ANNs for the successful discrimination of *Fuligo septica*, *Oudemansiella radicata*, *Megacollybia platyphyll* and *Tylophilus felleus* with an accuracy of 78%, 94%, 86% and 96%, respectively. With respect to bacterial identification there have been few studies; Boddy & Morris (1993b) have alluded to some preliminary results that analysed a group of 15 species of pathogenic bacteria, ANNs could not be trained to identify un-equivocally these bacteria and the authors suggested that the use of more flow cytometry parameters, most notably DNA fluorescence, may allow better classifi-cation. However, given that this publication was in 1993 and, at the time of writing of this chapter, nothing has been published yet it seems unlikely that they were successful. More recently, Davey & Kell (1995, 1997) have exploited flow cytomet-ric techniques with neural networks to detect *Bacillus globigii* spores against a background of other vegetative bacteria (*Micrococcus luteus* and *Escherichia coli*) and *Saccharomyces cerevisiae*. The parameters used as the input to back-propaga-tion ANNs were from a 'cocktail' of three fluorescent stains, together with forward and wide-angle light scattering; the single output node in their 6–3–1 ANNs was encoded so that *B. globigii* scored 1 and non-*B. globigii* scored 0. After training the ANN was interrogated with an independent test set of 50 of each of the four cell types and was able to assess whether the cell under scrutiny was *B. globigii* or not; they typically found 2% false negatives and 3% false positives.

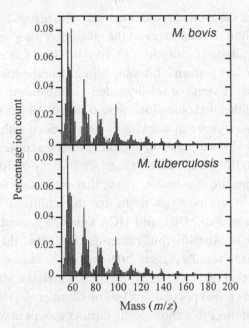

Figure 7.6. Normalized pyrolysis mass spectra of *Mycobacterium bovis* and *Mycobacterium tuberculosis*.

Although the above examples have been aimed at the analysis of eukaryotes or for the specific purpose of detecting target pathogens in high biological backgrounds, it would seem that there is no technical reason why, after a wider range of fluorescence stains are found, this technology cannot be transferred to the clinical laboratory for the rapid identification of pathogens at the single cell level.

Pyrolysis mass spectrometry

PyMS involves the thermal degradation of non-volatile complex molecules (such as bacteria) in a vacuum, causing their cleavage to smaller, volatile fragments separable by a mass spectrometer on the basis of their mass-to-charge ratio (m/z) (Meuzelaar et al. 1982). PyMS allows the (bio-)chemically based discrimination of microbial cells and produces complex biochemical fingerprints (i.e. pyrolysis mass spectra) that are distinct for different bacteria. It is the automation of the instrumentation and ease of use that has led to the widespread exploitation of PyMS as a taxonomic tool for whole-organism fingerprinting (Magee 1993; Goodacre 1994). The analytically useful multivariate data (see Figure 7.6 for an example) are typically constituted by a set of 150 normalized intensities versus m/z in the range 51 to 200 and these are applied to the nodes on the input layers of back-propagation ANNs.

The first demonstration of the ability of ANNs to discriminate between biological samples from their pyrolysis mass spectra was the qualitative assessment of the adulteration of extra virgin olive oils with various seed oils (Goodacre et al. 1992, 1993); in this study, which was performed double-blind, neural networks were trained with the spectra from 12 virgin olive oils, coded 1 at the output node, and with the spectra from 12 adulterated oils, which were coded 0. All oils in the test were correctly identified; in a typical run, the virgins were assessed with a code of 0.99976 ± 0.000146 (range 0.99954 to 1.00016) and the adulterated olive oils in the test set with a code of 0.001079 ± 0.002838 (range 0.00026 to 0.01009). This permitted their rapid and precise assessment, a task that previously was labour intensive and very difficult. It was most significant that the traditional 'unsupervised' multivariate analyses of PCA, DFA and HCA failed to separate the oils according to their virginity or otherwise but rather discriminated them on the basis of their cultivar (that is to say, the biggest difference in the mass spectra was due to the *type* of olive tree that the fruit came from, rather than the adulterant).

The first application to microbial populations was by Chun et al. (1993b) who studied 16 representatives of three morphologically distinct groups of *Streptomycetes* recovered from soil. Duplicated batches of the 16 strains were examined by PyMS and the first data set used for training 150–8–3 ANNs; the second duplicate set was used to test the model. All of the test strains were correctly identified using the ANN, whereas only 15 of the 16 strains were assigned to the correct group using the conventional operational fingerprinting procedure. It was, however, not surprising that the second set was correctly identified, since the same strains were used to train the ANN; indeed all their system was measuring was the reproducibility between the phenotypes of the cultures grown on two batches of the same media. These authors have subsequently extended their approach to a real unknown test set containing over 100 strains representing six other actinomycete genera (Chun et al. 1993a). All of the streptomycetes were correctly identified but many of the other actinomycetes were misidentified, because the ANN had not been exposed to their spectral fingerprints. A modified network topology was then developed to recognize the mass spectral patterns of the non-streptomycete strains.

Several studies have now shown that this combination of PyMS and ANNs is also very effective for the rapid identification of a variety of bacterial strains of clinical and veterinary importance. For example, this approach has allowed the propionibacteria isolated from dogs to be correctly identified as human *Propionibacterium acnes* (Goodacre et al. 1994c), for detecting *Escherichia coli* isolates that produced verocytotoxins (Sisson et al. 1995), and for distinguishing between *Mycobacterium tuberculosis* and *M. bovis* (Freeman et al. 1994). The latter study trained 150–8–1 ANNs with 16 spectra and was challenged with the spectra from 27 other mycobacterial isolates of the *M. tuberculosis* complex (MTBC). *Mycobacterium tuberculosis* could easily be differentiated from *M. bovis* irrespective of their susceptibility to anti-tuberculosis agents. This was significant because at the time it was not possible using DNA probes to differentiate between all species of the *M. tuberculosis* complex.

Another recent study has exploited PyMS and ANNs for the identification and discrimination of oral asaccharolytic *Eubacterium* spp. (Goodacre et al. 1996a). This study illustrated the need for numerical methods that allow easy direct interpretation of the identification of bacteria from their pyrolysis mass spectra, since ANNs can be encoded simply and the results read off in a tabulated format, compared with the more complex examination of three-dimensional ordination plots and dendrograms. Twenty-nine oral asaccharolytic *Eubacterium* strains, and six abscess isolates previously identified as *Peptostreptococcus heliotrinreducens* were analysed by PyMS. The spectra from eight different *Eubacterium* spp. type strains, and the type strain of *P. heliotrinreducens* were used to train 150–8–9 ANNs. In the test set all *Eubacterium* strains were correctly identified and the abscess isolates were identified as unnamed *Eubacterium* taxon C_2 and were distinct from *P. heliotrinreducens*. It was also significant that the test set contained three oral abscess isolates that did not belong to any of the nine classes used to train the ANN; rather than misidentify these the model gave 0 scores at all nine output nodes, indicating that the ANN has not been exposed to these types of spectrum. This is perhaps the exception rather than the rule and ANNs will often give incorrect identities for spectra outside of their knowledge base (i.e. outliers). A possible way to circumvent this problem is to include suitable outliers in the training set and a corresponding 'dummy' output variables in the training set; Goodacre et al. (1994a) have exploited this practice for discriminating non-propionibacteria from three *Propionibacterium* spp.

Probably one of the clearest examples of ANNs for fine discrimination is a recent study on the differentiation between methicillin-susceptible (MSSA) and methicillin-resistant *Staphylococcus aureus* (MRSA) (Goodacre et al. 1998a). In this study, PyMS spectra were obtained from 15 MRSA and 22 MSSA strains. Cluster analysis showed that the major source of variation between the pyrolysis mass spectra was due to the phage group of the bacteria (Figure 7.7) and not to their resistance or susceptibility to methicillin (Figure 7.8). By contrast, ANNs could be trained to recognize those aspects of the pyrolysis mass spectra that differentiated methicillin-resistant from methicillin-sensitive strains. The trained neural network could then use pyrolysis mass spectral data to assess whether or not an unknown strain was resistant to methicillin. The conclusion of this study is that the application of ANNs can be used to extend the role of PyMS analyses to more subtle physiological differences between strains of the same species of

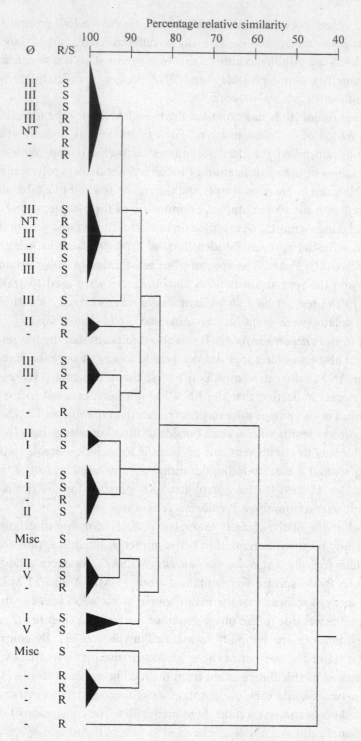

Figure 7.7. The natural relationship between some *Staphylococcus aureus* isolates depicted as a dendrogram. Lytic (ϕ) type is shown. 'S' refers to methicillin-susceptible *Staphylococcus aureus* and 'R' to methicillin-resistant *S. aureus*. NT, not typeable; Misc., miscellaneous. (Adapted from Goodacre et al. 1998.)

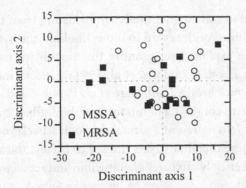

Figure 7.8. Discriminant function analysis biplot based on PyMS data showing the relationship between some *Staphylococcus aureus* strains. MSSA, methicillin-susceptible *S. aureus*; MRSA, methicillin-resistant *S. aureus*. (Adapted from Goodacre et al. 1998.)

bacteria, and in this case provides a very rapid and accurate antibiotic susceptibility testing technique.

With regard to neural network architecture other than the gradient descent algorithms illustrated above, Harrington (1993a,b) has compared minimal neural networks (MNN) with BP-ANNs (back-propagation ANNs) for the analysis of pyrolysis tandem mass spectrometry data. MNNs differ from BP-ANNs in that they use localized processing and build classification trees with branches composed of multiple processing units. A global entropy minimization may be achieved at a branch by combining the processing logic using principles from fuzzy set theory. Weight vectors are adjusted using an angular coordinate system and gradients of the fuzzy entropy function. The branches are optimal with respect to fuzziness and can accommodate non-linearly separable or ill-conditioned data. The most significant advantage of the MNNs is that relations among the training data and the mechanism of inference may be directly observed. Thus rule-based classification trees have been constructed from the mass spectral daughter ions to discriminate between diesel smoke, dry yeast, *Escherichia coli*, MS-2 coliphage, grass pollen, *Bacillus subtilis*, fog oil, wood smoke, aldolase and *Bacillus globigii* (Harrington 1993a).

All the above studies have been classification problems but perhaps the most significant application of ANNs to the analysis of PyMS data is to gain accurate and precise *quantitative* information about the chemical constituents of microbial samples. For example, it has been shown that it is possible using this method to measure the concentrations of binary and tertiary mixtures of cells of the bacteria *Bacillus subtilis*, *Escherichia coli* and *Staphylococcus aureus* (Goodacre et al. 1994b, 1996b; Timmins & Goodacre 1997). Goodacre et al. (1994b) also demonstrated that other supervised learning methods relying on linear regression, such as PLS and PCR, could also be used to extract quantitative information from the spectra of the tertiary bacterial mixtures. With regard to biotechnology, the combination of PyMS and ANNs can be exploited to quantify the amount of mammalian cytochrome b_5 expressed in *E. coli* (Goodacre et al. 1994a), and to measure the level of metabolites in fermentor broths (Goodacre et al. 1994d; Goodacre & Kell 1996b). Initially, model systems consisting of mixtures of the antibiotic ampicillin with either *E. coli* or *S. aureus* (to represent a variable biological background) were studied. It was especially interesting that ANNs trained to predict the amount of ampicillin in *E. coli* having seen only mixtures of ampicillin and *E. coli* were able to generalize so as to predict the concentration of ampicillin in a *S. aureus* background to approximately 5%, illustrating the very great robustness of ANNs to rather substantial variations in the biological background. Samples from fermentations of a single organism in a complex production medium were also analysed quantitatively for a drug of commercial interest, and the drug could also be quantified in a variety of mutant-producing strains cultivated in the same medium, thus effecting a rapid screening for the high-level production of desired substances (Goodacre et al. 1994d). In related studies *Penicillium chrysogenum* fermentation broths were analysed quantitatively for penicillins using PyMS and ANNs (Goodacre et al. 1995), and to monitor *Gibberella fujikuroi* fermentations producing gibberellic acid (Goodacre & Kell 1996b).

Vibrational spectroscopy

Fourier transform infrared spectroscopy (FT-IR) and dispersive Raman microscopy are physicochemical methods that measure predominantly the vibrations of bonds within functional groups, either through the absorbance of electromagnetic radiation (FT-IR; Figure 7.9) or from the inelastic scattering of light (Raman shift, Figure 7.10) (Griffiths & de Haseth 1986; Colthup et al. 1990; Drennen et al. 1991; Graselli & Bulkin 1991; Hendra et al. 1991; Ferraro & Nakamoto 1994; Schrader 1995). Therefore, like PyMS, these hyperspectral methods (Goetz et al. 1985; Abousleman et al. 1994; Wilson et al. 1995; Winson et al. 1997) also give quantitative information about the total biochemical composition of a sample.

Naumann and co-workers (e.g. Helm et al. 1991; Naumann et al. 1991) have shown that FT-IR absorbance spectroscopy (in the mid-IR range, usually defined as 4000 to 400 cm^{-1}) provides a powerful tool with sufficient resolving power to distinguish microbial cells at the strain level. However, the interpretation of the FT-IR spectra has conventionally been by the application of unsupervised pattern recognition methods of correspondence analysis maps and cluster analysis (Naumann et al. 1991), and is often subjective because it relies upon the interpretation of complicated scatter plots and dendrograms.

More recently, we (Goodacre et al. 1996c) have used diffuse reflectance–

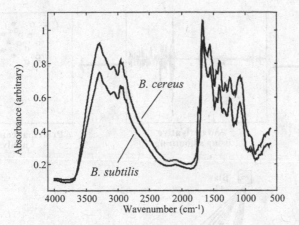

Figure 7.9. Fourier transform infrared diffuse reflectance–absorbance spectra of *Bacillus cereus* and *B. subtilis*.

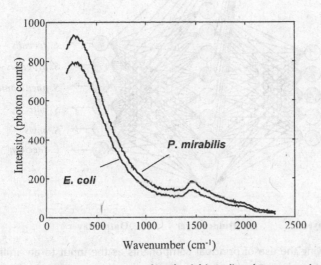

Figure 7.10. Dispersive Raman spectra of *Escherichia coli* and *Proteus mirabilis*.

absorbance FT-IR to analyse 19 hospital isolates that had been identified by conventional means as one of *Enterococcus faecalis*, *E. faecium*, *Streptococcus bovis*, *S. mitis*, *S. pneumoniae* or *S. pyogenes*. PCA of the FT-IR spectra showed that this unsupervised learning method failed to form six separable clusters (one for each species) and thus could not be used to identify these bacteria based on their FT-IR spectra. The normalized FT-IR spectra were applied to the input nodes of 882–10–6 ANNs and these failed to identify all spectra in the independent test set. To remove the effects of visible baseline shifts in the FT-IR spectra, the first and second derivative spectra were then used as inputs to ANNs; it was found that the second derivative gave better results, although only four out of the nine test set

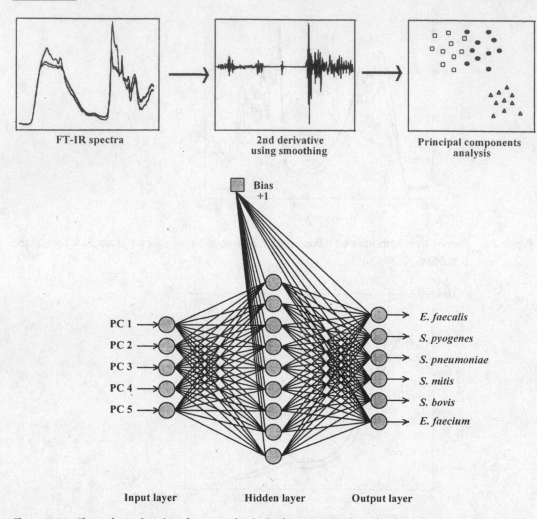

FT-IR spectra   2nd derivative using smoothing   Principal components analysis

Bias +1

PC 1
PC 2
PC 3
PC 4
PC 5

E. faecalis
S. pyogenes
S. pneumoniae
S. mitis
S. bovis
E. faecium

Input layer   Hidden layer   Output layer

Figure 7.11. Flow chart showing the use of principal components as the input to an artificial neural network. In the chart shown the first five principal components are based on the smoothed second derivative of FT-IR data. (Adapted from Goodacre et al. 1996c.)

spectra were identified correctly. Moreover, training to 0.01 root mean-squared error typically took between 5.10^3 and 1.10^4 epochs and because of the large network topology took 5 to 6 hours. To obey the parsimony principle (Seasholtz & Kowalski 1993) the number of inputs to the ANN was then reduced to the first five principal components scores (this accounted for 91.3% of the total variance) from the second derivative FT-IR spectra. These 5–9–6 ANNs took only 2 to 3 minutes to train (350 to 600 epochs) and correctly identified both the training and test sets unequivocally (Figure 7.11).

Further studies, which also included the first application of dispersive Raman microscopy to the identification of bacteria, have shown that it is also possible to use ANNs and radial basis functions (RBFs) to discriminate between common infectious agents associated with urinary tract infection (Goodacre et al. 1998b). One of the most important findings in this study was that the ANNs for the very high dimensional Raman spectra (where 2283 wave numbers were used as inputs) took a long time to train, and for the full spectral MLPs this was 30 hours. In contrast, when full spectral RBFs were trained with the same input data the training time was massively reduced to only 2 minutes, with equivalent perform-ance compared to the full spectral MLPs. This is because RBFs do not perform the rather slow computationally intense gradient descent methods used in MLPs. By contrast, RBFs comprise two stages: the first is the unsupervised clustering of the mass spectra, typically using *k*-means (Dillon & Goldstein 1984) followed by the linear regression of the outputs from the Gaussian kernel functions in the RBF's hidden layer onto the identities of the bacteria.

Instrument reproducibility

For the analytical tools discussed above to be used for the routine identification of microorganisms new (spectral) fingerprints must be able to be compared with those previously collected. However, the major problem with most analytical instruments is that long-term reproducibility is poor and inter-laboratory repro-ducibility abysmal, and so the biochemical or genetical fingerprints of the same material analysed at two different times are different. Because of the uncertainties over the long-term reproducibility of the PyMS system (as defined as > 30 days), PyMS has really been limited within clinical microbiology to the typing of short-term outbreaks where all microorganisms are analysed in a single batch (Magee 1993; Goodfellow 1995).

After tuning the instrument, to correct for drift one would need to analyse the *same* standards at the two different times and use some sort of mathematical correction method. This could simply be subtracting the amount of drift from new spectra collected; however, this assumes that the drift is uniform (linear) with time, which is obviously not the case. This method also relies on the variables (characters) being void of noise, which is also not the case. An alternative method would be to *transform* the spectra to look like the spectra of the same material previously collected using a method that was (a) robust to noisy data and (b) able to perform non-linear mappings. ANNs carry out non-linear mappings, whilst still being able to map the linearities, and are purported to be robust to noisy data. These mathematical methods are therefore ideally suited to be exploited for the correction of mass spectral drift.

Smits et al. (1993) have implemented a drift correction for pattern recognition using neural networks with *simulated* flow cytometry data. These data sets contained only two variables and the amount of drift was included in neural networks as an *extra* input variable (three input nodes in total). It is, however, often difficult to measure the amount of drift accurately in real systems, especially if the number of input variables is high (typically 150 for PyMS, and > 800 for FT-IR data), and it is neither monotonic with time nor does it have a variable index.

Freeman and colleagues (1995) studied a model of three bacteria (two subcultures of the same *E. coli* and a serologically distinct *E. coli*) and subcultivated these for 5 weeks; the 15 cultures were then analysed by PyMS. PCA and DFA were unable to identify the *E. coli* from multiple batches and in contrast five 150–8–2 ANNs could be trained with data from each batch to improve identification of the two serologically distinct *E. coli*; between 90% and 100% of the samples were identified correctly. However, the authors made a fundamental mistake in their comparison between ANNs and DFA; the coding for the ANN was to separate only the two different *E. coli* strains but the DFA was encoded to distinguish all 15 cultures. It was hardly surprising that DFA failed to cluster the *E. coli* strains, since the objective of DFA is to minimize the within-group variance and maximize the between-group variance; that is to say, split the 15 groups apart. A better comparison would have been to carry out five DFA analyses (one for each batch) with the same groupings as the ANN analyses and then to project the test set into the canonical variates space.

A far more elegant approach would be to *transform* the spectra collected today to be like those collected previously. Goodacre & Kell (1996a,c) have found that neural networks can be used successfully to correct for instrumental drift: identical materials were analysed by PyMS at dates from 4 to 20 months apart, but neural network models produced at *earlier* times could not be used to give accurate estimates of determinand concentrations or bacterial identities. Calibration samples common to the two data sets were run at the two times, and ANNs set up in which the inputs were the 150 'new' calibration masses and the outputs were the 150 calibration masses from the 'old' spectra. Such associative nets could thus be used as signal-processing elements to effect the transformation of data acquired in one day to those that would have been acquired on a later date. With regard to bacterial identification, 19 isolates representing three strains of human *P. acnes* were analysed; on the day 150–8–3 ANNs could be trained to identify all 19 strains; however, when new PyMS data collected 125 days later were used to challenge this model, 6 of the 19 bacteria were incorrectly identified. After using an associative ANN the transformed PyMS spectra were then used to challenge the old ANN model and now 18 of the 19 bacteria were correctly identified; the misclassified bacterium was scored as 0.5 at the correct identity and 0.6 and 0 elsewhere. These results show clearly that for the first time PyMS can be used to acquire spectra that could be compared with those previously collected and held in a database. It should seem obvious that this approach is not limited solely to PyMS but is generally applicable to any analytical tool prone to instrumental drift (which cannot be compensated for by tuning), such as FT-IR, GC and flow cytometry.

Conclusions

The exploitation of novel multivariate analysis techniques employing ANNs based on *supervised* learning, rather than *unsupervised* methods, has permitted even better discrimination of industrially and medically important bacteria from the increasing number of analytical tools that are being 'highjacked' by the modern microbial taxonomist.

ANNs clearly present themselves as extremely powerful and valuable tools. However, an ANN will only perform as well as the data that are given to it (Kell & Sonnleitner 1995); as in all other data analysis techniques these supervised learning methods are not immune from sensitivity to badly chosen initial data. Therefore the exemplars for the training set *must* be carefully chosen; the golden rule is 'garbage in – garbage out' (Zupan & Gasteiger 1993). This is also very true for the unknown interrogation set; if these are outside the knowledge base of the ANN then they will obviously be misidentified.

Training a neural network is not at all cumbersome, since there exists a number of user-friendly packages that are readily available; in the future it will be possible to devise automated cross-validation techniques so that the network decides when it is optimally trained without user interference.

Probably the biggest problem with using analytical tools for identifying microbes is that they are prone to drift and perform differently in different laboratories. However, our own studies have shown that, at least for mass spectra, both intra- and inter-instrument drift can be corrected for (Goodacre & Kell 1996a,c; Goodacre et al. 1997). Therefore, it is becoming increasingly possible to take the spectra of unknown microorganisms and challenge them against libraries of spectra previously collected and held in a central database.

The future

Raman microscopy, like flow cytometry, has the major advantage over PyMS and FT-IR in that it is possible to analyse single cells (Puppels & Greve 1993); but in contrast to flow cytometry, the information content in a Raman spectrum is immense as inelastic scattering will be measured from many biochemical species and not just those stained with a fluorescent marker. However, only 1 in 10^8 interrogating photons typically experience Raman scattering, this means that the signal is very weak and thus reliable filtering methods still need to be developed (Collthup et al. 1990; Williams et al. 1994; Schrader 1995).

Recently within mass spectrometry there has been an explosion of interest in the use of soft ionization methods such as matrix-assisted laser desorption ionization (MALDI) (Guilhaus 1995; Siuzdak 1996) and electrospray ionization (ESI) (Cole 1997; Gaskell 1997) for the analysis of biomacromolecules, as well as of small molecules, and such mass spectrometric methods are now essential tools in proteomics (Fenselau 1997) and functional genomics (Roepstorff 1997). It has been demonstrated using MALDI-MS that characteristic profiles of intact microorganisms can be obtained by mixing the microbes with a suitable matrix (Claydon et al. 1996; Holland et al. 1996; Krishnamurthy & Ross 1996; Krishnamurthy et al. 1996; Easterling et al. 1998; Welham et al. 1998). ESI-MS has also been shown to be a valuable tool for the reproducible analysis of complex biological samples, either by the introduction of bacteria via specific cell fractions or lysates (Gibson et al. 1994; Smith et al. 1995; Black & Fox 1996; Snyder 1996; Black et al. 1997; Wunschel et al. 1997; Fang & Barcelona 1998; Li et al. 1998; Liu et al. 1998; Krishnamurthy et al. 1999) or by the introduction of *intact* bacteria (Goodacre et al. 1999).

As the realization that miniaturization of instrumentation is assuming increasing importance (McClennen et al. 1994), as computers become more powerful, as our understanding of complex spectroscopies and their (chemometric) interpretation deepens, and as we enter the third millennium, perhaps we are witnessing the reality of the diagnostician's dream: a rapid, reagentless, accurate, robust 'intelligent' microbial identification tool.

Acknowledgements

I am indebted to the Wellcome Trust (grant number 042615/Z/94/Z), and to my colleague Professor Douglas Kell for kind reading of a draft of the manuscript. I am also very grateful to Dr Hazel Davey for the flow cytometry data shown in Figure 7.5.

REFERENCES

Abousleman, G. P., Gifford, E. & Hunt, B. R. (1994). Enhancement and compression techniques for hyperspectral data. *Optical Engineering* **33**, 2562–2571.

Amann, R. I., Ludwig, W. & Schleifer, K. H. (1995). Phylogenetic identification and in-situ detection of individual microbial cells without cultivation. *Microbiology Reviews* **59**, 143–169.

Austin, B. & Preist, F. G. (1986). *Modern Bacterial Taxonomy*. Van Nostrand Reinhold, Wokingham.

Balfoort, H. W., Snoek, J., Smits, J. R. M., Breedveld, L. W., Hofstraat, J. W. & Ringelberg, J. (1992). Automatic identification of algae: neural network analysis of flow cytometric data. *Journal of Plankton Research* **14**, 575–589.

Baxt, W. G. (1995). Application of artificial neural networks to clinical medicine. *Lancet* **346**, 1135–1138.

Bishop, C. M. (1995). *Neural Networks for Pattern Recognition.* Clarendon Press, Oxford.

Black, G. E. & Fox, A. (1996). Liquid chromatography with electrospray ionization tandem mass spectrometry – profiling carbohydrates in whole bacterial cell hydrolysates. *ACS Symposium Series* **619**, 81–105.

Black, G. E., Snyder, A. P. & Heroux, K. S. (1997). Chemotaxonomic differentiation between the *Bacillus cereus* group and *Bacillus subtilis* by phospholipid extracts analyzed with electrospray ionization tandem mass spectrometry. *Journal of Microbiological Methods* **28**, 187–199.

Boddy, L. & Morris, C. W. (1993a). Analysis of flow cytometry data – a neural network approach. *Binary* **5**, 17–22.

Boddy, L. & Morris, C. W. (1993b). Neural network analysis of flow cytometry data. In D. Lloyd, ed., *Flow Cytometry in Microbiology*, Springer-Verlag, London, pp. 159–169.

Boddy, L., Morris, C. W., Wilkins, M. F., Tarran, G. A. & Burkill, P. H. (1994). Neural network analysis of flow cytometric data for 40 marine phytoplankton species. *Cytometry* **15**, 283–293.

Brereton, R. G. (1990). *Chemometrics: Applications of Mathematics and Statistics to Laboratory Systems.* Ellis Horwood, New York.

Brereton, R. G. (1992). *Multivariate Pattern Recognition in Chemometrics.* Elsevier, Amsterdam.

Broomhead, D. S. & Lowe, D. (1988). Multivariable functional interpolation and adaptive networks. *Complex Systems* **2**, 312–355.

Brown, S. D., Blank, T. B., Sum, S. T. & Weyer, L. G. (1994). Chemometrics. *Analytical Chemistry* **66**, R315–R359.

Chatfield, C. & Collins, A. J. (1980). *Introduction to Multivariate Analysis.* Chapman & Hall, London.

Chauvin, Y. & Rumelhart, D. E. (1995). *Backpropagation: Theory, Architectures, and Applications.* Erlbaum, Hove, Kent.

Chun, J., Atalan, E., Kim, S. B., Kim, H. J., Hamid, M. E., Trujillo, M. E., Magee, J. G., Manfio, G. P., Ward, A. C. & Goodfellow, M. (1993a). Rapid identification of streptomycetes by artificial neural network analysis of pyrolysis mass spectra. *FEMS Microbiology Letters* **114**, 115–119.

Chun, J., Atalan, E., Ward, A. C. & Goodfellow, M. (1993b). Artificial neural network analysis of pyrolysis mass spectrometric data in the identification of *Streptomyces* strains. *FEMS Microbiology Letters* **107**, 321–325.

Claydon, M. A., Davey, S. N., Edwardsjones, V. & Gordon, D. B. (1996). The rapid identification of intact microorganisms using mass spectrometry. *Nature Biotechnology* **14**, 1584–1586.

Cole, R. B. (1997). *Electrospray Ionization Mass Spectrometry: Fundamentals, Instrumentation and Applications.* Wiley, New York.

Colthup, N. B., Daly, L. H. & Wiberly, S. E. (1990). *Introduction to Infrared and Raman Spectroscopy.* Academic Press, New York.

Davey, H. M. & Kell, D. B. (1995). Rapid flow cytometric detection and identification of microbial particles using multiple stains and neural networks. In *Scientific Conference on*

Chemical and Biological Defense Research, Edgewood, Baltimore, MD, pp. 393–399.

Davey, H. M. & Kell, D. B. (1996). Flow cytometry and cell sorting of heterogeneous microbial populations – the importance of single cell analyses. *Microbiology Reviews* **60**, 641–696.

Davey, H. M. & Kell, D. B. (1997). Fluorescent brighteners: novel stains for the flow cytometric analysis of microorganisms. *Cytometry* **28**, 311–315.

Dillon, W. R. & Goldstein, M. (1984). *Multivariate Analysis: Methods and Applications.* John Wiley & Sons, New York.

Drennen, J. K., Kraemer, E. G. & Lodder, R. A. (1991). Advances and perspectives in near-infrared spectrophotometry. *Critical Reviews in Analytical Chemistry* **22**, 443–475.

Dybowski, R. & Gant, V. (1995). Artificial neural networks in pathological and medical laboratories. *Lancet* **346**, 1203–1207.

Easterling, M. L., Colangelo, C. M., Scott, R. A. & Amster, I. J. (1998). Monitoring protein expression in whole bacterial cells with MALDI time-of-flight mass spectrometry. *Analytical Chemistry* **70**, 2704–2709.

Everitt, B. S. (1993). *Cluster Analysis.* Edward Arnold, London.

Fang, J. & Barcelona, M. J. (1998). Structural determination and quantitative analysis of bacterial phospholipids using liquid chromatography electrospray ionization mass spectrometry. *Journal of Microbiological Methods* **33**, 23–35.

Fenselau, C. (1997). MALDI MS and strategies for protein analysis. *Analytical Chemistry* **69**, A661–A665.

Ferraro, J. R. & Nakamoto, K. (1994). *Introductory Raman Spectroscopy.* Academic Press, London.

Forsström, J. J. & Dalton, K. J. (1995). Artificial neural networks for decision support in clinical medicine. *Annals of Medicine* **27**, 509–517.

Frankel, D. S., Olson, R. J., Frankel, S. L. & Chisholm, S. W. (1989). Use of a neural net computer system for analysis of flow cytometric data of phytoplankton populations. *Cytometry* **10**, 540–550.

Freeman, R., Goodacre, R., Sisson, P. R., Magee, J. G., Ward, A. C. & Lightfoot, N. F. (1994). Rapid identification of species within the *Mycobacterium tuberculosis* complex by artificial neural network analysis of pyrolysis mass spectra. *Journal of Medical Microbiology* **40**, 170–173.

Freeman, R., Sisson, P. R. & Ward, A. C. (1995). Resolution of batch variations in pyrolysis mass spectrometry of bacteria by the use of artificial neural networks. *Antonie van Leeuwenhoek* **68**, 253–260.

Gaskell, S. J. (1997). Electrospray: principles and practice. *Journal of Mass Spectrometry* **32**, 677–688.

Gibson, B. W., Phillips, N. J., John, C. M. & Melaugh, W. (1994). Lipooligosaccharides in pathogenic *Haemophilus* and *Neisseria* species – mass spectrometric techniques for identification and characterization. *ACS Symposium Series* **541**, 185–202.

Goetz, A. F. H., Vane, G., Solomon, J. & Rock, B. N. (1985). Imaging spectrometry for earth remote sensing. *Science* **228**, 1147–1153.

Goodacre, R. (1994). Characterisation and quantification of microbial systems using pyrolysis mass spectrometry: introducing neural networks to analytical pyrolysis. *Microbiology Europe* **2**, 16–22.

Goodacre, R. & Kell, D. B. (1993). Rapid and quantitative analysis of bioprocesses using pyrolysis mass spectrometry and neural networks – application to indole production. *Analytica Chimica Acta* **279**, 17–26.

Goodacre, R. & Kell, D. B. (1996a). Correction of mass spectral drift using artificial neural networks. *Analytical Chemistry* **68**, 271–280.

Goodacre, R. & Kell, D. B. (1996b). Pyrolysis mass spectrometry and its applications in biotechnology. *Current Opinion in Biotechnology* **7**, 20–28.

Goodacre, R. & Kell, D. B. (1996c). Composition analysis. International Patent no. WO 96/42058, 27 December.

Goodacre, R., Kell, D. B. & Bianchi, G. (1992). Neural networks and olive oil. *Nature* **359**, 594–594.

Goodacre, R., Kell, D. B. & Bianchi, G. (1993). Rapid assessment of the adulteration of virgin olive oils by other seed oils using pyrolysis mass spectrometry and artificial neural networks. *Journal of the Science of Food and Agriculture* **63**, 297–307.

Goodacre, R., Karim, A., Kaderbhai, M. A. & Kell, D. B. (1994a). Rapid and quantitative analysis of recombinant protein expression using pyrolysis mass spectrometry and artificial neural networks – application to mammalian cytochrome B5 in *Escherichia coli. Journal of Biotechnology* **34**, 185–193.

Goodacre, R., Neal, M. J. & Kell, D. B. (1994b). Rapid and quantitative analysis of the pyrolysis mass spectra of complex binary and tertiary mixtures using multivariate calibration and artificial neural networks. *Analytical Chemistry* **66**, 1070–1085.

Goodacre, R., Neal, M. J., Kell, D. B., Greenham, L. W., Noble, W. C. & Harvey, R. G. (1994c). Rapid identification using pyrolysis mass spectrometry and artificial neural networks of *Propionibacterium acnes* isolated from dogs. *Journal of Applied Bacteriology* **76**, 124–134.

Goodacre, R., Trew, S., Wrigley-Jones, C., Neal, M. J., Maddock, J., Ottley, T. W., Porter, N. & Kell, D. B. (1994d). Rapid screening for metabolite overproduction in fermentor broths using pyrolysis mass spectrometry with multivariate calibration and artificial neural networks. *Biotechnology and Bioengineering* **44**, 1205–1216.

Goodacre, R., Trew, S., Wrigley-Jones, C., Saunders, G., Neal, M. J., Porter, N. & Kell, D. B. (1995). Rapid and quantitative analysis of metabolites in fermentor broths using pyrolysis mass spectrometry with supervised learning: application to the screening of *Penicillium chrysogenum* fermentations for the overproduction of penicillins. *Analytica Chimica Acta* **313**, 25–43.

Goodacre, R., Hiom, S. J., Cheeseman, S. L., Murdoch, D., Weightman, A. J. & Wade, W. G. (1996a). Identification and discrimination of oral asaccharolytic *Eubacterium* spp. using pyrolysis mass spectrometry and artificial neural networks. *Current Microbiology* **32**, 77–84.

Goodacre, R., Neal, M. J. & Kell, D. B. (1996b). Quantitative analysis of multivariate data using artificial neural networks: a tutorial review and applications to the deconvolution of pyrolysis mass spectra. *Zentralblatt für Bakteriologie* **284**, 516–539.

Goodacre, R., Timmins, É. M., Rooney, P. J., Rowland, J. J. & Kell, D. B. (1996c). Rapid identification of *Streptococcus* and *Enterococcus* species using diffuse reflectance–absorbance Fourier transform infrared spectroscopy and artificial neural networks. *FEMS Microbiology Letters* **140**, 233–239.

Goodacre, R., Timmins, É. M., Jones, A., Kell, D. B., Maddock, J., Heginbothom, M. L. & Magee, J. T. (1997). On mass spectrometer instrument standardization and interlaboratory calibration transfer using neural networks. *Analytica Chimica Acta* **348**, 511–532.

Goodacre, R., Rooney, P. J. and Kell, D. B. (1998a). Discrimination between methicillin-resistant and methicillin-susceptible *Staphylococcus aureus* using pyrolysis mass spectrometry and artificial neural networks. *Journal of Antimicrobial Chemotherapy* **41**, 27–34.

Goodacre, R., Timmins, É. M., Burton, R., Kaderbhai, N., Woodward, A., Kell, D. B. & Rooney, P. J. (1998b). Rapid identification of urinary tract infection bacteria using hyperspectral, whole organism fingerprinting and artificial neural networks. *Microbiology*, **144**, 1157–1170.

Goodacre, R., Heald, J. K. & Kell, D. B. (1999). Characterisation of intact microorganisms using electrospray ionization mass spectrometry. *FEMS Microbiology Letters* **176**, 17–24.

Goodfellow, M. (1995). Inter-strain comparison of pathogenic microorganisms by pyrolysis mass spectrometry. *Binary – Computing in Microbiology* **7**, 54–60.

Graselli, J. G. & Bulkin, B. J. (1991). *Analytical Raman Spectroscopy*. John Wiley, New York.

Griffiths, P. R. & de Haseth, J. A. (1986). *Fourier Transform Infrared Spectrometry*. John Wiley, New York.

Guilhaus, M. (1995). Principles and instrumentation in time-of-flight mass-spectrometry – physical and instrumental concepts. *Journal of Mass Spectrometry* **30**, 1519–1532.

Harrington, P. B. (1993a). Minimal neural networks – concerted optimization of multiple decision planes. *Chemometrics and Intelligent Laboratory Systems* **18**, 157–170.

Harrington, P. B. (1993b). Minimal neural networks: differentiation of classification entropy. *Chemometrics and Intelligent Laboratory Systems* **19**, 143–154.

Haykin, S. (1994). *Neural Networks*. Macmillan, New York.

Helm, D., Labischinski, H., Schallehn, G. & Naumann, D. (1991). Classification and identification of bacteria by Fourier transform infrared spectroscopy. *Journal of General Microbiology* **137**, 69–79.

Hendra, P., Jones, C. & Warnes, G. (1991). *Fourier Transform Raman Spectroscopy*. In M. Masson & J. F. Tyson, eds., Ellis Horwood Series in Analytical Chemistry. Ellis Horwood, Chichester.

Hertz, J., Krogh, A. & Palmer, R. G. (1991). *Introduction to the Theory of Neural Computation*. Addison-Wesley, Redwood City, CA.

Holland, R. D., Wilkes, J. G., Rafii, F., Sutherland, J. B., Persons, C. C., Voorhees, K. J. & Lay, J. O. (1996). Rapid identification of intact whole bacteria based on spectral patterns using matrix-assisted laser desorption/ionization with time-of-flight mass-spectrometry. *Rapid Communications in Mass Spectrometry* **10**, 1227–1232.

Howard, J. & Whitcombe, D. M. (1995). *Diagnostic Bacteriology Protocols*. Human Press Inc., Totowa, NJ.

Janssen, P., Coopman, R., Huys, G., Swings, J., Bleeker, M., Vos, P., Zabeau, M. & Kersters, K. (1996). Evaluation of the DNA fingerprinting method AFLP as a new tool in bacterial taxonomy. *Microbiology* **142**, 1881–1893.

Jolliffe, I. T. (1986). *Principal Component Analysis.* Springer-Verlag, New York.

Kell, D. B. & Sonnleitner, B. (1995). GMP – Good Modelling Practice: an essential component of good manufacturing practice. *Trends in Biotechnology* 13, 481–492.

Krishnamurthy, T. & Ross, P. L. (1996). Rapid identification of bacteria by direct matrix-assisted laser desorption/ionization mass spectrometric analysis of whole cells. *Rapid Communications in Mass Spectrometry* 10, 1992–1996.

Krishnamurthy, T., Ross, P. L. & Rajamani, U. (1996). Detection of pathogenic and non-pathogenic bacteria by matrix-assisted laser desorption/ionization time-of-flight mass-spectrometry. *Rapid Communications in Mass Spectrometry* 10, 883–888.

Krishnamurthy, T., Davis, M. T., Stahl, D. C. & Lee, T. D. (1999). Liquid chromatography microspray mass spectrometry for bacterial investigations. *Rapid Communications in Mass Spectrometry* 13, 39–49.

Li, J., Thibault, P., Martin, A., Richards, J. C., Wakarchuk, W. W. & van der Wilp, W. (1998). Development of an on-line preconcentration method for the analysis of pathogenic lipopolysaccharides using capillary electrophoresis–electrospray mass spectrometry – application to small colony isolates. *Journal of Chromatography A* 817, 325–336.

Liu, C. L., Hofstadler, S. A., Bresson, J. A., Udseth, H. R., Tsukuda, T., Smith, R. D. & Snyder, A. P. (1998). On line dual microdialysis with ESI-MS for direct analysis of complex biological samples and microorganism lysates. *Analytical Chemistry* 70, 1797–1801.

Magee, J. T. (1993). Whole-organism fingerprinting. In M. Goodfellow & A. G. O'Donnell, eds., *Handbook of New Bacterial Systematics.* Academic Press, London, pp. 383–427.

Mango, L. J. (1994). Computer assisted cervical cancer screening using neural networks. *Cancer Letters* 77, 155–162.

Manly, B. F. J. (1994). *Multivariate Statistical Methods: A Primer.* Chapman & Hall, London.

Martens, H. and Næs, T. (1989). *Multivariate Calibration.* John Wiley, Chichester.

Massart, D. L., Vandeginste, B. G. M., Deming, S. N., Michotte, Y. & Kaufmann, L. (1988). *Chemometrics: A Textbook.* Elsevier, Amsterdam.

McClennen, W. H., Arnold, N. S. & Meuzelaar, H. L. C. (1994). Field-portable hyphenated instrumentation – the birth of the tricorder. *Trends in Analytical Chemistry* 13, 286–293.

Meuzelaar, H. L. C., Haverkamp, J. & Hileman, F. D. (1982). *Pyrolysis Mass Spectrometry of Recent and Fossil Biomaterials.* Elsevier, Amsterdam.

Moody, J. & Darken, C. J. (1989). Fast learning in networks of locally-tuned processing units. *Neural Computation* 1, 281–294.

Morris, C. W., Boddy, L. & Allman, R. (1992). Identification of basidiomycete spores by neural network analysis of flow cytometry data. *Mycological Research* 96, 697–701.

Naumann, D., Helm, D., Labischinski, H. & Giesbrecht, P. (1991). The characterization of microorganisms by Fourier-transform infrared spectroscopy (FT-IR). In W. H. Nelson, ed., *Modern Techniques for Rapid Microbiological Analysis.* VCH Publishers, New York, pp. 43–96.

Nelson, W. H., Manoharan, R. & Sperry, J. F. (1992). UV resonance Raman studies of bacteria. *Applied Spectroscopy Reviews* 27, 67–124.

Park, J. & Sandberg, I. W. (1991). Universal approximation using radial basis function networks. *Neural Computation* 3, 246–257.

Puppels, G. J. & Greve, J. (1993). Raman microspectroscopy of single whole cells. *Advances in*

Spectroscopy **20A**, 231–265.

Richard, M. D. & Lippmann, R. P. (1991). Neural network classifiers estimate Bayesian a posteriori probabilities. *Neural Computation* 3, 461–483.

Ripley, B. D. (1994). Neural networks and related methods for classification. *Journal of the Royal Statistical Society Series B – Methodology* 56, 409–437.

Ripley, B. D. (1996). *Pattern Recognition and Neural Networks.* Cambridge University Press, Cambridge.

Roepstorff, P. (1997). Mass spectrometry in protein studies from genome to function. *Current Opinion in Biotechnology* **8**, 6–13.

Rumelhart, D. E., McClelland, J. L. & The PDP Research Group (1986). *Parallel Distributed Processing, Experiments in the Microstructure of Cognition,* vols. I and II. MIT Press, Cambridge, MA.

Schrader, B. (1995). *Infrared and Raman Spectroscopy: Methods and Applications.* Verlag Chemie, Weinheim.

Seasholtz, M. B. & Kowalski, B. (1993). The parsimony principle applied to multivariate calibration. *Analytica Chemica Acta* **277**, 165–177.

Simpson, P. K. (1990). *Artificial Neural Systems.* Pergamon Press, Oxford.

Sisson, P. R., Freeman, R., Law, D., Ward, A. C. & Lightfoot, N. F. (1995). Rapid detection of verocytotoxin production status in *Escherichia coli* by artificial neural network analysis of pyrolysis mass spectra. *Journal of Analytical and Applied Pyrolysis* **32**, 179–185.

Siuzdak, G. (1996). *Mass Spectrometry for Biotechnology.* Academic Press, London.

Smith, P. B. W., Snyder, A. P. & Harden, C. S. (1995). Characterization of bacterial phospholipids by electrospray ionization tandem mass spectrometry. *Analytical Chemistry* **67**, 1824–1830.

Smits, J. R. M., Breedveld, L. W., Derksen, M. W. J., Kateman, G., Balfoort, H. W., Snoek, J. & Hofstraat, J. W. (1992). Pattern classification with artificial neural networks: classification of algae, based upon flow cytometer data. *Analytica Chimica Acta* **258**, 11–25.

Smits, J. R. M., Melssen, W. J., Derksen, M. W. J. & Kateman, G. (1993). Drift correction for pattern classification with neural networks. *Analytica Chimica Acta* **284**, 91–105.

Snyder, A. P. (1996). Electrospray: a popular ionization technique for mass spectrometry. *ACS Symposium Series* **619**, 1–20.

Sokal, R. R. & Sneath, P. H. A. (1963). *Principles of Numerical Taxonomy.* W. H. Freeman & Co., San Francisco.

Timmins, É. M. & Goodacre, R. (1997). Rapid quantitative analysis of binary mixtures of *Escherichia coli* strains using pyrolysis mass spectrometry with multivariate calibration and artificial neural networks. *Journal of Applied Microbiology* **83**, 208–218.

Wasserman, P. D. (1989). *Neural Computing: Theory and Practice.* Van Nostrand Reinhold, New York.

Welham, K. J., Domin, M. A., Scannell, D. E., Cohen, E. & Ashton, D. S. (1998). The characterization of micro-organisms by matrix-assisted laser desorption/ionization time-of-flight mass spectrometry. *Rapid Communications in Mass Spectrometry* **12**, 176–180.

Werbos, P. J. (1994). *The Roots of Back-propagation: From Ordered Derivatives to Neural Networks and Political Forecasting.* John Wiley, Chichester.

White, H. (1992). *Artificial Neural Networks: Approximation and Learning Theory*. Blackwell, Oxford.

Wilkins, M. F., Morris, C. W. & Boddy, L. (1994). A comparison of radial basis function and backpropagation neural networks for identification of marine phytoplankton from multivariate flow cytometry data. *CABIOS* **10**, 285–294.

Wilkins, M. F., Boddy, L., Morris, C. W. & Jonker, R. (1996). A comparison of some neural and non-neural methods for identification of phytoplankton from flow cytometry data. *CABIOS* **12**, 9–18.

Williams, J. G. K., Kubelik, A. R., Livak, K. J., Rafalski, J. A. & Tingey, S. V. (1990). DNA polymorphisms amplified by arbitrary primers are useful as genetic markers. *Nucleic Acids Research* **18**, 6531–6535.

Williams, K. P. J., Pitt, G. D., Batchelder, D. N. & Kip, B. J. (1994). Confocal Raman microspectroscopy using a stigmatic spectrograph and CCD detector. *Applied Spectroscopy* **48**, 232–235.

Wilson, T. A., Rogers, S. K. & Myers, L. R. (1995). Perceptual-based hyperspectral image fusion using multiresolution analysis. *Optical Engineering* **34**, 3154–3164.

Winson, M. K., Goodacre, R., Woodward, A. M., Timmins, É. M., Jones, A., Alsberg, B. K., Rowland, J. J. & Kell, D. B. (1997). Diffuse reflectance absorbance spectroscopy taking in chemometrics (DRASTIC). A hyperspectral FT-IR-based approach to rapid screening for metabolite overproduction. *Analytica Chimica Acta* **348**, 273–282.

Wunschel, D. S., Fox, K. F., Fox, A., Nagpal, M. L., Kim, K., Stewart, G. C. & Shahgholi, M. (1997). Quantitative analysis of neutral and acidic sugars in whole bacterial cell hydrolysates using high-performance anion-exchange liquid chromatography electrospray ionization tandem mass spectrometry. *Journal of Chromatography A* **776**, 205–219.

Zupan, J. & Gasteiger, J. (1993). *Neural Networks for Chemists: An Introduction*. VCH Verlagsgesellschaft, Weinheim.

Part II

Prospects

8

Recent advances in EEG signal analysis and classification

Charles W. Anderson and David A. Peterson

Introduction

Electrical signals recorded from the scalp of human subjects, or electroencephalographic (EEG) signals, were first studied extensively by Berger (1929). Since these initial experiments, investigators in many branches of science, including physics, medicine, neuroscience, and psychology, have searched for meaningful patterns in EEG signals (Pilgreen 1995). For example, the analysis of patterns in EEG has for some time been extremely useful in the study and treatment of epilepsy (Kellaway & Petersen 1976).

Many of the traditional approaches to EEG pattern analysis that have been employed during the last six decades are based on visual inspection of graphs of voltage amplitude over time, or on the inspection of spectra showing the energy with which various frequencies appear in the signal. However, recent advances in signal analysis and classification using artificial neural networks have led to significant, new results in the filtering and interpretation of EEG signals. This chapter describes some of these new approaches as they are applied to EEG signals surrounding a response to a stimulus and to spontaneous EEG signals recorded while subjects perform mental tasks. Applications of these approaches include the study of sensory, motor and cognitive processing in the brain, and the development of brain–computer interfaces to provide a new avenue for communication with locked-in patients suffering from advanced anterolateral sclerosis (ALS).

Effect of attention on spectral dynamics of event related potentials

The event-related potential, or ERP, is simply the EEG recorded in response to a time-locked stimulus. The ERP is typically presented as the average over many identical trials characterized by the amplitude and poststimulus latency of its positive and negative peaks, or 'components'. Amplitudes of ERP components are modulated by attention; stimuli that receive greater attention produce ERP components with larger magnitude (Woldorff & Hillyard 1991). Thus ERPs can be used as a physiological measure of attention. There is also evidence that the frequency composition of the EEG is modulated by attention (Gomez et al. 1998). This suggests that EEG frequencies could also be used as a physiological measure of attention.

We conducted an exploratory study to combine these measures to see whether temporal dynamics in ERP frequency composition also had correlations with attention. In other words, are the temporal dynamics of ERP frequency modulated by attention? We used data from an alternating dichotic listening task, modified from Hansen & Hillyard (1983) and Fujiwara et al. (1998). The task is a type of auditory selective attention task. High (1000 Hz) and low (800 Hz) tones of 50-millisecond duration were presented in a sequence that was random both within and between ears. High tones were presented with 20% probability and low tones with 80%. Participants were instructed to respond to the high tones in only one ear. Thus, for each session, there is one attended tone and one attended ear. EEG data (128-channel) were recorded during each section.

Although signal frequencies are usually analysed with Fourier transforms, we used wavelet transforms (Strang & Nguyen 1996), because Fourier transforms discard the temporal information that we want to preserve. Time-windowed Fourier transforms preserve some temporal information, but only to the resolution of the window.

Like most signal transformation methods, the wavelet transformation is simply a basis transformation, converting a time-domain signal to a scale and shift domain (Daubechies 1990). Scales correspond to frequencies, although only roughly, because wavelet basis functions are not smooth sinusoids. The shift corresponds to the signal's time axis. Instead of amplitude as in the ERP, the wavelet transformation gives a measure of energy in the signal at each time and frequency. Thus the wavelet transform provides a systematic method for spectral analysis of non-stationary signals. The specific wavelet basis we used was the popular Daubechies order-4 wavelet.

We call the wavelet transform of an ERP an event-related wavelet, or ERW. The temporal dynamics of ERP frequency, as depicted with the ERW, are modulated by attention. ERPs and ERWs in Figure 8.1 depict the difference between the amplitudes (for ERP) and the wavelet coefficients (for ERW). On the left are shown differences between the attended and unattended tones for the attended ear, and on the right is shown differences between attended and unattended ears, for the attended tone. The ERW plots illustrate that ERP frequency compositions are temporally dynamic. Thus, frequency-based ERP analyses that discard temporal information, such as non-windowed Fourier transform-based methods, might miss important information in the ERP. Furthermore, the dynamics of low-frequency energy appears to be similar across the two ERW plots. This

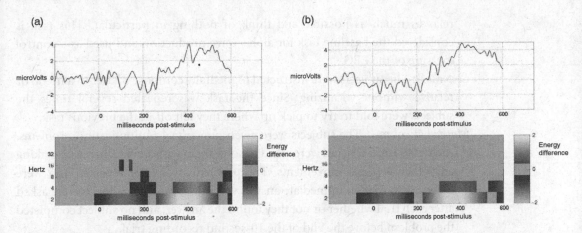

Figure 8.1.   Differences in event-related potential (ERP) (upper row) and event-related wavelet (ERW) (lower row). The graphs on the left show the differences between attended and unattended tones, for the attended ear. The graphs on the right show the differences between attended and unattended ears, for the attended tone.

suggests that the differential effect of selective auditory attention may have similar spectral dynamics in the ERP regardless of whether it is attention to a particular ear or a particular tone.

Brain–computer interface based on spontaneous EEG

New EEG recording and analysis methods are having a very strong impact on the body of work that seeks a brain–computer interface (BCI). In fact, in June of 1999, J. Wolpaw and T. Vaughan of the Wadsworth Center of the New York State Department hosted an international meeting called Brain–Computer Interface Technology: Theory and Practice, funded by the National Institutes of Health and other organizations. At this meeting, a number of approaches to using EEG patterns in a BCI were discussed. In the rest of this section, we summarize our work towards a brain–computer interface using spontaneous EEG.

Mental tasks and signal representations

In our current work, subjects do not attempt to exert control over some device. They are simply asked to perform various mental tasks. Our objective is to find patterns in their spontaneous EEG that reliably appear while they are performing one of the tasks. The detection of these patterns could be used to move a cursor or select a choice on a computer screen, or even control a wheelchair.

Subjects were asked to perform the following five mental tasks.

Baseline task: The subjects were not asked to perform a specific mental task, but to relax as much as possible and think of nothing in particular. This task is considered the baseline task for alpha-wave production and used as a control measure of the EEG.

Letter task: The subjects were instructed to mentally compose a letter to a friend or relative without vocalizing. Since the task was repeated several times the subjects were told to try to pick up where they left off in the previous task.

Mathematical task: The subjects were given non-trivial multiplication problems, such as 49 times 78, and were asked to solve them without vocalizing or making any other physical movements. The problems were not repeated and were designed so that an immediate answer was not attainable. Subjects were asked after each trial whether or not they found the answer, and no subject completed the problem before the end of the 10-second recording trial.

Visual counting: The subjects were asked to imagine a blackboard and to visualize numbers being written on the board sequentially, with the previous number being erased before the next number was written. The subjects were further instructed not to verbally read the numbers but to visualize them, and to pick up counting from the previous task rather than starting over each time.

Geometric figure rotation: The subjects were given 30 seconds to study a drawing of a complex three-dimensional block figure after which the drawing was removed and the subjects instructed to visualize the object being rotated about an axis.

Data were recorded for 10 seconds during each task and each task was repeated five times per session. Most subjects attended two such sessions recorded on separate weeks, resulting in a total of 10 trials for each task.

EEG from six electrodes at C3, C4, P3, P4, O1 and O2 (from the 10–20 standard of electrode placement (Jasper 1958)), was sampled at 250 Hz and filtered to 0.1 to 100 Hz. These six time series were divided into half-second segments that overlap by one quarter-second, producing at most 39 segments per trial after discarding segments containing eye blinks, identified by large voltage changes in an electro-oculogram (EOG) channel.

Based on the success of others (Keirn & Aunon 1990), we focused on signal representations based on autoregressive (AR) models and on Fourier transforms. In choosing an AR model order, we found that Akaike's information criterion (AIC) is minimized for orders of 2 and 3 (Stolz 1995). However, based on previous results by Keirn & Aunon, an order of 6 was used. For one subject performing 10 trials of each of the five tasks, a total of 1385 half-second segments was collected, with 277 segments from each of the five tasks.

To compare with the performance of the AR representation, a power spectrum density (PSD) representation was implemented using the same data segment of 125 samples, or one half-second, with a quarter-second overlap. Data segments were windowed with the Hanning window and a 125-point fast-Fourier transform was applied, resulting in a 63-point power spectrum density spanning 0 to 125 Hz with a resolution of 2 Hz.

We also generated reduced-dimensionality versions of the AR and PSD representations via a Karhunen–Loève (KL) transformation (Jollife 1986), in which the eigenvectors of the covariance matrix of all AR or PSD vectors are determined and the AR or PSD vectors are projected onto a subset of the eigenvectors having the highest eigenvalues. The key parameter of this transformation is the number of eigenvectors onto which each vector is projected. A common way to choose this number is to set it equal to the global KL estimate, given by the smallest index i for which $\lambda_i/\lambda_{max} \leq 0.01$, where the λ_i are the eigenvalues in decreasing order for $i = 1, 2, \dots$.

For the AR representation of all segments from the five tasks, the global KL estimate is 31, a small reduction from the original 36 dimensions of the representation. For the PSD representation, the global KL estimate is 21. This is a large reduction from the 378 dimensions of the PSD representation.

Neural network classifier

The classifier implemented for this work is a standard, feedforward, neural network with one hidden layer and one output layer, trained with the error back-propagation algorithm (Rumelhart et al. 1986; Hassoun 1995). The output layer contains five units, corresponding to the five mental tasks. Their target values were set to 1,0,0,0,0 for the baseline task, 0,1,0,0,0 for the letter task, 0,0,1,0,0 for the math task, 0,0,0,1,0 for the counting task, and 0,0,0,0,1 for the rotation task. After trying a large number of different values, we found that a learning rate of 0.1 for the hidden layers and 0.01 for the output layer produced the best performance.

To limit the amount of overfitting during training, the following 10-fold, cross-validation procedure was performed. Eight of the ten trials were used for the training set, one of the remaining trials was selected for validation and the last trial was used for testing. The error of the network on the validation data was calculated after every pass, or epoch, through the training data. After 3000 epochs, the network state (its weight values) at the epoch for which the validation error is smallest was chosen as the network that will most likely perform well on novel data. This best network was then applied to the test set; the result indicates how well the network will generalize to novel data. With 10 trials, there are 90 ways of choosing the validation and test trials, with the remaining eight trials combined for the training set. Results described in the next section are reported as the average classification accuracy on the test set averaged over all 90 partitions of the data. Each of the 90 repetitions started with different, random, initial weights.

The neural networks were trained using a CNAPS Server II (Adaptive Solutions,

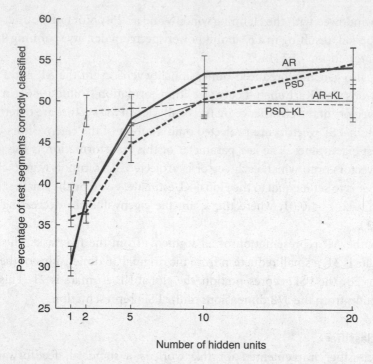

Figure 8.2.   Average percentage of test segments correctly classified. Error bars show 90% confidence intervals. AR, autoregressive; PSD, power spectrum density; KL, Karhunen–Loève transformation. (From Anderson 1999, Figure 2, p. 233, with permission; Springer-Verlag copyright 1999.)

Incorporated), a parallel computer with 128 20-MHz processors, upgradable to 512 processors. Training a neural network with a single hidden layer containing 20 hidden units (a 20–0 network) took an average of 3.2 minutes on the CNAPS, while, on a Sun SparcStation 20, the same experiment took an average of 20 minutes. An experiment of 90 repetitions required 4.8 hours on the CNAPS and 30 hours on the SparcStation.

Results

Figure 8.2 summarizes the average percentage of test segments classified correctly for various-sized networks using each of the four representations. For one hidden unit, the PSD representations perform better than the AR representations. With two hidden units, the PSD–KL representation performs about 10% better than the other three. With 20 hidden units, the KL representations perform worse than the non-KL representations, though the difference is not statistically significant.

Inspection of how the network's classification changes from one segment to the next suggests that better performance might be achieved by averaging the net-

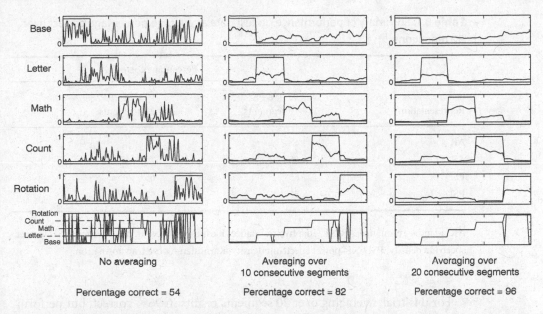

Base

Letter

Math

Count

Rotation

Rotation
Count
Math
Letter
Base

No averaging

Averaging over
10 consecutive segments

Averaging over
20 consecutive segments

Percentage correct = 54

Percentage correct = 82

Percentage correct = 96

Figure 8.3.   Network output values and desired values for one test trial. The first five rows of graphs show the values of the five network outputs over the 175 test segments. The sixth row of graphs plots the task determined by the network outputs and the true task. The first column of graphs is without averaging over consecutive segments, the second is for averaging the network output over 10 consecutive segments, while the third column is for averaging over 20 segments. (From Anderson 1999, Figure 3, p. 233, with permission; Springer-Verlag copyright 1999.)

work's output over consecutive segments. To investigate this, a 20-unit network trained with the AR representation is studied. The left column of graphs in Figure 8.3 show the output values of the network's five output units for each segment of test data from one trial. On each graph the desired value for the corresponding output is also drawn. The bottom graph shows the true task and the task predicted by the network. For this trial, 54% of the segments are classified correctly when no averaging across segments is performed. The other two columns of graphs show the network's output and predicted classification that result from averaging over 10 and 20 consecutive segments. Confusions made by the classifier are identified by the relatively high responses of an output unit for test segments that do not correspond to the task represented by that output unit. For example, in the third graph in the right column, the output value of the mathematical unit is high during mathematical segments, as it should be, but it is also relatively high during count segments. Also, the output of the count unit, shown in the fourth graph, is high during count segments, but is also relatively high during letter segments.

Table 8.1. Summary of performance on test data as average percentage correct over 90 repetitions

	Percentage correct	
Representation	Averaging over 10 segments	Averaging over 20 segments
AR	68	72
AR-KL	65	70
PSD	65	65
PSD-KL	55	57

AR, adaptive resonance; AR-KL, adaptive resonance–Karhunen–Loève transformation; PSD, power spectrum density; PSD-KL, power spectrum density–Karhunen–Loève transformation.

For this trial, averaging over 20 segments results in 96% correct, but performance is not improved this much on all trials. The best classification performance for the 20 hidden unit network, averaged over all 90 repetitions, is achieved by averaging over all segments. Table 8.1 summarizes the significant information, showing that the AR representation performs the best whether averaged over 10 or 20 segments, but when averaged over 20 segments, the AR and AR–KL representations perform equally well. The PSD and PSD–KL representations do consistently worse than the AR representations.

Removal of eye blinks using independent components analysis

EEG data are prone to significant interference from a wide variety of artefacts, particularly eye blinks. Most methods for classifying cognitive tasks with EEG data simply discard time-windows containing eye blink artefacts, typically detected by crude measures such as thresholds in the magnitude of the EEG or EOG signals. However, future applications of EEG-based cognitive task classification should not be hindered by eye blinks. The value of an EEG-controlled brain–computer interface, for instance, would be severely diluted if it did not work in the presence of eye blinks. Fortunately, recent advances in blind signal separation algorithms and their applications to EEG data mitigate the artefact contamination issue. In this section, we show how independent components analysis (ICA) and its extension for sub-Gaussian sources, extended ICA (eICA), can be applied to accurately classify cognitive tasks with eye blink-contaminated EEG recordings. See Peterson & Anderson (1999) for further details.

ICA is a method for blind source separation. It assumes that the observed signals are produced by a linear mixture of source signals. Thus the original source signals could, in principle, be recovered from the observed signals by running the observed signals back through the inverted mixing matrix. Computationally intensive matrix inversions can be avoided, with recent relaxation-based ICA algorithms (Bell & Sejnowski 1995). These algorithms derive maximally independent components by maximizing their joint entropy, which is equivalent to minimizing the components' mutual information. The result is a simple rule for evolving the inverse of the mixing matrix in an iterative, gradient-based algorithm.

It is reasonable to apply ICA to EEG data, because EEG signals measured on the scalp are the result of linear filtering of underlying cortical activity (Makeig et al. 1996; Jung et al. 1998). However, ICA assumes that all of the underlying sources have similar, super-Gaussian, probability density functions. It is unknown how well EEG 'sources' follow this assumption, but it is reasonable to assume that some may not. A recent extension to ICA, eICA, takes a first step towards addressing this issue.

Recently, Jung et al. (1998) have shown that various artefacts, including eye blinks, can be separated from the remaining EEG signals with eICA. Here we report on the effect of applying ICA and eICA to EEG data on classification performance using standard PSD signal representations and feedforward neural network classifiers.

Extended ICA provides the same type of source separation as ICA, but also allows some sources to have sub-Gaussian distributions. The learning rule for the inverse of the mixing matrix is modified to be a function of the data's normalized fourth order cumulant, or kurtosis. During the course of learning, the kurtosis is calculated and the learning rule adjusted according to the kurtosis sign. Positive kurtosis is indicative of super-Gaussian distributions, and negative kurtosis of sub-Gaussian distributions. By accommodating sub-Gaussian distributions in the data, eICA should provide a more accurate decomposition of multichannel EEG data, particularly if different underlying sources follow different distributions.

We considered only three of the five tasks described earlier, the baseline task, the letter-writing task, and the mathematical task. Despite instructions to avoid eye blinks, many of the trials contain one or more eye blinks. Two schemes were used for handling the eye blinks, the threshold approach and ICA. With the threshold approach, eye blinks were detected by at least a 100 µV change in less than 100 milliseconds in the EOG channel. The subsequent 0.5-second window of the trial was removed from further consideration.

With the ICA approach, eye blinks are 'subtracted' rather than explicitly detected, and no portion of the trials are thrown out. ICA is performed on the combination of the EOG and six EEG channels. The number of components specified was the same as the number of input channels: seven. As a result, activity in the EEG channels that is closely correlated with the activity of the EOG channel

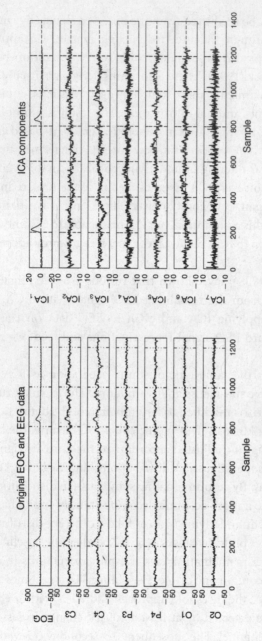

Figure 8.4. Separation of electro-oculogram (EOG) and electroencephalogram (EEG) (left) into independent components (right). (From Peterson & Anderson 1999, Figure 1, p. 265, with permission; Springer-Verlag copyright 1999.)

is separated and placed in one component, as illustrated in Figure 8.4 for the first 5 seconds of one trial of the base task. Notice that the eye blinks in the EOG channel influence even the most posterior EEG recordings at channels O1 and O2. The ICA activations show the eye blink activity in only one component.

Thus eye blink activity reflected in the EEG channels is effectively subtracted from the EEG channels. The component containing the EOG activity can be transparently detected, because it is the one with the highest correlation to the original EOG data. The remaining components are retained as the eye-blink-subtracted independent components of the EEG data. Thus, with the ICA approach, the full trial of EEG data is used for all trials, regardless of the number or distribution of eye blinks in those trials.

We compared three forms of ICA for eye blink removal: (a) ICA, (b) eICA, in which the algorithm chooses the number of sub-Gaussian components to use, and (c) extended ICA with fixed number of sub-Gaussian components. Thus a total of four different schemes was used to remove eye blinks and represent the 'blink-free' signals: thresh (for eye blink removal using threshold detection, as described above), ICA, eICA, and eICA_f (for eICA with fixed sub-Gaussian components). Our objectives were not only to see how cognitive task classification performance varies as a function of the eye blink-removal approach, but also to see how cognitive task classification performance varies as a function of the number of sub-Gaussians in the ICA representation.

Following eye blink removal with one of the four methods, the power spectral density of each channel in every window was computed and summed over the five primary EEG frequency bands: δ (0–4 Hz), θ (4–7 Hz), α (8–12 Hz), β (13–35 Hz), and γ (> 35 Hz). The PSD was used because it has been a popular and successful signal representation for many types of EEG analyses for decades. Finally, because the PSD values were so heavily weighted in the lower frequencies, the $\log_{10}$ of this vector was computed. Thus each window was represented by a feature vector of length 30 (i.e. six channels × five frequency bands).

The cognitive tasks were classified in two pairwise task comparisons: base versus mathematics and letter versus mathematics. By analysing two pairwise classifications we hoped to assess how well the classification scheme would generalize to different task pairs.

Supervised learning and simple feedforward neural networks were used to classify the feature vectors into one of the two tasks. The networks had one linear output node. The number of sigmoidal hidden nodes was varied over [0 1 2 3 5 10]. By including zero hidden nodes as one of the network architectures, we are effectively assessing how well a simple linear perceptron can classify the data. Network inputs were given not only to the hidden layer, but also to the output node, in a cascade-forward configuration. Thus network classifications

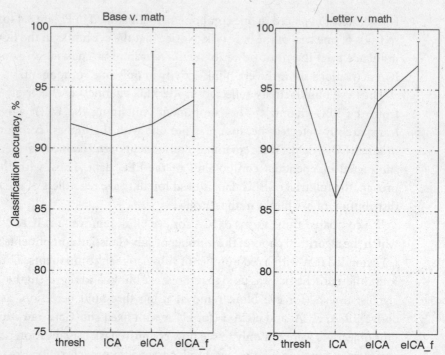

Figure 8.5.   Best classification performance as a function of eye blink removal schemes. (Error bars are one σ above and below mean.) For abbreviations, see the text. (From Peterson & Anderson 1999, Figure 2, p. 270, with permission; Springer-Verlag copyright 1999.)

were based on a combination of the non-linear transformation of the input features provided by the hidden layer as well as a linear transformation of the input features given directly to the output node.

The networks were given input feature vectors normalized so that each feature has a $N(0, 1)$ distribution. The networks were trained with Levenberg–Marquardt optimized back-propagation (Hagan & Menjah 1994). Training was terminated with early stopping, with the data set partitioned into 80%, 10% and 10% portions for training, validation and test sets, respectively. The mean and standard deviation of classification accuracy reported in the results section reflect the statistics of 20 randomly chosen partitions of the data and initial network weights.

Results comparing methods for eye blink removal

The best classification accuracy for each different eye blink removal scheme over all network architectures is shown in Figure 8.5. For the eICA_f scheme, the performance shown is for the best number of sub-Gaussian components. The performance is statistically similar across the different schemes. In all cases except ICA on the letter v. mathematics pair, mean classification accuracies are over 90%.

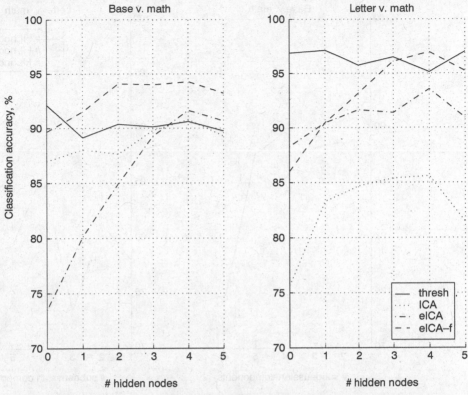

Figure 8.6.   Classification performance as a function of hidden layer size. (Error bars omitted for clarity. For most data points, $\sigma < 4$.) For abbreviations, see the text. (From Peterson & Anderson 1999, figure 3, p. 271, with permission; Springer-Verlag copyright 1999.)

For both task pairs, eICA and eICA_f perform statistically as well as the thresh scheme.

Figure 8.6 shows how classification accuracy varies with the size of the neural network's hidden layer. For the thresh scheme, the linear neural networks (i.e. zero non-linear hidden layer nodes) perform about as well as the non-linear networks. Thus the simple thresh scheme seems to represent the data's features in a linearly separable fashion. However, with all three of the ICA-based schemes, performance tends to improve with the size of the hidden layer, then decrease again as the number of hidden nodes is increased from 5 to 10. Notice that eICA and eICA_f perform about as well as thresh when networks of sufficient hidden layer size are used for the classification. Apparently the eICA representations produce feature vectors whose class distinctions fall along non-linear feature space boundaries. Notice that for the base v. mathematics task pair, the mean performance with eICA_f is greater than that of thresh for all of the non-linear networks.

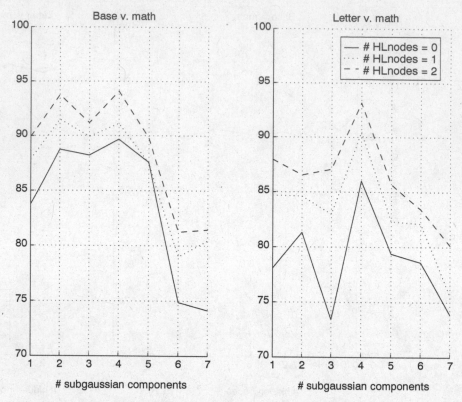

Figure 8.7. Classification performance as a function of number of sub-Gaussian components. (Results were similar for larger networks, and not plotted here for clarity.) HL, hidden layer. (From Peterson & Anderson, Figure 4, p. 271, with permission; Springer-Verlag copyright 1999.)

So are there specific numbers of sub-Gaussian components for which perform-ance is better than others? We explored this question, analysing task pair classifica-tion accuracy while varying the number of fixed sub-Gaussian components used in the eICA_f scheme. The results are summarized in Figure 8.7. Notice that for both task pairs, classification performance is indeed a function of the number of sub-Gaussian components. Also, the variability in performance is consistent across different size networks. For both task pairs, performance is about maxi-mum when the number of sub-Gaussians is four, and decreases steadily with additional sub-Gaussian components. However, the classification performance differs markedly between the task pairs when the number of sub-Gaussian compo-nents is fewer than four. Perhaps with the base task the underlying sources have fewer sub-Gaussian components, making the choice of fewer fixed sub-Gaussian components in our representation helpful for classification.

We have shown that eICA can be used to subtract eye blinks from EEG data and still provide a signal representation conducive to accurate cognitive task classification. We have also provided preliminary evidence that eICA-based schemes can generalize across different cognitive tasks. In both cases, however, it was necessary to use non-linear neural networks to achieve the same performance as was attained with a simple thresholding eye blink removal scheme and linear neural network classifiers. Further work needs to be done to assess the sensitivity of these results to different cognitive tasks.

By using a combination of ICA and artefact-correlated recording channels (e.g. the EOG channel) for artifact removal, eye blinks were removed without a hard-coded definition of eye-blink such as magnitude thresholds. This approach could generalize to other artefact sources. If, for example, specific muscle activity is interfering with EEG signals in a specific cognitive task monitoring setting, then this approach could be used to subtract the myographic activity from the EEG signals by including the appropriate electromyographic (EMG) reference channel in the ICA decomposition.

Next steps

Our current work has three objectives. The only results summarized here that include information about how EEG changes over time is our work on wavelets. One of our objectives is better classification accuracy through increased emphasis on representations that include such temporal information. Therefore, we are continuing our exploration of various signal representations, including wavelets, independent component analysis, desynchronization, coherence, and combinations thereof.

A second objective to our work is to develop tools to analyse and visualize what the neural networks are learning. We have found that by inverting the neural network, we can determine a set of fictitious EEG signals that the trained neural network would most strongly classify as one or another task. This gives us a sense of the discriminations the trained nets are making.

A third objective of our work is a portable EEG acquisition and analysis system that will provide the type of classification results described here in real time. This would lead to an exciting biofeedback protocol in which the subject can modify how he or she performs a mental task while observing the system's classification confidence. Our hope is that even a small bit of training with such a system will result in increased classification accuracy, providing a better channel of communication for locked-in patients of advanced anterolateral sclerosis.

The analysis methods summarized here and other recent developments are very general and can be applied to any EEG and MEG (magnetoencephalogram) data.

They show promise in aiding our understanding of and potential interventions in central nervous system disorders.

Acknowledgements

EEG data from the selective auditory attention experiments, background on the experiments, and assistance with the data interpretation were provided by Dr Jane M. Mende and Kristen S. Cardinal, University of Colorado Health Sciences Center. EEG data for the BCI experiments were collected by Keirn and Aunon (Keirn & Aunon 1990). We used the Salk Institute's Matlab toolbox for ICA (http://www.cnl.salk.edu/~scott/) for the ICA analyses. Research classifying the mental tasks was supported by the National Science Foundation through grants IRI-9202100 and CISE-9422007.

REFERENCES

Anderson, C. W. (1999). Identifying mental tasks from spontaneous EEG: signal representation and spatial analysis. In J. Mira & J. V. Sandrez-Andres, eds., *Proceedings of the International Work Conference on Neural Networks*, IWANN '99, Springer-Verlag, Berlin, pp. 228–237.

Bell, A. J. & Sejnowski, T. J. (1995). An information-maximization approach to blind separation and blind deconvolution. *Neural Computation* 7, 1129–1159.

Berger, H. (1929). Über das elektrenkephalogramm des menschen. *Archiv für Psychiatrie* 87, 527.

Daubechies, I. (1990). The wavelet transform, time-frequency localization and signal analysis. *IEEE Transactions on Information Theory* 36, 961–1005.

Fujiwara, N., Nagamine, T., Imai, M., Tanaka, T. & Shibasaki, H. (1998). Role of the primary auditory cortex in auditory selective attention studied by whole-head neuromagnetometer. *Cognitive Brain Research* 7, 99–109.

Gomez, C. M., Vazquez, M., Vaquero, E., López-Mendoza, D. & Cardoso, M. J. (1998). Frequency analysis of the EEG during spatial selective attention. *International Journal of Neuroscience* 1–2, 17–32.

Hagan, M. T. & Menjah, M. (1994). Training feedforward networks with the marquardt algorithm. *IEEE Transactions on Neural Networks* 5, 989–993.

Hansen, J. & Hillyard, S. (1983). Selective attention to multidimensional auditory stimuli. *Journal of Experimental Psychology: Human Perception and Performance* 9, 1–19.

Hassoun, M. H. (1995). *Fundamentals of Artificial Neural Networks*. MIT Press, Cambridge, MA.

Jasper, H. (1958). The ten twenty electrode system of the international federation. *Electroencephalography and Clinical Neurophysiology* 10, 371–375.

Jollife, I. T. (1986). *Principal Component Analysis*. Springer-Verlag, New York.

Jung, T.-P., Humphries, C., Lee, T. W., Makeig, S., McKeown, M. J., Iragui, V. & Sejnowski, T. J.

(1998). Extended ICA removes artifacts from electroencephalographic recordings. In M. Jordan, M. Kearns & S. Solla, eds., *Advances in Neural Information Processing Systems*, vol. 10. MIT Press, Cambridge, MA, pp. 894–900.

Keirn, Z. A. & Aunon, J. I. (1990). A new mode of communication between man and his surroundings. *IEEE Transactions on Biomedical Engineering* **37**, 1209–1214.

Kellaway, P. & Petersen, I. (1976). *Quantitative Analytic Studies in Epilepsy.* Raven Press, New York.

Makeig, S., Bell, A. J., Jung, T.-P. & Sejnowski, T. J. (1996). Independent component analysis of electroencephalographic data. In D. S. Touretzky, M. C. Mozer & M. E. Hasselmo, eds., *Advances in Neural Information Processing Systems*, vol. 8. MIT Press, Cambridge, MA, pp. 145–151.

Peterson, D. A. & Anderson, C. W. (1999). EEG-based cognitive task classification with ica and neural networks. In J. Mira & J. V. Sanchez-Andres, eds., *Proceedings of the International Work Conference on Neural Networks, IWANN '99*, Springer-Verlag, Berlin, pp. 265–272.

Pilgreen, K. L. (1995). Physiologic, medical, and cognitive correlates of electroencephalography. In *Neocortical Dynamics and Human EEG Rhythms.* Oxford University Press, Oxford, pp. 195–248.

Rumelhart, D. E., Hinton, G. E. & Williams, R. W. (1986). Learning internal representations by error propagation. In D. E. Rumelhart, J. L. McClelland & T. P. R. Group, eds., *Parallel Distributed Processing: Explorations in the Microstructure of Cognition*, vol. 1. Bradford, Cambridge, MA, pp. 318–362.

Stolz, E. (1995). Multivariate autoregressive models for classification of spontaneous electroencephalogram during mental tasks. Master's thesis, Electrical Engineering Department, Colorado State University.

Strang, G. & Nguyen, T. (1996). *Wavelets and Filter Banks.* Wellesley-Cambridge Press, Wellesley, MA.

Woldorff, M. G. & Hillyard, S. A. (1991). Modulation of early auditory processing during selective listening to rapidly presented tones. *Electroencephalography and Clinical Neurophysiology* **79**, 170–191.

9

Adaptive resonance theory: a foundation for 'apprentice' systems in clinical decision support?

Robert F. Harrison, Simon S. Cross, R. Lee Kennedy,
Chee Peng Lim and Joseph Downs

Introduction

apprentice *n*. Learner of a craft. [Old French *apprendre*]

In the field of clinical decision-making, a decision aid that is able to continue to learn from 'experience' is likely to have an advantage over one which is not. For instance, a system that is developed from data gathered at one location should be able, safely, to tune in to local conditions, for example demography elsewhere. Similarly, as practice or technology changes, such changes should be accommodated by the device itself, rather than by having to involve statisticians, knowledge engineers, etc. to rederive algorithms. After all, when doctors change hospital they are not subjected to complete retraining. Neither should a computerized decision aid have to be. Of course, this assumes the need for such systems in the first place, which is a wider question not addressed here. We use the analogy of an apprentice to motivate development of systems that learn in perpetuity.

Expert systems are characterized by the processes of rule elicitation, rule-base development and inference. Knowledge, in the form of rules, is built into the system a priori and, once embedded, remains unchanged throughout the lifetime of the system, unless a knowledge engineer intervenes. Conclusions are drawn by a deductive process. As a model of human expert behaviour this has some drawbacks because it presupposes that once individuals have achieved expert status they no longer continue to learn from their experience. In reality, experts are primed with knowledge, via schools, universities, on-the-job training, etc., but ultimately become known as experts for what they know over and above what they have been taught, i.e. what experience has taught them or what they are able to deduce from their earlier knowledge. Indeed, expertise might well be thought of as that knowledge which does not exist in our primary repositories of knowledge (textbooks, lecture courses, etc.). Furthermore, it is well recognized that, even for a static expert system, the knowledge acquisition process is difficult and time-consuming (Hayes-Roth et al. 1983).

In contrast, we propose the idea of an 'apprentice' system, which attempts to model the human knowledge acquisition and inference process more closely, either by refining in-built, prior, knowledge or by developing a model of the problem domain from scratch and from example (i.e. by induction). In either case, the key feature is an ability to adapt, over time, in the light of experience. The ability of systems to 'learn', incrementally, in this way is not something that expert systems in general possess. Neural networks, on the other hand, hold much promise for machine learning.

Looked at from a different perspective, expert systems have the advantage of being able to provide an explanation of their reasoning processes – an attractive property for the end-user – while neural networks have proved, in the main, unwilling to reveal the knowledge embedded within them, making potential beneficiaries of the technology wary of its adoption and raising a number of potential legal questions (Brahams & Wyatt 1989). Some inroads have been made in addressing both of these problems: rule induction systems such as those based on 'information gain' open the way towards automatic knowledge acquisition and update (Quinlan 1986, 1990, 1993), while rule extraction techniques attempt to 'open the black box' of neural networks (Saito & Nakano 1990; Shavlik et al. 1991; Towell & Shavlik 1993; Andrews & Geva 1995; Ma & Harrison 1995a).

As models of apprentice behaviour, mainstream rule induction and neural network techniques are hampered by the need, artificially, to suppress learning at some point prior to making the system operational. Thus the system, although apparently 'learning' to solve the problem, in fact does not continue to learn into the future; that is, any learning that takes place is acausal (offline). This is of course the conventional way of developing decision aids such as logistic regression models. Should, therefore, the problem characteristics change, perhaps owing to a change in practice (non-stationarity) or owing to differences between populations at different locations (inhomogeneity), or had there been an insufficient amount of representative information available at the time the system was established, the performance of these mainstream techniques may be severely compromised. Retraining on a new information set comprising both the original data, and any additional knowledge remains, by and large, the only solution, although tech- niques for incremental learning for both paradigms are beginning to emerge. The desirability of a system that can learn to improve its performance in situ and causally (online), without the intervention of a systems engineer, is evident.

The reason that learning must be suppressed derives from the so-called stabil-ity-plasticity dilemma (Carpenter & Grossberg 1987a). This makes explicit the conflict between the need to retain previously learned knowledge (stability) and the ability to adapt to new information (plasticity), i.e. how can we prevent existing knowledge from being overwritten or corrupted by new information or noise? This problem is known as 'catastrophic forgetting' (Sharkey & Sharkey 1995) and besets the majority of machine learning paradigms.

Of those approaches that attempt to address this dilemma, the adaptive reson-ance theory (ART) family of neural networks offers a number of significant advantages over the more common feedforward and competitive networks for the establishment of apprentice systems. These are:

an ability to discriminate novelty from noise, and familiar (statistical) events from rare but important (outlier) ones,

rapid learning based on predictive success rather than on predictive failure (mismatch),

self-organization, with few arbitrary parameters to tune, and automatic structure determination,

linear rather than exponential scaling with problem size,

straightforward revelation of embedded rule sets, and

inherently parallel implementation.

This is not to say that the establishment of ART-based systems is without its own problems, or indeed that ART is yet a mature technology. ART is under continual development and at present provides a way forward in this area. We shall explore some of ART's shortcomings at the appropriate points in the text.

Feedforward neural networks

Advances in neurocomputing have opened the way for the establishment of decision-support systems that are able to learn complex associations by example. The main thrust of work in this area has been in the use of the feedforward networks (e.g. the multilayer perceptron (MLP) (Rumelhart et al. 1986) or the radial basis function networks (RBFN); Moody & Darken 1989) to learn the association between evidence and outcome. Theoretical work in this area has led to the discovery of two important properties of feedforward networks:

for one-from-many classification, their learning rules lead to an interpretation of their outputs as estimates of the posterior (class conditional) probability distribution, conditioned on a set of evidence, provided that 'optimality' is attained (Wan 1990; Richard & Lippman 1991);

architectures such as the MLP or the RBFN have been shown to be rich enough in structure to be able to approximate any (sufficiently smooth) function with arbitrary accuracy (Cybenko 1989; Park & Sandberg 1991).

It can be inferred from these facts that, given sufficient data, computational resources[1] and time,[2] it is possible, using a feedforward network, to estimate the Bayes-optimal classifier to any desired degree of accuracy, directly and with no prior assumptions on the probabilistic structure of the data (e.g. independence). This is an attractive scenario and has been extensively exploited, although in the absence of a concrete set of design and validation criteria the establishment of such systems relies heavily on trial and error and cross-validation. Indeed, it can be argued that the establishment of networks of the feedforward class is nothing other than non-linear regression, but, in the main, without the advantage of the extensive body of design, analysis and validation tools that have been developed within that branch of statistics, although this situation is changing (Bishop 1995; Ripley 1996). However, contrasted with this must be the fact that the feedforward paradigm is intuitively appealing, straightforward to implement and has been taken up by a much wider community than has ever adopted non-linear statistics.

The inherent adaptability of feedforward neural networks may make it easier to tune in to local conditions but would still require significant intervention and additional effort in data capture, retraining and revalidation. Indeed, the process of establishing such a system is precisely the same as that of establishing any other statistical classifier.

Feedforward networks are static devices in operation, and fail to cope with the stability-plasticity dilemma other than by suppressing learning after an acceptable performance is attained. The system is then put into operation. Implicit in this is the assumption that a trained network both represents the problem adequately at the time of development and continues to do so into the future, or in remote locations. Should learning remain continuously active in feedforward networks, new data will be learned indiscriminately,[3] with the attendant risk of serious performance degradation (Sharkey & Sharkey 1995).

Adaptive resonance theory

An entirely different approach, utilizing a network comprising both feedforward and feedback components has been taken by Carpenter and Grossberg and colleagues (Carpenter & Grossberg 1987a,b, 1988, 1990; Carpenter et al. 1991a), which overcomes the stability-plasticity dilemma. This has resulted in the ART family of architectures, which seek to model biological and psychological properties of the brain, rather than being derived from a data-processing perspective. In their earliest manifestations these were unsupervised systems that autonomously learned to recognize categories of their own devising.

A schematic of a single ART module is shown in Figure 9.1. Here the intention is simply to describe the ART architectures in an informal way; the references

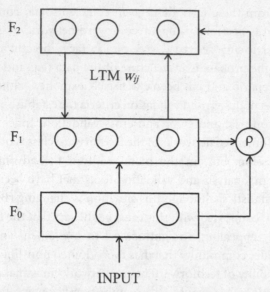

F_2

LTM w_{ij}

F_1

ρ

F_0

INPUT

Figure 9.1.   A single ART module comprising three layers, F_0, F_1 and F_2. F_1 and F_2 are fully interconnected in both directions via weighted links (w_{ij}) which form the long-term memory (LTM). ρ is the vigilance parameter that governs the coarseness of categorization. F_0 buffers the input patterns so that they remain present during processing.

(Carpenter & Grossberg 1987a,b, 1988, 1990; Carpenter et al. 1991a) provide complete details. ART modules use feedback to compare the existing state of knowledge or long-term memory (LTM or weights) of the system with the current set of evidence and either (a) adjust the LTM that codes for a particular category, to account for the current situation if this is 'similar' enough to other patterns in that category, or (b) initiate a new category that codes for the unrecognized (current) pattern. Similarity is measured by comparing the stored representation of the class (prototype) with the current input pattern to ascertain how close they are, according to some measure of distance. This has a major advantage from a design viewpoint in that there is no off-line 'hand crafting' of network architecture to be done, i.e. one autonomous network can address any problem or, indeed, many problems simultaneously. Also, commonly occurring patterns have the effect of reinforcing their category's ability to recognize like examples, while categories representing spurious events are rarely, if ever, excited again and so do not corrupt previously learned information. Conversely, should a rare but valid event occur, it will reside in LTM until next recalled.

The ART architectures of interest here comprise two layers of nodes, fully interconnected in both directions, together with a layer that serves to distribute the input signal to the active components. These are the input/comparison field (F_1) and the output/recognition field (F_2), the latter implementing a 'winner-take-all' competition. F_0 acts merely as a buffer to register the current input during processing and comparison. Together F_1 and F_2 form an *attentional* subsystem, which is complemented by an *orienting* subsystem, which initiates search. ART takes its name from the interplay between learning and recall whereby signals reverberate between the two layers. When an input pattern is recognized, a stable oscillation (resonance) ensues and learning (adaptation) takes place. Categories are coded by the formation of templates in the competitive (F_2) layer (represented by the weight vector for a particular node) and these are refined as new information becomes available. During recall, when a given node is excited, a template is fed back to the F_1 layer for comparison with the current input. The degree of match is assessed against the vigilance parameter (ρ), which is used to control the coarseness of categorization. If the degree of match is not sufficiently good, parallel search is initiated until either an acceptable match is found (resonance) or the pattern is assigned to a new category (F_2) node.

ARTMAP

Single ART modules are restricted to unsupervised learning. This means that the autonomously selected categories are unlikely to correspond to meaningful categories in the problem domain. The so-called ARTMAP (Carpenter et al. 1991b, 1992) family of architectures resolves this problem by providing a *mapping* network capable of supervised learning whilst retaining the desirable properties of the earlier ART networks. These networks comprise two ART modules (ART_a and ART_b) coupled via a *map* field. Each ART module individually self-organizes into categories representing data (evidence) and supervisory signal (target or outcome) and the association between categories is formed by the map field. Figure 9.2 presents the general ARTMAP configuration.

In addition to the individual vigilance tests carried out for ART_a and ART_b, a further test is performed at the map field when both the ART modules are active (resonant). In this situation, a category prediction is sent from the winning node of the ART_a F_2 layer to the F_2 layer of ART_b and the so-called map field vigilance test is performed, which determines whether or not the predicted class is equal to the actual class. If so, learning is permitted throughout ARTMAP (i.e. at ART_a and ART_b, and in the map field). If not, an activity called *match tracking* will be triggered, which initiates a search cycle in ART_a. The baseline ART_a vigilance is raised by this process by just enough to ensure that the ART_a vigilance test fails and the currently active node is thus deselected. A new winning node is selected from ART_a and a fresh prediction is sent to the map field. Match tracking therefore provides a means of selecting a node that satisfies both the ART_a and map field vigilance tests. If no such node exists the input is ignored. Full details of the ARTMAP learning procedure are given in Carpenter et al. (1991b, 1992).

INPUT

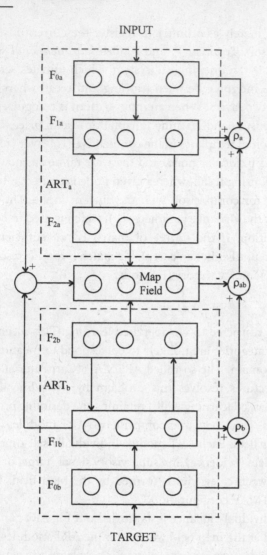

Figure 9.2.   General ARTMAP configuration. This comprises two ART modules, labelled a and b, which self-organize the input and target data streams, respectively. Categories formed for each of these are associated via the map field. Category size is determined for each module by its own vigilance parameter, and incorrect associations between ART_a and ART_b categories are handled via the match-tracking process, governed by the map field vigilance, ρ_{ab}.

The basic ART and ARTMAP algorithms accept only binary valued inputs. However, by replacing the operations of bivalent logic (AND, OR) that take place in these networks, with their counterparts from fuzzy logic, a generalization is obtained that accepts data on the interval zero to one. These networks are known as fuzzy ART and fuzzy ARTMAP (FAM), respectively (Carpenter et al. 1991c,

1992). Further developments that provide a Bayesian interpretation of ARTMAP operation in the sense that the outputs may be regarded as predictions of posterior or class conditional probabilities have recently been conducted (Lim & Harrison 1996b,c).

For computational efficiency, a simplified ARTMAP architecture results from noting that in one-from-many classification there is no need to self-organize the supervisory signal at ART_b because classes are predefined (Kasuba 1993).

/ ARTMAP networks are able to learn to improve their predictive performance on-line in non-stationary environments, using their entire memory capacities. Learning is driven by approximate (soft) match and takes place very rapidly, as does recall or recognition – the basic theory, as opposed to the computational models, allows for a full parallel implementation. Contrast this with the feedforward architectures. These learn offline and assume a stationary environment. Learning must be suppressed to overcome the stability-plasticity dilemma and: is very slow, driven by mismatch; is prone to spurious solutions; may scale poorly (e.g. exponentially) with problem size; often requires lengthy cycles of 'train and test' to arrive at a satisfactory solution. Recall, however, is very fast.

Two principal difficulties arise with the use of existing ART models: a local (as opposed to distributed) representation of information that arises through the adoption of a winner-take-all strategy in the competitive layer, and a sensitivity to the order in which stimulus data are encountered. The first is due to the assumptions made in deriving algorithms that are easily computed and owes nothing to the underlying theory. Indeed, a fully distributed ART model, dART, and its mapping equivalent has recently been proposed but its utility has yet to be evaluated (Carpenter 1996). The second is not, in fact, peculiar to ART but is rather a feature of all causal learning systems and is often present even in off-line training of feedforward networks, hence the need to 'shuffle' the order of data presentation.

ARTMAP presents the prospect of an autonomous system capable of learning stably to categorize data whilst protecting the user from spurious predictions. This means that the system can safely continue learning in situ, whilst providing useful support. Thus, in clinical diagnosis, evidence would be presented and should it excite a recognition category (from previous training) a prediction is returned. Update of LTM can then be initiated if and when diagnosis is confirmed. If the current pattern is not recognized the user is so informed. Again adjustment of LTM is initiated only upon confirmation of the diagnosis. Provided diagnosis remains unconfirmed, no LTM adjustment takes place. This is a crucial issue in the development of a portable decision aid, which should be able to adapt to local practice and to changing procedures, in much the same way as humans do.

Any decision-making or diagnostic procedure where evidence is to be associated either with an objective outcome or with expert (subjective) opinion, is a potential application area for this approach and, most importantly, it can put development (via, say, a fourth-generation language) of decision aids into the hands of the domain expert, rather than the computing expert. This capability can be seen as crucial in overcoming resistance to the use of computational decision aids – the domain expert assumes 'ownership'.

Practical strategies

Voting strategy

As stated above the formation of category clusters in ARTMAP is affected by the order of presentation of input data items (Carpenter et al. 1992). Thus the same data presented in a different order to different ARTMAP networks can lead to the formation of quite different clusters within the two networks. This subsequently leads to differing categorizations of novel data, and thus different performance scores. The effect is particularly marked with small training sets and/or high-dimensional input vectors.

A voting strategy can be used to compensate for the ordering problem (see Carpenter et al. 1992). A number of ARTMAP networks are trained on different orderings of the training data. During testing, each individual network makes its prediction for a test item in the normal way. The number of predictions made for each category is then totalled and the one with the highest score (majority votes) is the final predicted category outcome. The voting strategy can provide improved performance in comparison with that of the individual networks. In addition it also provides an indication of the confidence of a particular prediction, since the larger the voting majority, the more certain is the prediction. Clearly, strategies other than a simple majority can be used depending on the desired effect. Furthermore, recent work has indicated the effectiveness of other ways of combining outputs from multiple classifiers (Lim & Harrison 1997a,c; Lim et al. 1997) such as via the Bayesian formalism (Xu et al. 1992) or the so-called behaviour–knowledge space approach (Huang & Suen 1995).

Symbolic rule extraction

Most neural networks suffer from the opaqueness of their learned associations (Towell & Shavlik 1993). In medical domains, this 'black-box' nature may make clinicians reluctant to use an artificial neural network-based application, no matter how well it performs in a statistical sense. Thus there is a need to supplement artificial neural networks with symbolic rule extraction capabilities in order to provide explanatory facilities for the network's reasoning. ARTMAP provides such a capability (Carpenter & Tan 1993) as a result of its localized knowledge representation. Thus what is seen as a shortcoming from one angle becomes an advantage from another.

Rule extraction from feedforward networks has proved to be a difficult problem and, although some progress has been made (Towell & Shavlik 1993; Andrews & Geva 1995; Ma & Harrison 1995; Ma et al. 1995; Setiono 1996), it seems that the feedforward paradigm is not a natural one for semantic interpretation. The act of rule extraction is a straightforward procedure in ARTMAP, compared with that required for feedforward networks, since there are no hidden units with implicit meaning. In essence, each category cluster in ART_a represents a symbolic rule whose antecedents are the category prototype weights, and whose consequent is the associated ART_b category (indicated by the map field).

ARTMAP's symbolic rules also differ from those of conventional expert systems as regards the way they are matched to input features. Expert system rules are 'hard' – an input must match to each and every feature in a rule's antecedent before the consequent will be asserted. In ARTMAP the rules are 'soft'. Recall that they are derived from prototypical category clusters that are in competition with each other to match to the input data. Exact matching between inputs and categories is not necessary, merely a reasonably close fit suffices. (The degree of inexactness that is tolerated being determined by the value of the ART_a vigilance parameter.) This provides greater coverage of the state space for the domain using fewer rules.

A drawback of the approach is that the rules are 'correlational' rather than causal, since ARTMAP possesses no underlying theory of the domain but simply associates conjunctions of input features with category classes. Of course, this problem is not specific to ARTMAP but occurs with artificial neural networks generally, being based upon an inductive rather than a deductive mechanism. Nonetheless, useful diagnostic performance can often be achieved from correlational features without recourse to any 'deep' knowledge of the domain.

Category pruning

An ARTMAP network often becomes overspecified to the training set, generating many low-utility ART_a category clusters that represent rare but unimportant cases, and subsequently provide poor-quality rules. The problem is particularly acute when a high ART_a baseline vigilance level is used during training. To overcome this difficulty, rule extraction involves a preprocessing stage known as category pruning (Carpenter & Tan 1993). This involves the deletion of these low utility nodes. Pruning is guided by the calculation of a confidence factor (CF) between 0 and 1 for each category cluster, based equally upon a node's usage (proportion of training set exemplars it encodes) and accuracy (proportion of correct predictions it makes on a separate data sample known as the prediction set). All nodes with a confidence factor below a user-set threshold are then excised.

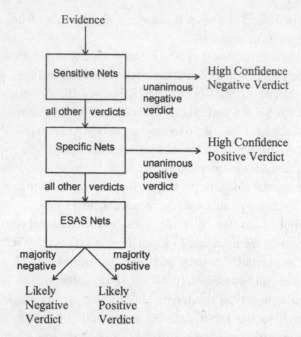

Evidence

Sensitive Nets → High Confidence Negative Verdict

unanimous negative verdict

all other | verdicts

Specific Nets → High Confidence Positive Verdict

unanimous positive verdict

all other | verdicts

ESAS Nets

majority negative   majority positive

Likely Negative Verdict   Likely Positive Verdict

Figure 9.3.   Cascaded ARTMAP voting strategy showing how high confidence decisions can be made by allowing cases to percolate through a pair of stringent voting systems tuned for high sensitivity and specificity, respectively. Those cases for which a unanimous decision cannot be made are treated by a majority voting system whose degree of confidence can be estimated from the relative numbers of votes for each diagnosis. (Adapted from Downs et al. 1995b.)

The pruning process can provide significant reductions in the size of a network. In addition, it also has the very useful side-effect that a pruned network's performance is usually superior to the original, unpruned net on both the prediction set and on entirely novel test data.

In the original formulation of the pruning process, a uniform CF threshold is used to select nodes for deletion, irrespective of their category class (Carpenter & Tan 1993). We have since generalized the pruning process to allow separate CF thresholds for nodes belonging to different category classes (Downs et al. 1995b, 1996). This allows us to vary the proportion of the state-space covered by different categories and is useful for medical domains, since it allows an ARTMAP network to be pruned so as to trade sensitivity for specificity and vice versa.

Generalization of the category pruning process enabled us to devise a novel 'cascaded' variant of the voting strategy to be employed, as shown in Figure 9.3 (Downs et al. 1995b, 1996). This comprises three layers, a set of voting networks pruned so as to maximize sensitivity, another set pruned so as to maximize specificity, and a third set of voters pruned so as to have approximately equal sensitivity and specificity (ESAS). The first two layers are intended to identify those cases that have a very high certainty of being classified correctly, with the sensitive networks being used to 'trap' the negative cases and the specific networks capturing the positive cases. The intuition behind this is that a set of networks displaying very high sensitivity will rarely make false negative predictions and so any negative predictions made by the networks are very likely to be correct. Conversely, highly specific networks will make very few false positive predictions, and so their positive predictions have a high certainty of being correct.

The cascaded voting strategy therefore operates as follows. An input data vector is first presented to the sensitive voting networks. If these yield a unanimous negative verdict, this is taken as the final category prediction. If not, the data item is next presented to the specific voting nets. If these yield a unanimous positive verdict, this is taken as the ultimate category prediction. Otherwise the final prediction of the category class of the input is obtained by majority verdict from the ESAS nets, with a lower certainty of the prediction being correct than with the previous two layers.

Case studies in clinical decision support

Early diagnosis of myocardial infarction

The early identification of patients with acute ischaemic heart disease remains one of the great challenges of emergency medicine. The electrocardiograph (ECG) only shows diagnostic changes in about one-half of acute myocardial infarction (AMI) patients at presentation (Stark & Vacek 1987; Adams et al. 1993b). None of the available biochemical tests becomes positive until at least 3 hours after symptoms begin, making such measurements of limited use for the early triage of patients with suspected AMI (Adams et al. 1993a). The early diagnosis of AMI, therefore, relies on an analysis of clinical features along with ECG data. A variety of statistical and computer-based algorithms has been developed to assist with the analysis of these factors (for a review, see Kennedy et al. 1993), including the use of feedforward neural networks (Baxt 1990; Hart & Wyatt 1990; Harrison et al. 1991). Although none of these has yet found widespread usage in clinical practice, this remains an important area of research, not only owing to its clear potential to improve triage practices for the commonest of all medical problems but also because of the light it may shed on techniques for the development of decision aids for use in other areas of medicine.

Patients and clinical data

The data used in this study were derived from consecutive patients attending the Accident and Emergency Department of the Royal Infirmary, Edinburgh,

Scotland, with non-traumatic chest pain as the major symptom. The relevant clinical and ECG data (see below) were entered onto a purpose-designed proforma at, or soon after, the patient's presentation. The study included patients who were admitted and those who were discharged. Nine hundred and seventy patients were recruited during the study period (September to December 1993). The final diagnosis for these patients was assigned independently by a Consultant Physician, a Research Nurse and a Cardiology Registrar. This diagnosis made use of follow-up ECGs, cardiac enzyme studies and other investigations, as well as clinical history obtained from review of the patient's notes. Patients discharged from Accident and Emergency were contacted directly regarding further symptoms and, where necessary, their General Practitioners were also contacted and the notes of any further hospital follow-up reviewed. The final diagnosis in the 970 patients was Q-wave AMI in 146 cases, non-Q-wave AMI in 45, unstable angina in 69, stable angina in 271 and other diagnoses in 439 cases. The patients were 583 men and 387 women, with a mean age of 58.2 years (range 14–92). Unstable angina was defined as either more than two episodes of pain lasting more than 10 minutes in a 24-hour period or more than three episodes in a 48-hour period, or as angina associated with the development of new ECG changes of ischaemia (either at diagnosis or in the subsequent 3 days).

The input data items for the ARTMAP model were all derived from data available at the time of the patient's presentation. In all, 35 items were used, coded as 37 binary inputs. The full list of the inputs is given in Appendix 9.1, together with their feature names, used for symbolic rule extraction from the networks. For the purposes of this application, the final diagnoses were collapsed into two classes: 'AMI' (Q-wave AMI and non-Q-wave AMI) and 'not-AMI' (all other diagnoses). AMI cases were taken as positive, and not-AMI cases as negative, diagnoses. Informed consent was obtained from all patients participating in the study which was approved by the local Medical Ethics Committee.

Method

The 970 patient records were divided into three data sets: 150 randomly selected records formed the prediction set, a further 150 randomly chosen records formed the test set, and the remaining 670 comprised the training data. The prediction set consisted of 28 cases of AMI and 122 not-AMI; the test set of 30 AMI and 120 not-AMI.

The training data were randomly ordered in ten different ways, and each ordering applied to a different ARTMAP network using single-epoch training. The ART_a baseline vigilance was set to a medium level (0.6) for training, all other parameters were set to their standard values (Kasuba 1993). The performance of the 10 trained ARTMAP networks was then measured on both the prediction and test sets. During this testing phase the ART_a baseline vigilance was relaxed slightly (to 0.5) in order to ensure that all test items were matched to an existing category cluster (i.e. forced choice prediction).

The performance of the trained networks on the prediction set alone was then used to calculate accuracy scores for the category nodes in each network, as a prerequisite of the category pruning process.

The 'standard' form of category pruning (Carpenter & Tan 1993) was performed on the original networks, such that all nodes with a CF below 0.5 were deleted from the networks in order to improve predictive accuracy. Performance of the resultant pruned networks was then measured on the prediction and test sets. Vigilance was further relaxed to 0.4 for testing these (and all other) pruned networks, again to ensure forced choice prediction.

The original networks were then pruned using different CF thresholds for the AMI and not-AMI nodes in order to produce pruned networks that maximized sensitivity. CF thresholds of 0.2 for AMI nodes and 0.95 for not-AMI nodes were employed, the criterion for setting the CF thresholds being to produce a mean sensitivity greater than 95% on the prediction set for the 10 pruned networks. Performance of the resultant nets was recorded for both the prediction and test sets. A similar procedure was then conducted to produce 10 networks that maximized specificity. CF thresholds of 0.7 AMI and 0.5 not-AMI were sufficient to yield a mean specificity greater than 95% on the prediction set.

The final pruning procedure was to produce 10 networks with approximately equal sensitivity and specificity, the criterion for setting the CF thresholds being a performance on the prediction set where sensitivity and specificity were within 5% of each other. The performance of the pruned networks was again recorded on both the prediction and test sets.

Performance results using the voting strategy were then obtained for the unpruned networks and all classes of pruned network. Three voters were used with all network types, except the ESAS class, where five voters were used. Voters for the unpruned, uniformly pruned, and ESAS network classes were selected on the basis of the networks with the highest accuracy on the prediction set. Selection criteria for the set of sensitive networks was maximum specificity, while maintaining a minimum sensitivity of 95% on the prediction set. The converse criteria were used for the set of specific networks.

Last, the cascaded variant of the voting strategy was employed utilizing three sensitive nets, two specific nets and five ESAS nets (see Figure 9.3). The number of networks in each stage was chosen arbitrarily. The cascade operated as follows: data items were first applied to the sensitive voting nets. If these yielded a unanimous (3–0) verdict that the category prediction was not-AMI, this was taken as the final category prediction. If not, the input was presented to the specific

Table 9.1. Mean performance of 10 differently pruned networks

Pruning type	Prediction set (%)			Test set (%)		
	Acc	Sens	Spec	Acc	Sens	Spec
None	80.9	51.8	87.5	80.9	59.0	86.3
Uniform	88.2	60.7	94.5	83.6	52.0	91.5
Sensitivity	50.0	96.4	39.3	47.3	94.3	35.5
Specificity	86.9	41.8	97.2	84.7	39.7	96.0
ESAS	76.6	76.1	76.7	75.6	80.0	74.5

Adapted from Downs et al. 1995b.

Acc, accuracy; Sens, sensitivity; Spec, specificity; ESAS, equal sensitivity and specificity.

voting nets. If these yielded a unanimous (2–0) verdict of AMI, this was taken as the final prediction. Otherwise the final prediction of the category class of the test item was obtained by majority verdict from the ESAS nets.

Results

The mean performance on the prediction and test sets for all classes of ARTMAP networks is shown in Table 9.1. As a baseline for comparisons, the expert diagnoses showed an accuracy, sensitivity and specificity of 83.0%, 81.3% and 83.5%, respectively, over the entire data set.

Average accuracy for the unpruned networks can be seen to be only slightly below this baseline. However, this is largely an artefact of the unequal prior probabilities of the category distributions – specificity accounts for the majority of accuracy – and, although the networks' sensitivity is much poorer than that of the humans, this is compensated for by the superior specificity.

As expected, the uniformly pruned networks show an across-the-board increase in accuracy over the unpruned nets, with a 2.7% increase on the test set, and a 7.3% increase on the prediction set. (The greater increase in performance on the prediction set is explained by the fact that pruning utilized the accuracy scores for this data, and the networks are consequently optimized for this data.) However, the increase in accuracy arises largely from an overall improvement in specificity rather than sensitivity, which actually drops on the test set.

Figures for the sensitive nets show that almost all AMI cases can be diagnosed by the network, while approximately 36% of the not-AMI cases are detected. Conversely, with the sensitive nets, almost all not-AMI cases are trapped, while approximately 40% of the AMI cases are detected.

The performance of the ESAS class networks is most directly comparable with

Table 9.2. Voting strategy performance of differently pruned networks

Pruning type	Prediction set (%)			Test set (%)		
	Acc	Sens	Spec	Acc	Sens	Spec
None	86.0	64.3	91.0	83.3	56.7	90.0
Uniform	92.0	78.6	95.1	88.0	56.7	95.8
Sensitivity	55.3	96.4	45.9	51.3	96.7	40.0
Specificity	88.7	46.4	98.4	84.7	33.3	97.5
ESAS	82.0	82.1	82.0	81.3	83.3	80.8

Adapted from Downs et al. 1995b.

Acc, accuracy; Sens, sensitivity; Spec, specificity; ESAS, equal sensitivity and specificity.

that of the expert diagnoses, since they are not unduly biased towards specificity or sensitivity. It can be seen that the mean individual accuracy of such networks is approximately 7% worse than that of the human diagnoses.

When the voting strategy is employed the accuracy of all network types except the specific nets is improved, as shown in Table 9.2. Furthermore, unlike pruning, performance improvements owing to the voting strategy almost always result from increases in both sensitivity and specificity.

Accuracy for the ESAS nets is now much closer to that of the expert diagnoses and sensitivity is slightly better. Accuracy for the unpruned and uniformly pruned networks is now higher than that of the human diagnoses, particularly with the latter network class. However, this again results from the networks' very high specificity, while their sensitivity remains relatively poor.

Use of the voting strategy with the sensitive networks on the test set results in increased coverage of the not-AMI cases, while trapping more AMI cases than previously. However, the converse is not true for the specific nets, where a gain in not-AMI coverage is offset by poorer coverage of the AMI cases in comparison with the individual network means.

The best overall network performance was achieved by the cascaded voting strategy, shown in Table 9.3. The cascade's overall performance can be seen to be almost identical with that of the expert diagnoses. Moreover, the cascade provides a partitioning of input items into those with a higher and a lower certainty of a correct diagnosis. Unanimous not-AMI decisions by the highly specific networks (i.e. the first stage of the cascade) are almost certain to be correct, similarly unanimous AMI decisions by the highly sensitive networks (the second stage of the cascade) are also almost certain to be correct. The ESAS class voters then provide lower certainty predictions for the remaining data items at the bottom of

Table 9.3. Performance of the cascaded voting strategy

	Prediction set (%)			Test set (%)		
Pruning type	Acc	Sens	Spec	Acc	Sens	Spec
High-certainty voters	100.0	100.0	100.0	96.3	88.9	97.8
Lower-certainty voters	71.0	73.7	70.3	72.9	81.0	70.7
Overall	82.0	82.1	82.0	82.7	86.7	81.7

Adapted from Downs et al. 1995b.

Acc, accuracy; Sens, sensitivity; Spec, specificity.

the cascade. High-certainty predictions accounted for 38% of items in the prediction set and 36% of items in the test set.

Perfect performance by the high-certainty voters on the test set was prevented by the occurrence of one false positive case and one false negative case. The false positive case displays most of the 'barn-door' features of AMI, including ST-segment elevation, new pathological Q-waves and ST-segment or T-wave changes suggestive of ischaemia, while the false negative case displays almost no typical features (although the presence of old Q-waves should mean that a doctor would not entirely rule out AMI).

Symbolic rule extraction

The ability to extract symbolic rules from neural networks is an important enhancement to their use as decision-support tools in medical domains. Such symbolic rules provide two advantages that, taken collectively, should help to overcome reluctance to use an artificial neural network decision support tool.

Firstly, a domain expert can examine the complete rule set in order to validate that the network has acquired an appropriate mapping of input features to category classes. Secondly, the symbolic rules provide explanatory facilities for the network's predictions during online operation. In the case of ARTMAP this corresponds to displaying the equivalent rule for the ART_a cluster node that was activated to provide a category decision. (In the case of the voting strategy, a number of such rules, one per voting network, would be displayed.) The diagnosing doctors are then able to decide whether or not to concur with the network's prediction, based upon how valid they believe that rule to be.

In this domain, each network retained, on average, 49 cluster nodes after uniform CF pruning. Space limitations therefore preclude the display of a typical complete rule set here. Instead, we provide a list of all rules for diagnosing AMI from nodes with a CF greater than 0.8 from the 10 original networks. In order to

Table 9.4. Symbolic rules for AMI diagnosis extracted from ARTMAP networks

IF retro THEN ami	IF retro sweat sttwave THEN ami	IF age = 45–65 retro stelev THEN ami
IF age > 65 retro sweat THEN ami	IF smokes retro sttwave THEN ami	IF retro newq sttwave THEN ami
IF age > 65 retro sttwave THEN ami	IF age > 65 retro alltight sweat THEN ami	IF age > 65 retro larm sttwave THEN ami
IF retro larm sweat sttwave THEN ami	IF smokes retro alltight sttwave THEN ami	IF age = 45–65 retro newq sttwave THEN ami
IF age > 65 retro sweat likemi THEN ami	IF age = 45–65 smokes retro sttwave THEN ami	IF age = 45–65 smokes sweat nausea sttwave THEN ami
IF smokes retro larm nausea stelev THEN ami	IF age > 65 retro alltight sweat nausea sttwave THEN ami	IF smokes retro alltight sweat nausea sttwave THEN ami

Adapted from Downs et al. 1995b.

See Appendix 9.1 for definitions of terms: ami, acute myocardial infarction.

pass such a high threshold a node must encode a large proportion of the training exemplars and possess high predictive accuracy. Hence these nodes are best in the sense of being the most useful to their originating networks for the purpose of diagnosing AMI. In all, 18 such nodes occurred, their equivalent rules are shown in Table 9.4. See Appendix 9.1 for definitions of the terms in the rules.

Examination of the rules as a whole allows the following picture of a typical AMI case to be constructed. The patient is likely to be a smoker, aged over 45 (and most likely over 65), exhibiting central chest pain which possibly radiates to the left arm. The pain itself is likely to be described as 'tight' or 'heavy'. Other physical symptoms may include sweating and nausea. ECG readings are very likely to show ST-segment or T-wave changes suggestive of ischaemia, and perhaps also new ST-segment elevation and/or new pathological Q-waves.

This picture closely corresponds to a 'textbook' example of AMI, although it has been discovered by ARTMAP through self-organization of the input data without any prespecified knowledge of the domain. Thus the ARTMAP decision support tool encodes rules that provide valid classifications for the domain, while bypassing the difficult and time-consuming knowledge-acquisition process found with rule-based expert systems (Hayes-Roth et al. 1983).

Causal (online) learning

We now demonstrate the applicability of the ARTMAP variant, fuzzy ARTMAP (FAM) to the problem of the early diagnosis of AMI (Harrison et al. 1994). FAM achieves a synthesis of fuzzy logic and ART that enables it to learn and to recognize arbitrary sequences of analogue or binary input pairs, which may represent fuzzy or crisp sets of features. Here only 26 features were abstracted from each patient record and these were coded into a binary-valued vector excepting real-valued data such as age, duration of pain, etc., which was normalized in the range 0 to 1 (Lim 1993; Harrison et al. 1994). The need for FAM rather than its purely binary predecessor, ARTMAP, is evident, because interval data are now present and must be handled by the network.

In the assessment of online performance, a subset of 474 data was used both to train and to test the system; statistics being gathered prior to the verification of diagnosis at each stage. Thus the neural network starts out in a completely naive state. The statistics of interest here are again the accuracy, sensitivity and specificity of diagnosis.

It should be noted that, whereas it is usual to select optimal decision thresholds by analysis of the receiver operating characteristic (ROC) curve (Meistrell 1990), this technique is not appropriate here owing to the 'all-or-nothing' predictions made by FAM. It will be seen that this inability to select optimal thresholds, and hence counteract the effects of bias in the data, can result in an imbalance in the values of accuracy, sensitivity and specificity. Subsequent work has introduced a modification to FAM that has the capacity to achieve, online, very close to Bayes-optimal classification rates for strongly biased data, and to deliver accurate estimates of the Bayesian (posterior or class conditional) probabilities (Lim & Harrison 1997b,c).

Figure 9.4 indicates the online performance of FAM for two separate cases. The first uses the technique of 'sample replacement'. Here, samples are drawn at random and are returned after use. Thus any individual sample may be chosen repeatedly. The second case is analogous to in situ or real-time learning, when samples are taken in the order in which they occur and are not returned to the pool. Average values over 10 runs are plotted with an indication of their standard deviations. There are three important points to note pertaining to online processing.

1. Sometimes FAM fails to make a prediction (recognize a pattern). This is especially true in the early stages of learning when insufficient prototypes have been created. We have chosen to count such non-predictions as errors so that the performance indicators are biased downwards slightly.
2. Because statistics are gathered sequentially for each run, frequent poor (or non-) predictions in the early stages are included in the long-run results. Again this has the effect of biasing the results downwards.
3. Although any given problem may itself be stationary, the learning procedure is inherently non-stationary, owing to the build-up of knowledge. Thus, to obtain

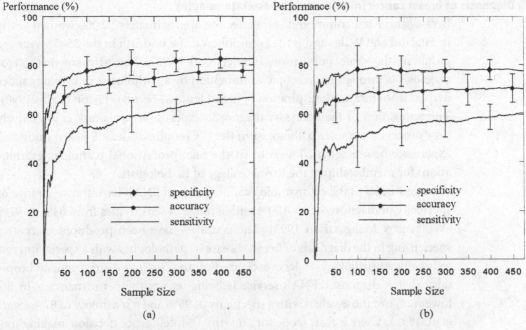

Figure 9.4.   Online fuzzy ARTMAP performance. (Adapted from Harrison et al. 1994.)

truly statistically valid results, averages should be taken over the ensemble of all possible realizations. For real problems this is often not feasible, as is the case here. To overcome this we have artificially created a small ensemble (of 10) by training 10 networks using different orderings of the data and averaging both across those, and also with time (see (2) above).

In both cases the qualitative behaviour of FAM is as expected: broadly speaking, a monotone improvement in performance as the number of samples increases. Peaks and troughs in the early stages result from initial formation of poor templates and more frequent non-predictions. Sample replacement yields a better result owing to the relatively small sample size (relatively large probability of repetition).

This set of data comprises approximately equal proportions of infarction, angina and non-ischaemic heart disease sufferers and has a bias towards excluding a diagnosis of myocardial infarction of 2.2 : 1. This bias manifests itself as favouring specificity over sensitivity. Clearly, the ability to predict a probability of class membership (as presented by Lim & Harrison (1997b)) rather than the simpler binary decision would enable a user to control the types of misclassification to suit the domain, for example high sensitivity for initial screening, high specificity when deciding whether or not to thrombolyse.

Diagnosis of breast cancer from fine needle aspirate samples

Breast cancer is a common disease affecting approximately 22 000 women yearly in England and Wales and is the commonest cause of death in the 35–55-year age group of the same population (Underwood 1992). The primary method of diagnosis is through microscopic examination by a pathologist of cytology slides derived from fine needle aspiration of breast lesions (FNAB) (Elston & Ellis 1990). The acquisition of the necessary diagnostic expertise for this task is a relatively slow process. (A trainee pathologist in the UK requires at least 5 years' study and experience before being allowed to sit the final professional pathology examinations for membership of the Royal College of Pathologists.)

Large studies of the cytopathological diagnosis of FNAB have shown a range of specificity of diagnosis of 90–100% with a range of sensitivities from 84% to 97% (Wolberg & Mangasarian 1993). These studies have been produced in centres specializing in the diagnosis of breast disease by pathologists with a special interest in breast cytopathology. In less specialized centres, such as district general hospitals, when a diagnostic FNAB service is being set up, the performance is in the lower range of those values with a specificity of 95% and a sensitivity of 87% (Start et al. 1992). There is thus scope for an artificial intelligence decision-making tool for this domain to assist in training junior pathologists and to improve the performance of experienced pathologists.

Data and method

The data set consisted of 413 patient records, each comprising 10 binary-valued features recorded from human observation of breast tissue samples, together with the actual outcome for each case (i.e. whether a lesion proved to be malignant or benign) (Downs et al. 1995a). The distribution of categories within the data was fairly even – 53% of cases were malignant, 47% benign. The features themselves are all claimed to have predictive value for the diagnosis task (Trott 1991; Koss 1992). The following abbreviations: DYS, ICL, 3D, NAKED, FOAMY, NUCLEOLI, PLEOMORPH, SIZE, NECROTIC and APOCRINE are used here: full definitions of the features are provided in Appendix 9.2.

As with almost all information gathered from a medical domain, the data set possesses a degree of 'noise'. Specifically, some feature-states do not always have the same outcome in every case. Analysis of the data set revealed the existence of 12 such states, which collectively account for 188 cases. Assuming that the most frequent outcome should always be chosen when an ambiguous feature-state occurs will result in 17 of these cases being misclassified. This represents approximately 4% of the data set, and thus optimal performance in the domain is a diagnostic accuracy of 96%.

On this particular data set, assigning malignant cases as 'positive' and benign

Table 9.5. Performance of 10 ARTMAP networks on a 100 item test set

No. ART nodes	No. false +ve DX	No. false −ve DX	Accuracy (%)	Sensitivity (%)	Specificity (%)
60	5	2	93	96.2	89.6
61	4	4	92	92.3	91.7
59	3	1	96	98.1	93.8
58	3	2	95	96.2	93.8
58	5	2	93	96.2	89.6
60	5	1	94	98.1	89.6
61	5	2	93	96.2	89.6
60	3	2	95	96.2	93.8
68	2	4	94	92.3	95.8
65	5	1	94	98.1	89.6

Adapted from Downs et al. 1995a.

+ve, positive; −ve, negative; DX, diagnosis.

cases as 'negative', an expert human pathologist (of consultant status with 10 years' experience in the field) performed with accuracy 91%, sensitivity 83%, and specificity 100%, while a Senior House-Officer with 18 months' experience achieved an accuracy of 71%, a sensitivity of 57% and a specificity of 98%.

Notice that these figures are biased towards specificity. The pathologist's prime concern is to avoid false positive predictions (i.e. diagnosing benign tumours as malignant), since these may result in unnecessary mastectomies. The resultant increase in false negatives (diagnosing malignant tumours as benign) is tolerated because, if the clinical suspicion of malignancy remains, the surgeon will then take further samples to be sent to the pathologist for additional testing.

One hundred records were randomly selected from the data to serve as test items in the evaluation of ARTMAP for the task. The remaining 313 records served as the teaching data. Ten ARTMAP networks were trained, each on a different random ordering of the teaching data. During training, the ART_a baseline vigilance parameter was set to 0.9 to ensure narrow category clustering; during testing this was relaxed to 0.6 to ensure that a category prediction (diagnosis) was made for all data items. (High vigilance during testing can lead to items failing to match sufficiently to any existing category clusters.)

Results

The subsequent performance of the 10 networks on the test set is shown in Table 9.5. The mean performance of the 10 networks gives an accuracy of 94%, a sensitivity of 96% and a specificity of 92%. The five most accurate individual networks were then tested collectively, using the voting strategy described above (Carpenter et al. 1992).

In this particular domain the voting strategy yields performance figures of accuracy 95%, sensitivity 96% and specificity 94%. Although this may seem to be only a slight improvement on the individual ARTMAP results, it should be noted that diagnostic accuracy with the voting strategy is almost at the maximum possible for the domain.

Furthermore, when unanimous voting decisions only were considered, performance becomes near-perfect on a large subset of the test cases. Five-nil category decisions accounted for 91% of the test set and showed an accuracy of 99%, a sensitivity of 100% and a specificity of 98% on this subset of the data. Thus the voting strategy can provide a useful partitioning between data items with high and low certainty of outcome.

Symbolic rule extraction

Symbolic rule extraction (Carpenter & Tan 1993) was then performed upon all 10 of the previously trained ARTMAP networks.

Severe pruning was performed upon the 10 trained ARTMAP networks, using a threshold confidence level of 0.7. The number of category cluster nodes remaining for each individual network after pruning ranged from three to nine. Thus the networks were reduced to a small number of ART_a category nodes of strong predictive power from which rules could be extracted. Before doing so, however, the test data were reapplied to each of the pruned networks to check that pruning had not adversely affected performance. Since pruning necessarily reduces ARTMAP's coverage of the feature-space, the baseline ART_a vigilance was this time relaxed further to 0.5. Despite this, some pruned networks were still unable to generate category predictions for all test set items. The mean performance of the 10 networks after pruning gave an accuracy of 94%, a sensitivity of 90% and a specificity of 99%.

It can be seen that pruning has virtually no effect upon overall diagnostic accuracy but has led to increased specificity and reduced sensitivity. The five most accurate pruned networks (excluding those which did not generate predictions on all test set items) were then tested using the voting strategy. This resulted in an accuracy of 95%, a sensitivity of 92% and a specificity of 98%, again confirming that the voting strategy allows the optimum accuracy for the domain to be closely approached.

Rule extraction from the 10 pruned nets yielded 14 distinct rules, 12 for malignant outcomes and 2 for benign. The full list of rules is shown in Table 9.6, ranked by how many of the 10 pruned networks a rule occurred in.

Table 9.6. Symbolic rules for FNAB diagnosis

Rule 1 (*10 occurrences*)	Rule 2 (*8 occurrences*)	Rule 3 (*8 occurrences*)
if no symptoms *then* benign	*if* 3D NUCLEOLI PLEOMORPH SIZE *then* malignant	*if* 3D FOAMY NUCLEOLI PLEOMORPH SIZE *then* malignant
Rule 4 (*7 occurrences*)	Rule 5 (*4 occurrences*)	Rule 6 (*4 occurrences*)
if FOAMY *then* benign	*if* ICL 3D NUCLEOLI PLEOMORPH SIZE *then* malignant	*if* DYS NUCLEOLI PLEOMORPH SIZE *then* malignant
Rule 7 (*3 occurrences*)	Rule 8 (*3 occurrences*)	Rule 9 (*2 occurrences*)
if FOAMY NUCLEOLI PLEOMORPH size *then* malignant	*if* NUCLEOLI PLEOMORPH SIZE *then* malignant	*if* 3D FOAMY NUCLEOLI PLEOMORPH SIZE NECROTIC *then* malignant
Rule 10 (*2 occurrences*)	Rule 11 (*2 occurrences*)	Rule 12 (*1 occurrence*)
if 3D FOAMY PLEOMORPH SIZE NECROTIC *then* malignant	*if* DYS ICL NUCLEOLI PLEOMORPH SIZE *then* malignant	*if* ICL NUCLEOLI PLEOMORPH SIZE *then* malignant
Rule 13 (*1 occurrence*)	Rule 14 (*1 occurrence*)	
if FOAMY NUCLEOLI PLEOMORPH SIZE NECROTIC *then* malignant	*if* ICL 3D PLEOMORPH SIZE *then* malignant	

Adapted from Downs et al. 1995a.

For definitions of terms, see Appendix 9.2.

It can be seen that an absence of features, or the FOAMY feature present in isolation, leads to a benign diagnosis. PLEOMORPH and SIZE are found in all rules for malignant diagnoses, and NUCLEOLI is additionally present in all but two of these same rules (both of which have low frequency of occurrence). Thus these three features in combination seem to be the strongest indicators of malignancy. Other features are weaker indicators of malignancy, and indeed two input features, NAKED and APOCRINE, are conspicuous by their absence from any of the rules. We would conclude therefore that these two features are the least useful in forming a diagnosis, at least for this particular data set.

An expert human pathologist confirmed the relative importance of the features listed above in making his own diagnoses, with the exception that he places no value on the presence or absence of the FOAMY feature. It should be noted that this feature has a somewhat ambiguous status within the ARTMAP rules. In isolation, it is indicative of a benign diagnosis. However, when it occurs in combination with other features, a malignant diagnosis results.

There is some disagreement between different domain experts as to the relative

Table 9.7. Relative performance of human pathologists and ARTMAP

	Accuracy (%)	Sensitivity (%)	Specificity (%)
Human expert	91	83	100
Human novice	71	57	98
Unpruned ARTMAP (mean)	94	96	92
Unpruned ARTMAP (voting)	95	96	94
Pruned ARTMAP (mean)	94	90	99
Pruned ARTMAP (voting)	95	92	98

Adapted from Downs et al. 1995a.

importance of the features in making diagnoses. Thus another pathologist states 'I think the presence of bipolar naked nuclei and foamy macrophages can be taken as indicative of benignancy. This is not to say, however, that when these features are combined with cells showing obvious features of malignancy, malignancy should not be diagnosed'. This accords with the self-discovered ARTMAP rules for the FOAMY feature.

Table 9.7 summarizes the performance figures for ARTMAP in comparison with human pathologists in this domain. It can be seen that in terms of diagnostic accuracy ARTMAP always performs at least as well as the human expert and much better than the novice. However, the weak spot in the unpruned ARTMAP networks' performance is the lower specificity in comparison with the human pathologists. As pointed out earlier, it is vital that false positive cases (which reduce specificity) are avoided in this domain.

The pruning procedure achieves this goal, by increasing specificity at the expense of sensitivity without changing overall diagnostic accuracy. The reason for this is that the category clusters formed at ART_a predominantly indicate positive (malignant) cases. (On average, 70% of ART_a category nodes in the unpruned networks denote malignant outcomes.) Pruning therefore mostly deletes nodes with malignant outcomes, and so coverage of these cases in the state space is reduced disproportionately more than for benign cases. This effect of biasing the trade-off between sensitivity and specificity was achieved naturally in this domain as a side-effect of the rule extraction process, although such an effect can be achieved purposely in other domains by use of the generalized pruning procedure discussed earlier.

Conclusions

ART-based systems are clearly one candidate for providing the knowledge acquisition and inference engine in apprentice systems. Our studies have shown that in two different medical problem domains the ARTMAP neural network architecture provides solutions with performance that at least equals that of human experts and provides explicit rules agreeing with those given by human experts. Continued online learning is possible and the networks can be implemented to run on standard personal computers. All these factors provide a suitable environment for the development of apprentice systems that can be used for clinical decision support. The use of such technology is in its very early stages and much research and development is needed to establish a truly autonomously learning decision aid that can operate safely in a medical environment.

NOTES

1. The MLP, in particular, does not scale well with problem size.
2. Non-linear optimization which is non-linear in the parameters may be time consuming to perform numerically, and much trial and error may be required in deriving an adequate network architecture.
3. More recent developments that enable feedforward networks to 'grow' their own architectures and to learn causally are emerging although these do not in general overcome the problem of catastrophic forgetting and thus are not well suited to pattern recognition.

Appendix 9.1. Coding for AMI data

Input Code	Meaning	Input Code	Meaning
age < 45	Age less than 45 years	alltight	Pain described as 'tight'
age = 45–65	Age 45–65 years	allsharp	Pain described as 'sharp'
age > 65	Age greater than 65 years	sweat	Sweating
smokes	Smokes	s_o_breath	Short of breath
ex_smoker	Ex-smoker	nausea	Nausea
fam_ihd	Family history of IHD	vomit	Vomiting
diabetes	Diabetes mellitus	syncope	Syncope
hypertense	Hypertension	epis	Episodic pain
hyperlipid	Hyperlipidaemia	likemi	Worse than usual angina/similar to previous AMI
retro	Central chest pain	lvf	Fine crackles suggestive of pulmonary oedema
lchest	Pain in left side of chest	added_hs	Added heart sounds
rchest	Pain in right side of chest	hypoperf	Signs of hypoperfusion
back	Pain radiates to back	stelev	New ST-segment elevation
larm	Pain radiates to left arm	newq	New pathological Q-waves
jaw	Pain radiates to neck or jaw	sttwave	ST-segment or T-wave changes suggestive of ischaemia
rarm	Pain radiates to right arm	bbb	Bundle branch block
breathing	Pain is worse on inspiration	old_q	Old ECG features of myocardial infarction
posture	Pain related to posture	old_st	ECG signs of ischaemia known to be old
tender_cw	Chest wall tenderness		

IHD, ischaemic heart disease; AMI, acute myocardial infarction; ECG, electrocardiograph.

Appendix 9.2. FNAB feature definitions

DYS: True if majority of epithelial cells are dyhesive; false if majority of epithelial cells are in cohesive groups.

ICL: True if intracytoplasmic lumina are present; false if absent.

3D: True if some clusters of epithelial cells are not flat (more than two nuclei thick) and this is not due to artefactual folding; false if all clusters of epithelial cells are flat.

NAKED: True if bipolar 'naked' nuclei in background; false if absent.

FOAMY: True if 'foamy' macrophages present in background; false if absent.

NUCLEOLI: True if more than three easily visible nucleoli in some epithelial cells; false if three or fewer easily visible nucleoli in epithelial cells.

PLEOMORPH: True if some epithelial cell nuclei with diameters twice that of other epithelial cell nuclei; false if no epithelial cell nuclei twice the diameter of other epithelial cell nuclei.

SIZE: True if some epithelial cells with nuclear diameters at least twice that of lymphocyte nuclei; false if all epithelial cell nuclei with nuclear diameters less than twice that of lymphocyte nuclei.

NECROTIC: True if necrotic epithelial cells present; false if absent.

APOCRINE: True if apocrine change present in all epithelial cells; false if not present in all epithelial cells.

REFERENCES

Adams, J. E., Abendschein, D. R. & Jaffe, A. S. (1993a). Biochemical markers of myocardial injury. Is MB creatine kinase the choice for the 1990s? *Circulation* **88**, 750–763.

Adams, J. E., Trent, R. & Rawles, J. (1993b). Earliest electrocardiographic evidence of myocardial infarction: implications for thrombolytic treatment. *British Medical Journal* **307**, 409–413.

Andrews, R. & Geva, S. (1995). RULEX & CEBP networks as the basis for a rule refinement system. In J. Hallam, ed. *Hybrid Problems, Hybrid Solutions: 10th Biennial Conference on AI and Cognitive Science.* IOS Press, Amsterdam, pp. 1–12.

Baxt, W. G. (1990). Use of an artificial neural network for data analysis in clinical decision-making: the diagnosis of acute coronary occlusion. *Neural Computation* **2**, 480–489.

Bishop, C. M. (1995). *Neural Networks for Pattern Recognition.* Clarendon Press, Oxford.

Brahams, D. & Wyatt, J. (1989). Decision aids and the law. *Lancet* **2**, 632–634.

Carpenter, G. (1996). Distributed learning, recognition and prediction by ART and ARTMAP neural networks. Research Report CAS/CNS-96-004, Boston University, Boston, MA.

Carpenter, G. & Grossberg, S. (1987a). A massively parallel architecture for a self-organizing neural pattern recognition machine. *Computer Vision, Graphics and Image Processing* **37**, 54–115.

Carpenter, G. & Grossberg, S. (1987b). ART 2: self-organization of stable category recognition codes for analog input patterns. *Applied Optics* **26**, 4919–4930.

Carpenter, G. & Grossberg, S. (1988). The ART of adaptive pattern recognition by a self-organising neural network. *Computer* **21**, 77–88.

Carpenter, G. & Grossberg, S. (1990). ART3: hierarchical search using chemical transmission in self-organising pattern recognition architectures. *Neural Networks* **3**, 129–152.

Carpenter, G. & Tan, A. (1993). Rule extraction, fuzzy ARTMAP and medical databases. In *Proceedings of the World Congress on Neural Networks*, pp. 501–506.

Carpenter, G., Grossberg, S. & Reynolds, J. (1991a). ARTMAP: supervised real-time learning and classification of nonstationary data by a self-organizing neural network. *Neural Networks* **4**, 565–588.

Carpenter, G., Grossberg, S. & Rosen, D. (1991b). ART2-A: an adaptive resonance algorithm for rapid category learning and recognition. *Neural Networks* **4**, 493–504.

Carpenter, G., Grossberg, S. & Rosen, D. (1991c). Fuzzy ART: fast, stable learning and categorisation of analogue patterns by an adaptive resonance system. *Neural Networks* **4**, 759–771.

Carpenter, G., Grossberg, S., Markuzon, S., Reynolds, J. & Rosen, D. (1992). Fuzzy ARTMAP: a neural network architecture for incremental supervised learning of analog multi-dimensional maps. *IEEE Transactions on Artificial Neural Networks* **3**, 698–712.

Cybenko, G. (1989). Approximations by superpositions of a sigmoidal function. *Mathematics of Control, Signals and Systems* **2**, 303–314.

Downs, J., Harrison, R. F. & Cross, S. S. (1995a). A neural network decision support tool for the diagnosis of breast cancer. In J. Hallam, ed., *Hybrid Problems, Hybrid Solutions: 10th Biennial Conference on AI and Cognitive Science.* IOS Press, Amsterdam, pp. 51–60.

Downs, J., Harrison, R. F. & Kennedy, R. L. (1995b). A prototype neural network decision-support tool for the diagnosis of acute myocardial infarction. In P. Barahona, M. Stefanelli & J. Wyatt, eds., *Proceedings of the 5th European Conference on Artificial Intelligence in Medicine, AIME-95, Pavia, Italy.* Springer-Verlag, Berlin, pp. 355–366.

Downs, J., Harrison, R. F., Kennedy, R. L. & Cross, S. S. (1996). Application of the fuzzy ARTMAP neural network model to medical pattern classification tasks. *Artificial Intelligence in Medicine* **8**, 403–428.

Elston, C. W. & Ellis, I. O. (1990). Pathology and breast screening. *Histopathology* **16**, 109–118.

Harrison, R. F., Marshall, S. J. & Kennedy, R. L. (1991). A connectionist aid to the early diagnosis of myocardial infarction. In M. Stefanelli, A. Hasman, M. Fieschi & J. Talman, eds., *Proceedings of the 3rd European Conference on Artificial Intelligence in Medicine, Maastricht.* Springer-Verlag, Berlin, pp. 119–128.

Harrison, R. F., Lim, C. P. & Kennedy, R. L. (1994). Autonomously learning neural networks for clinical decision support. In E. C. Ifeachor & R. G. Rosen, eds., *Proceedings of the The International Conference on Neural Networks and Expert Systems in Medicine and Healthcare.* University of Plymouth, Plymouth, pp. 15–22.

Hart, A. & Wyatt, J. (1990). Evaluating black-boxes as medical decision aids: issues arising from a study of neural networks. *Medical Informatics* **15**, 229–236.

Hayes-Roth, F., Waterman, D. A. & Lenat, D.B. (1983). *Building Expert Systems.* Addison Wesley, London.

Huang, Y.S. & Suen, C.Y. (1995). A method of combining multiple experts for the recognition of unconstrained handwritten numerals. *IEEE Transactions on Pattern Analysis and Machine Intelligence* **17**, 90–94.

Kasuba, T. (1993). Simplified fuzzy ARTMAP. *AI Expert* **8**, 18–25.

Kennedy, R. L., Harrison, R. F. & Marshall, S. J. (1993). Do we need computer-based decision support for the diagnosis of acute chest pain? *Journal of the Royal Society of Medicine* **86**, 31–34.

Koss, L. G. (1992). *Diagnostic Cytology and its Histopathologic Basis.* Lippincott Williams & Wilkins, New York.

Lim, C. P. (1993). An autonomous-learning system. MSc dissertation, University of Sheffield.

Lim, C. P. & Harrison, R. F. (1997a). A multiple neural network architecture for sequential evidence aggregation and incomplete data classification. In *Proceedings of the World Multiconference on Systemics, Cybernetics and Informatics:* SCT '97/ISAS '97, Caracas, pp. 332–339.

Lim, C. P. & Harrison, R. F. (1997b). An incremental adaptive network for on-line, supervised learning and probability estimation. *Neural Networks* 10, 925–939.

Lim, C. P. & Harrison, R. F. (1997c). Modified fuzzy ARTMAP approaches Bayes optimal classification rates: an empirical demonstration. *Neural Networks* 10, 755–774.

Lim, C. P. & Harrison, R. F. (2000). ART-based autonomous learning systems. Part I: Architectures and algorithms. In K. K. Jain, B. Lazzerini & U. Halici, eds., *Innovations in ART Neural Networks.* Springer-Verlag, Berlin, pp. 133–166.

Lim, C. P., Harrison, R. F. & Kennedy, R. L. (1997). Application of autonomous neural network systems to medical pattern classification tasks. *Artificial Intelligence in Medicine* 11, 215–240.

Ma, Z. & Harrison, R. F. (1995). GR2: a hybrid knowledge-based system using general rules. In C. S. Mellish, ed., *Proceedings of the 14th International Joint Conference on Artificial Intelligence,* Montreal, Morgan Kaufmann, San Mateo, CA, pp. 488–493.

Ma, Z., Harrison, R. F. & Kennedy, R. L. (1995). A heuristic for general rule extraction from a multilayer Perceptron. In J. Hallam, ed., *Hybrid Problems, Hybrid Solutions. 10th Biennial Conference on AI and Cognitive Science.* IOS Press, Amsterdam, pp. 133–144.

Meistrell, M. L. (1990). Evaluation of neural network performance by receiver operating characteristic (ROC) analysis: examples from the biotechnology domain. *Computer Methods and Programs in Biomedicine* 32, 73–80.

Moody, J. & Darken, C. (1989). Fast learning in networks of locally-tuned processing units. *Neural Computation* 1, 281–294.

Park, J. & Sandberg, I. (1991). Universal approximation using radial basis function networks. *Neural Computation* 3, 246–257.

Quinlan, J.R. (1986). Induction of decision trees. *Machine Learning* 1, 81–106.

Quinlan, J. R. (1990). Decision trees and decision making. *IEEE Transactions on Systems, Man and Cybernetics* 20, 339–346.

Quinlan, J. R. (1993). *C4.5: Programs for Machine Learning.* Morgan Kauffman, San Mateo, CA.

Richard, M. & Lippman, R. (1991). Neural network classifiers estimate Bayesian a posteriori probabilities. *Neural Computation* 3, 461–483.

Ripley, B.D. (1996). *Pattern Recognition and Neural Networks.* Cambridge University Press, Cambridge.

Rumelhart, D., Hinton, G. & Williams, R. (1986). Learning representations by back-propagating errors. *Nature* 323, 533–536.

Saito, K. & Nakano, R. (1990). Rule extraction from facts and neural networks. In N. Thellier, ed., *Proceedings of the International Neural Network Conference.* Kluwer, Dordrecht, pp. 379–382.

Setiono, R. (1996). Extracting rules from pruned neural networks for breast cancer diagnosis. *Artificial Intelligence in Medicine* 8, 37–51.

Sharkey, N. E. & Sharkey, A. J. C. (1995). An analysis of catastrophic interference. *Connection Science* 7, 301–329.

Shavlik, J. W., Mooney, R. J. & Towell, G.G. (1991). Symbolic and neural learning algorithms: an experimental comparison. *Machine Learning* 6, 111–143.

Stark, M. E. & Vacek, J. L. (1987). The initial electrocardiogram during admission for myocardial infarction. *Archives of Internal Medicine* 147, 843–847.

Start, R. D., Silcocks, P. B., Cross, S. S. & Smith, J. H. F. (1992). Problems with audit of a new fine-needle aspiration service in a district general hospital. *Journal of Pathology* 167, 141A (Abstract).

Towell, G. G. & Shavlik, J. W. (1993). Extracting refined rules from knowledge-based neural networks. *Machine Learning* 13, 71–101.

Trott, P. A. (1991). Aspiration cytodiagnosis of the breast. *Diagnostic Oncology* 1, 79–87.

Underwood, J. C. E. (1992). Tumours: benign and malignant. In J. C. E. Underwood, ed., *General and Systematic Pathology*. Churchill Livingstone, Edinburgh, pp. 223–246.

Wan, E. A. (1990). Neural network classification: a Bayesian interpretation. *IEEE Transactions on Neural Networks* 1, 303–305.

Wolberg, W. H. & Mangasarian, O. L. (1993). Computer-designed expert systems for breast cytology diagnosis. *Analytical and Quantitative Cytology and Histology* 15, 67–74.

Xu, L., Krzyzac, A. & Suen, C. Y. (1992). Methods of combining multiple classifiers and their applications to handwriting recognition. *IEEE Transactions on Systems, Man and Cybernetics* 22, 418–435.

10

Evolving artificial neural networks

V. William Porto and David B. Fogel

Introduction

Artificial neural networks (or simply *neural networks*) are computer algorithms loosely based on modelling the neuronal structure of natural organisms. They are stimulus–response transfer functions that accept some input and yield some output, and are typically used to learn an input–output mapping over a set of examples. For example, the input can be radiographic features from mammograms, with the output being a decision concerning the likelihood of malignancy.

Neural networks are parallel processing structures consisting of non-linear processing elements interconnected by fixed or variable weights. They are quite versatile, for they can be constructed to generate arbitrarily complex decision regions for stimulus–response pairs. That is, in general, if given sufficient complexity, there exists a neural network that will map every input pattern to its appropriate output pattern, so long as the input–output mapping is not one-to-many (i.e. the same input having varying output). Neural networks are therefore well suited for use as detectors and classifiers. The classic pattern recognition algorithms require assumptions concerning the underlying statistics of the environment. Neural networks, in contrast, are non-parametric and can effectively address a broader class of problems (Lippmann 1987).

Multilayer perceptrons, also sometimes described as *feedforward networks*, are probably the most common architecture used in supervised learning applications (where exemplar patterns are available for training). Each computational node sums N weighted inputs, subtracts a threshold value and passes the result through a logistic (e.g. sigmoid) function. Single-layer perceptrons form decision regions separated by a hyperplane. If the input from the given different data classes are linearly separable, a hyperplane can be positioned between the classes by adjusting the weights and bias terms. If the inputs are not linearly separable, containing overlapping distributions, a least mean square (LMS) solution is typically generated to minimize the mean squared error between the calculated output of the network and the actual desired output. While perceptrons can generate hyperplane boundaries, perceptrons with a hidden layer of processing nodes have been proved to be capable of approximating any measurable function (Hornik et al. 1989), indicating their broad utility for addressing general pattern recognition problems.

Another versatile neural network architecture is the *radial basis function network*. Rather than partitioning the available data using hyperplanes, the radial basis function network clusters available data, often with the use of approximate Gaussian density functions. The network comprises an input layer of nodes corresponding to the input feature dimension, a single hidden layer of nodes with computational properties described as Gaussian density functions, and output nodes that perform linear combinations on the hidden nodes. Each connection between an input node and hidden node carries two variable parameters corresponding to a mean and standard deviation. Poggio & Girosi (1990) proved that linear combinations of these near-Gaussian density functions can be constructed to approximate any measurable function. Therefore, like the multilayer perceptron, radial basis functions are universal function approximators.

Given a network architecture (i.e. type of network, the number of nodes in each layer, the connections between the nodes, and so forth), and a training set of input patterns, the collection of variable weights determines the output of the network to each presented pattern. The error between the actual output of the network and the desired target output defines a response surface over an n-dimensional hyperspace, where there are n parameters (e.g. weights) to be adapted. Multilayer feed forward perceptrons are the most commonly selected architecture. Training these networks is typically accomplished through a *back-propagation* algorithm, which implements a gradient search over the error response surface for the set of weights that minimizes the sum of the squared error between the actual and target values.

Although the use of back-propagation is common in neural network applications, it is quite limiting. This procedure is mathematically tractable and provides guaranteed convergence, but only to a locally optimal solution that may be neither globally optimal nor sufficient. Even if the network's topology provides sufficient complexity to completely solve the given pattern recognition task, the back-propagation method may be incapable of discovering an appropriate set of weights to accomplish the task. When this occurs, the operator has several options: (a) accept suboptimal performance; (b) restart the procedure and try again; (c) use ad hoc tricks, such as adding noise to the exemplars; (d) collect new data and retrain; or (e) add degrees of freedom to the network by increasing the number of nodes and/or connections.

Adding more degrees of freedom to the network will eventually allow back-propagation to demonstrate adequate performance on the training set, provided sufficient nodes and layers are available. Yet this also presents problems to the designer of the network, for any function can map any measurable domain to its corresponding range if given sufficient degrees of freedom. Unfortunately, such overfit functions generally provide very poor performance during validation on independently acquired data. Such anomalies are commonly encountered in regression analysis, statistical model-building, and system identification. Assessing the proper trade-off between the goodness-of-fit to the data and the required degrees of freedom requires information criteria (e.g. Akaike's information criterion, minimum description length principle, predicted squared error, or others). By relying on the back-propagation method, the designer almost inevitably accepts that the resulting network will not satisfy the maxim of parsimony, simply because of the defective nature of the training procedure itself. The problems of local convergence with the back-propagation algorithm indicate the desirability of training with stochastic optimization methods such as simulated evolution, which can provide convergence to globally optimal solutions.

Evolutionary computation and neural networks

Natural evolution is a population-based optimization process. Simulating this process on a computer results in stochastic optimization algorithms that can often outperform classical methods of optimization when applied to difficult real-world problems. There are currently three main avenues of research in simulated evolution: evolution strategies, evolutionary programming, and genetic algorithms (Fogel 1995; Bäck 1996; Michalewicz 1996). The methods are broadly similar in that each maintains a population of trial solutions, imposes random changes to those solutions and incorporates the use of selection to determine which solutions to maintain into future generations and which to remove from the pool of trials. The methods differ in the types of random change that are used (e.g. mutation and/or recombination) and the methods for selecting successful trials (e.g. proportional, tournament, or other selection mechanisms). Fogel (1995) provides a review of the similarities and differences between these procedures. The methods have been shown to possess asymptotic global convergence properties (Rudolph 1994), and in some cases the techniques can be shown to have geometric rates of error convergence (Bäck et al. 1993).

The procedures generally proceed as follows. A problem to be solved is cast in the form of an objective function that describes the worth of alternative solutions. Without loss of generality, suppose that the task is to find the solution that minimizes the objective function. A collection (population) of trial solutions is selected at random from some feasible range across the available parameters. Each solution is scored with respect to the objective function. The solutions (parents) are then mutated and/or recombined with other solutions in order to create new trials (offspring). These offspring are also scored with respect to the objective function and a subset of the parents and offspring are selected to become parents of the next iteration (generation) based on their relative performance. Those with superior performance are given a greater chance of being selected than are those of inferior quality. Bäck et al. (1997) detailed examples of evolutionary algorithms applied to a wide range of problems, including designing neural networks.

Optimizing neural networks through simulated evolution not only offers a superior search for appropriate network parameters, but also the evolution can be used to adjust the network's topology simultaneously. By mutating both the structure of the network and its associated parameters (weights), a very efficient search can be made for a truly robust design. This frees the operator from having to preselect a topology and then searching for the best weights under that constraint. This procedure was described by Fogel (1995) to evolve neural networks in mathematical games, and by Fogel & Simpson (1993), and Ghozeil & Fogel (1996) to evolve clusters based on fuzzy membership functions. Information criteria can be applied to design evolutionary networks in a manner similar to the construction of models in system identification (Fogel 1991). The self-design process is almost automatic; unlike traditional neural network paradigms that require the active participation of the user as part of the learning algorithm, an evolutionary neural network can adapt to unexpected feature inputs on its own, or with little operator intervention. The resulting system is more robust than traditional approaches in symbolic artificial intelligence, and is capable of machine learning.

The earliest attempts to use simulated evolution to train artificial neural networks go back at least to Mucciardi & Gose (1966), Klopf & Gose (1969), and others. More recently, however, the traditional methods in evolutionary computation were applied to training feedforward networks in the late 1980s and early 1990s (e.g. Montana & Davis 1989; Fogel et al. 1990). When simulated evolution has been used to train neural networks the results have often been superior to those from other methods. Porto et al. (1995) compared back propagation, simulated annealing, and evolutionary programming for training a fixed network topology to classify active sonar returns. The results indicated that stochastic search techniques such as annealing and evolution consistently outperform back propagation, yet can be executed more rapidly on an appropriately configured parallel processing computer. After sufficient computational effort, the most successful network can be put into practice. But the evolutionary process can be continued during application, so as to provide iterative improvements on the basis of newly acquired exemplars. The procedure is efficient because it can use the entire current population of networks as initial solutions to accommodate each

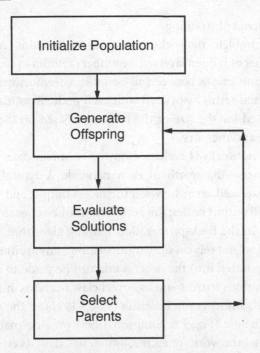

Figure 10.1. The flowchart of a basic evolutionary algorithm. An initial population of solutions to the problem at hand is constructed. For the sake of the current discussion, these take the form of neural networks. Often, individual solutions are selected uniformly at random from the space of all possible solutions; however, hints may be used to bias this initialization if they are available. The initial parents are used to generate offspring through random variation. This typically involves mutation and/or recombination of existing individual solutions. All solutions (parents and offspring) are evaluated in the light of a performance index. A selection operation then determines which solutions to keep as parents for the next generation, and the process iterates. The loop is usually halted when a solution of sufficient worth has been discovered or a preset number of generations have transpired.

newly acquired datum. There is no need to restart the search procedure in the face of new data, in contrast with many classic search algorithms, such as dynamic programming.

When addressing a typical problem of pattern recognition, as might be found in medical diagnosis, designing neural networks through simulated evolution follows an iterative procedure (see Figure 10.1):

1. A specific type of neural network is selected. The number of input nodes corresponds to the amount of input data to be analysed. The number of classes of concern (i.e. the number of output classification types of interest) determines the number of output nodes.

2. Exemplar data are selected for training.
3. A population of P complete networks is selected at random. A network incorporates the number of hidden layers, the number of nodes in each of these layers, the weighted connections between all nodes in a feedforward or other design, and all of the bias terms associated with each node. Reasonable initial bounds must be selected for the size of the networks, based on the available computer architecture and memory.
4. Each of these 'parent' networks is evaluated on the exemplar data. A pay-off function is used to assess the worth of each network. A typical objective function is the mean squared error between the target output and the actual output summed over all output nodes; this technique is often chosen because it simplifies calculations in the back-propagation training algorithm. As evolutionary computation does not rely on similar calculations, any arbitrary pay-off function can be incorporated into the process and can be made to reflect the operational worth of various correct and incorrect classifications. Information criteria such as Akaike's information criterion (Fogel 1991) or the minimum description length principle (Fogel & Simpson 1993) provide mathematical justification for assessing the worth of each solution, based on its classification error and the required degrees of freedom.
5. 'Offspring' are created from these parent networks through random mutation and/or recombination. Simultaneous variation may be applied to the number of layers and nodes, and to the values for the associated parameters (e.g. weights and biases of a multilayer perceptron, weights, biases, means and standard deviations of a radial basis function network). A probability distribution function is used to determine the likelihood of selecting combinations of these variations. The probability distribution can be preselected a priori by the operator or can be made to evolve along with the network (i.e. self-adaptation), providing for nearly completely autonomous evolution.
6. The offspring networks are scored in a manner similar to that of their parents.
7. A selection operation is applied to determine which networks survive into the next generation, and which are removed. One possible method for accomplishing this is to conduct a probabilistic round-robin competition to determine the relative worth of each proposed network. Pairs of networks are selected at random. The network with superior performance is assigned a 'win'. Competitions are run to a preselected limit. Those networks with the most wins are selected to become parents for the next generation. In this manner, solutions that are far superior to their competitors have a corresponding high probability of being selected. The converse is also true. This function helps to prevent stagnation at local optima by providing a parallel biased random walk.
8. The process iterates by returning to step (5).

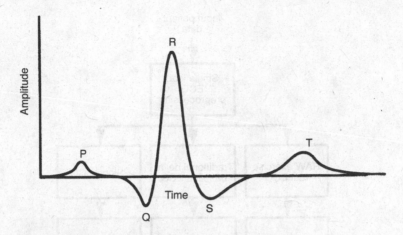

Figure 10.2. A sample ECG waveform (after Brotherton & Simpson 1995). The waveform describes the electrical activity of the heart over a beat. The significant segments of the waveform are labelled as P, Q, R, S, and T. Classic ECG waveform analysis relies on scalar parameters associated with these labelled segments.

Examples of evolving neural networks in medical applications

For the sake of space, only two examples of the application of evolutionary neural networks to medical diagnosis are described below, although the literature on such applications is growing rapidly.

Dynamic feature set training for classification

Brotherton & Simpson (1995) considered the problem of classifying the severity of coronary artery disease (CAD) from multiple-input electrocardiograph (ECG) waveform representations collected during exercise tests. Such attempts have a history of over 20 years, and have traditionally focused on the QRS-ST-T-segments of the ECG waveform (Figure 10.2). Brotherton & Simpson (1995) focused on a hierarchical approach to processing original and transformed waveforms in a series of neural networks (Figure 10.3). The goal was to develop neural networks that would minimize a function of the classification error:

$$E = \frac{m}{n} + aN + bF$$

where m is the number of misclassifications out of n total classifications, N is the number of nodes in a neural network, F is the number of features that are used, and a and b are scalar terms to weight the individual contribution of each concern. The neural architecture used was a 'fuzzy min–max' network (Figure 10.4).

Attention was given to 90 male patients randomly selected from a pool of 441

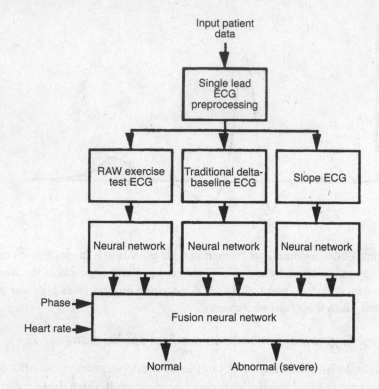

Figure 10.3. Hierarchical neural network flow diagram (after Brotherton & Simpson 1995). The hierarchical neural net processes the original ECG waveform and two transformations selected to highlight ECG features in the three first-layer nets. Outputs from the first layer, along with two scalar ECG measures (heart rate and exercise test phase), are fused together in the second or 'fusion' layer for the final classification.

patients who had undergone treadmill exercise ECG testing and coronary angiography. These 90 cases were then pruned down to 50, where 30 were angiographic normals (0-vessel disease) and 20 had severe 3-vessel disease (abnormal). Training was performed on 25 patients (50% from each category), and testing was performed on the remaining cases. Evolutionary programming was used to modify the weighted connections of the network as well as identify the suitable input features. The final result was a fusion network that had a sensitivity of 0.94 and specificity of 0.96 in training, and was completely correct when verified against the test set. Brotherton & Simpson (1995) noted that the task of classifying 0-vessel vs. 3-vessel disease is straightforward for a trained electrocardiologist; however, the effort demonstrated that the task could be automated and points towards future efforts for assisting in the discrimination of 1-vessel and 2-vessel disease.

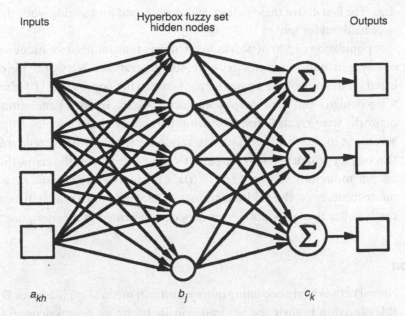

Figure 10.4. Topology of the fuzzy min–max classification neural network (after Brotherton & Simpson 1995). Inputs to the net are on the left. Those inputs are passed to the hyperboxes in the middle layer. The hyperboxes partition the input features into class-dependent clusters (this is similar to radial basis functions except that hyperboxes are selected instead of Gaussian density functions). Those hyperbox outputs are fuzzy class membership values for the features. The value for each of the classes is considered when making an overall classification. The variables *a, b, c* indicate the inputs, hidden nodes and outputs, respectively.

Computer-assisted diagnosis of breast cancer

There have been several recent efforts to use neural networks to assist radiologists in the diagnosis of breast cancer. Some of these have focused on automating the assessment of histological features of cells removed by fine needle aspiration (Wolberg et al. 1994, 1995) while others have developed systems to classify radiographic features of film screen mammograms (e.g. Wu et al. 1993; Floyd et al. 1994; Wilding et al. 1994).

Fogel et al. (1995) used evolutionary algorithms to design neural networks to classify histological data, archived in the machine learning database at the University of California at Irvine. There were 699 instances of parameterized histopathology from breast biopsies (65.5% benign), each having nine parameters: (1) clump thickness, (2) uniformity of cell size, (3) uniformity of cell shape, (4) marginal adhesion, (5) single epithelial cell size, (6) bare nuclei, (7) bland chromatin, (8) normal nucleoli, and (9) mitosis. Each of these parameters was rated on a 10-scale. Sixteen of the 699 data had missing values and were removed, leaving 683 data. The first 400 of these in the archive were used for training while the other 283 were held out for testing.

A population of 500 networks, each having nine inputs, two hidden nodes, and one output node, was evolved over 400 generations. Networks were evaluated based on the sum of the squared error between the target value (1 for malignancy, 0 for benign) and their output for each pattern. In each generation, offspring networks were created from surviving parents by mutating all of their weights according to a zero-mean Gaussian random variable, with a standard deviation that was set proportional to the parent's error (the greater the error, the larger the average mutation). In a series of 16 trials, the best evolved neural networks had a mean accuracy on the held-out test set of 98.05%, which was statistically significantly better than previous performance documented in the literature.

Discussion

Neural networks are becoming more routine in medical applications. One reasonable objection to their use has traditionally been that neural networks are 'black boxes' and therefore unexplainable. It appears difficult to trust the results from such a device. It would be useful to keep the networks used in operation as parsimonious as possible. Training methods that rely on gradient search suffer in this regard because they can stall in locally optimal configurations and it may therefore be necessary to increase the complexity of the networks in order to discover suitable weights. Evolutionary algorithms offer the potential to alleviate much of this problem because the stochastic search for optimal weight sets can overcome multiple minima on the error response surface and discover suitable solutions for simpler networks. These simpler models should be easier to explain, and therefore may be expected to have a greater practical impact on the field of computer-assisted medicine.

Acknowledgements

The authors thank R. Dybowski for his patience and encouragment, and T. W. Brotherton for permission to reprint figures.

REFERENCES

Bäck, T. (1996). *Evolutionary Algorithms in Theory and Practice*. Oxford University Press, New York.

Bäck, T., Rudolph, G. & Schwefel, H.-P. (1993). Evolution strategies and evolutionary programming: similarities and differences. In D. B. Fogel & W. Atmar, eds., *Proceedings of the 2nd*

Annual Conference on Evolutionary Programming. Evolutionary Programming Society, La Jolla, CA, pp. 11–22.

Bäck, T., Fogel, D. B. & Michalewicz, Z. (Eds.) (1997). *Handbook of Evolutionary Computation.* Oxford University Press, New York.

Brotherton T. W. & Simpson, P. K. (1995). Dynamic feature set training of neural networks for classification. In J. R. McDonnell, R. G. Reynolds & D. B. Fogel, eds., *Evolutionary Programming IV: Proceedings of the Fourth Annual Conference on Evolutionary Programming.* MIT Press, Cambridge, MA, pp. 79–90.

Floyd, C. E., Lo, J. Y., Yun, A. J., Sullivan, D. C. & Kornguth, P. J. (1994). Prediction of breast cancer malignancy using an artificial neural network. *Cancer* 74, 2944–2998.

Fogel. D. B. (1991). An information criterion for optimal neural network selection. *IEEE Transactions on Neural Networks* 2, 490–497.

Fogel, D. B. (1995). *Evolutionary Computation: Toward a New Philosophy of Machine Intelligence.* IEEE Press, New York.

Fogel, D. B. & Simpson, P. K. (1993). Experiments with evolving fuzzy clusters. In D. B. Fogel & W. Atmar, eds., *Proceedings of the 2nd Annual Conference on Evolutionary Programming.* Evolutionary Programming Society, La Jolla, CA, pp. 90–97.

Fogel, D. B., Fogel, L. J. & Porto, V. W. (1990). Evolving neural networks. *Biological Cybernetics* **63**, 487–493.

Fogel, D. B., Wasson, E. C. & Boughton, E. M. (1995). Evolving neural networks for detecting breast cancer. *Cancer Letters* **96**, 49–53.

Ghozeil, A. & Fogel, D. B. (1996). Discovering patterns in spatial data using evolutionary programming. In J. R. Koza, D. E. Goldberg, D. B. Fogel & R. L. Riolo, eds., *Genetic Programming 1996: Proceedings of the 1st Annual Conference,* MIT Press, Cambridge, MA, pp. 521–7.

Hornik, K., Stinchcombe, M. & White, H. (1989). Multilayer feedforward networks are universal approximators. *Neural Networks* 2, 359–366.

Klopf, A. H. & Gose, E. (1969). An evolutionary patterm recognition network. *IEEE Transactions on Systems Science and Cybernetics* **SSC-5**, 247–250.

Lippmann, R. P. (1987). An introduction to computing with neural nets. *IEEE ASSP Magazine,* April, pp. 4–22.

Michalewicz, Z. (1996). *Genetic Algorithms + Data Structures = Evolution Programs,* 3rd edn. Springer-Verlag, Berlin.

Montana, D. J. & Davis, L. (1989). Training feedforward neural networks using genetic algorithms. In *Proceedings of the 11th International Joint Conference on Artificial Intelligence.* Morgan Kaufmann, San Mateo, CA, pp. 762–767.

Mucciardi, A. N. & Gose, E. E. (1966). Evolutionary pattern recognition in incomplete nonlinear multithreshold networks. *IEEE Transactions on Electronic Computers* **EC-15**, 257–261.

Poggio, T. & Girosi, F. (1990). Networks for approximation and learning. *Proceedings of the IEEE* **78**, 1481–1497.

Porto, V. W., Fogel, D. B. & Fogel, L. J. (1995). Alternative neural network training methods. *IEEE Expert* **10**(3), 16–22.

Rudolph, G. (1994). Convergence analysis of canonical genetic algorithms. *IEEE Transactions on Neural Networks* **5**, 96–101.

Wilding, P., Morgan, M. A., Grygotis, A. E., Shoffner, M. A. & Rosato, E. F. (1994). Application of backpropagation neural networks to diagnosis of breast and ovarian cancer. *Cancer Letters*, **77**, 145–153.

Wolberg, W. H., Street, W. N. & Mangasarian, O. L. (1994). Machine learning techniques to diagnose breast cancer from image-processed nuclear features of fine needle aspirates. *Cancer Letters* **77**, 163–171.

Wolberg, W. H., Street, W. N., Heisey, D. M. & Mangasarian, O. L. (1995). Computerized breast cancer diagnosis and prognosis from fine-needle aspirates. *Archives of Surgery* **130**, 511–516.

Wu, Y. Z., Giger, M. L., Doi, K., Vyborny, C. J., Schmidt, R. A. & Metz, C. E. (1993). Artificial neural networks in mammography: application to decision making in the diagnosis of breast cancer. *Radiology* **187**, 81–87.

Part III

Theory

11

Neural networks as statistical methods in survival analysis

Brian D. Ripley and Ruth M. Ripley

Introduction

Artificial neural networks are increasingly being seen as an addition to the statistics toolkit that should be considered alongside both classical and modern statistical methods. Reviews in this light have been given by one of us (Ripley 1993, 1994a–c, 1996) and Cheng & Titterington (1994) and it is a point of view that is being widely accepted by the mainstream neural networks community. There are now many texts (Hertz et al. 1991; Haykin 1994; Bishop 1995; Ripley 1996) covering the wide range of artificial neural networks; we concentrate here on methods that we see as most appropriate generally in medicine, and in particular on methods for survival data that have not to our knowledge been reviewed in depth (although Schwarzer et al. (1997) reviewed a large number of applications in oncology). In particular, we point out the many different ways classification networks have been used for survival data, as well as their many flaws.

Most applications of artificial neural networks to medicine are classification problems; that is, the task is on the basis of the measured *features* to assign the patient (or biopsy or electroencephalograph or . . .) to one of a small set of classes. Baxt (1995) gave a table of applications of neural networks in clinical medicine that are almost all of this form, including those in laboratories (Dybowski & Gant 1995). Classification problems include diagnosis, some prognosis problems ('will she relapse within the next 3 years?'), establishing depths of anaesthesia (Watt et al., 1995) and classifying sleep state (Pardey et al. 1996). Other prognosis problems are sometimes converted to a classification problem with an ordered series of categories, for example time to relapse as 0–1, 1–2, 2–4 or 4 or more years (Ripley et al. 1998) and prognosis after head injury (Titterington et al. 1981; Lowe & Webb 1990; Mathieson 1997). We discuss neural networks for classification and their main competitors in the next section.

Regression problems are less common in medicine, especially those requiring sophisticated non-linear methods such as neural networks. We can envisage them being used for some calibration tasks in the laboratory, but a simpler example is to predict time to death of a patient with advanced breast cancer. As methods for regression can often be applied in a clever or modified way to solve classification or survival problems, we consider them in the second section. The general idea is to replace a linear function by a neural network, which can be done within many areas of statistics.

Most prognosis problems have the characteristic that for some patients in the study set the outcome has not yet happened (or they have been lost to follow-up or died from an unrelated cause). This is known as *censoring* and has generated much statistical interest (Cox 1972; Kalbfleisch & Prentice 1980; Andersen et al. 1993; Collett 1994) over the last three decades. Researchers have begun to consider how neural networks could be used within this framework, and we review this work and add some suggestions in the third section.

One important observation is that neural networks provide 'black-box' methods; they may be very good at predicting outcomes but are not able to provide explanations of, say, the diagnosis or prognosis. Some of the other modern methods are able to provide explanations, and one promising idea is to fit these to the predictions of the neural network and come up with an explanation. Neural networks also lack another of the characteristics of expert systems, the ability to incorporate (easily; there is some work on 'hints' (Abu-Mostafa 1995)) qualitative information provided by domain experts.

Neural networks are powerful, and like powerful cars are difficult to drive well. For many users the power will be an embarrassment, and they may do better to use the simpler tools from modern statistics. Because of the 'hype' surrounding artificial neural networks many expensive computer programs have been produced that have had much more effort (and understanding) devoted to the user interface than to the algorithms used. In the fourth section we point out a few of the pitfalls, but would-be users are advised to read a recommended book on the subject (or to consult an expert statistician). The statistical view has pointed out many ways to use neural networks better, but unfortunately these are still only very rarely implemented. We used the S-PLUS (MathSoft Data Analysis Products Division 1987–97) statistical environment on both a PC and a Unix workstation to compute the examples, but the code used to fit neural networks was written by ourselves. (The basic code is freely available as part of the on-line material for Venables & Ripley (1997).)

Examples

We use two cancer data sets to illustrate some of our points; note that their use here is purely illustrative and is not intended as an analysis of those sets of data. The first is on survival in months (up to 18 years, but with a median of 23 months) from advanced breast cancer, supplied by Dr J.-P. Nakache. There are 981 patients

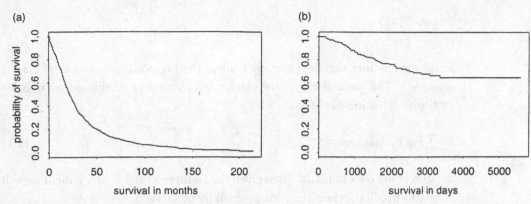

Figure 11.1. Plots of the Kaplan–Meier estimates of survival curves for the full (a) breast cancer and (b) melanoma data sets.

and 12 explanatory features all of which are categorical. We randomly divided this into a test set of size 500 and a training set of size 481, and assessed the methods on predictions of survival for 24 months; only 3% of the patients did not have complete follow-up to that time.

The second data set is of 205 patients with malignant melanoma following a radical operation, and has five explanatory features. This is taken from Andersen et al. (1993); it is the same data set that was analysed (with additional explanatory variables) in Liestøl et al. (1994). Figure 11.1 shows that there appears to be long-term survival (from melanoma) for 65% of patients, so the survival distribution does not follow any of the standard distributions. Only 57 of the patients died from the melanoma during the study. We assessed methods on their ability to predict survival to 2500 days, by which point 86 of the patients had incomplete follow-up; our analysis shows that we expect 82 of these to have survived for 2500 days.

Classification

Suppose for the moment that we wish to put a patient into one of two classes (e.g. survival for 5 years or not); for many purposes it will be more helpful to know the predicted probability of survival. A simple but much neglected method is logistic regression or discrimination (Ripley 1996), which is specified by

$$P(\text{class }2\,|\,x) = \frac{e^{\eta}}{1 + e^{\eta}}, \qquad \eta = \beta_0 + \beta_1 x_1 + \cdots + \beta_p x_p$$

$$P(\text{class }1\,|\,x) = 1 - P(\text{class }2\,|\,x) = \frac{1}{1 + e^{\eta}}$$

$$\frac{P(\text{class } 2 \mid x)}{P(\text{class } 1 \mid x)} = e^{\eta},$$

so the explanatory variables linearly control the log-odds η in favour of class 2 (survival). The parameters β are chosen by maximum likelihood, that is by maximizing the log-likelihood

$$L = \sum_i \log P(\text{class}_i \mid x_i), \tag{11.1}$$

the sum being over patients. Then given the features x on a future patient we will be able to predict $P(\text{class } 2 \mid x)$, her probability of survival.

There have been many non-linear extensions of logistic regression. There are several variants of *generalized additive models* (Hastie & Tibshirani 1990; Wahba 1990; Wahba et al. 1995) in which

$$\eta = \sum g_i(x_i)$$

where smooth functions g_i of one (or perhaps two) of the features are chosen as part of the estimation procedure, and classification trees (Breiman et al. 1984; Ripley 1996) in which the patients are divided into groups with a common η for each group.

The extension of logistic regression to neural network is straightforward; we take η to be the (linear) output of a neural network with inputs x and write $\eta = g(x; \theta)$ where the parameters θ are known as 'weights' in the neural network literature. (Note that we can also regard this as a neural network with a single logistic output unit giving $P(\text{class } 2 \mid x)$, but that is rather coincidental.) Fitting the neural network by maximum likelihood is known as 'entropy' fitting in that literature and is definitely not common (and supported by amazingly few packages). It is more common to use the regression methods we discuss in the next section, which may be adequate for predicting the class (survival or death) but will be less good for predicting probabilities.

The extension to $k > 2$ classes is even less well known, although it has a long history. The idea is to take the log-odds of each class relative to one class, so the model becomes

$$\frac{P(\text{class } j \mid x)}{P(\text{class } 1 \mid x)} = e^{\eta_j}, \quad j = 2, \ldots, k,$$

and so

$$P(\text{class } j \mid x) = \frac{e^{\eta_j}}{\sum_{c=1}^{k} e^{\eta_c}}, \quad \eta_1 \equiv 0. \tag{11.2}$$

With $\eta_j = \beta_j^T x$ this is known as multiple logistic regression (Ripley 1996). The parameters (β_j) are fitted by maximizing the log-likelihood L given in Eq. (11.1). There have been surprisingly few non-linear extensions in the statistics literature; there is some recent work on additive multiple logistic regression called *POLY-CLASS* models (Kooperberg et al. 1997). The extension to neural networks is easy; use Eq. (11.2) with $(\eta_1, \ldots, \eta_k)$ the k (linear) outputs of a neural network. (Only $k - 1$ outputs are needed, but for symmetry we do not insist that $\eta_1 = 0$.) Bridle (1990a,b) gave this the pretentious title of *softmax*. Once again, softmax networks are not implemented in most neural network packages; rather they provide networks with k logistic outputs, which amounts to using

$$P(\text{class } j \mid x) = \frac{e^{\eta_j}}{1 + e^{\eta_j}}, \quad j = 1, \ldots, k.$$

This is an appropriate model for diagnosis where a patient might have none, one or more out of k diseases, but not for general classification problems.

Classification for prognosis problems

It is surprising how often classification networks have been applied to prognosis problems, especially as it would seem that the methods we consider in the third section would often be more appropriate. (This is probably due to the ready availability of software for classification networks.) There are many variants. We usually have to take *censoring* into account; that is, that follow-up on some patients may end before the event (which we describe as 'death').

1. The simplest idea (Bugliosi et al. 1994; Burke et al. 1995; Tarassenko et al. 1996) considers survival for some fixed number of months or years, and ignores patients censored before that time, thereby giving a standard two-class classification problem. Omitting censored patients, however, may bias the result. Imagine a study of survival for 5 years after an operation where most deaths occur in the postoperative phase; all patients have been followed up for 3 years but few for the full 5 years. Then the censored patients are very likely to have survived for 5 years, and the estimates of the survival probabilities will be biased downwards. This bias may not be important in explaining the variations in survival from the explanatory features, but these studies are concerned with predicting not explaining.

   Ravdin & Clark (1992) gave an example of this effect: in their study 268 patients had known follow-up for 60 months, of whom 213 had died, although the Kaplan–Meier estimate of the survival probability was 50%. We can also see this in our melanoma example. Of those patients with complete follow-up to

10 years, 23 out of 80 survived, yet the Kaplan–Meier estimate of survival for this time is 64.5%.

2. A refinement is to divide the survival time into one of a set of non-overlapping intervals, giving an ordered series of k classes. (For definiteness let us take the classes 'death in year 1', 'death in year 2', 'death in year 3' and 'survive 3 or more years'.) This can be done in a number of ways. Perhaps the most natural is to use a proportional odds model (Mathieson 1996) for the ordered outcomes. It is much more common to ignore the ordering of the classes, and to use a k-class classification network (Lapuerta et al. 1995; Ohno-Machado 1997; Ripley et al. 1998). The perceived difficulty is how to handle censoring: sometimes all censored patients are ignored (but this causes a bias in the predictions). The remedy is in fact theoretically easy: for example, the contribution to the log-likelihood L for a patient who was lost to follow up after 2 years is

$$\log\{P(\text{death in year } 3 \mid x) + P(\text{survive 3 or more years} \mid x)\}.$$

This does, however, need modifications to the software, so standard methods for fitting classification networks cannot be used. If this is done there is only a small bias, due to the fact that censored patients will have survived some of the interval in which they were lost to follow-up.

These methods produce a crude estimate of the survivor curve $S(t) = P(\text{alive}$ at time $t)$ by taking 1 minus the cumulative probabilities across classes. If a prediction of prognosis is required we clearly should not take the class with the largest predicted probability (especially if the intervals are of unequal length); a good choice would be the interval over which the cumulative probability of death moves from below 50% to above 50%.

3. Other authors use k separate networks. This can be done in one of two ways: in our example we could use networks for either (a) the original four classes (Bottaci et al. 1997) or (b) the three classes (Kappen & Neijt 1993; Theeuwen et al. 1995; Ohno-Machado & Musen 1997) 'death in year 1', 'death in year 1 or 2' and 'death in years 1, 2 or 3'. In either case we can train each network on those patients with follow-up past the end of the interval, so that later networks are trained on fewer data, and once again there are problems of bias.

It is easy for networks trained with option (b) to give inconsistent answers, for example to give a higher predicted probability for 'death in year 1 or 2' than for 'death in years 1, 2 or 3'. This was reported by Ohno-Machado & Musen (1997), who tried to circumvent it by employing the output of one network (say 'death in year 1 or 2') as an input to the others. However, such difficulties are indicative of a wrong formulation of the problem. (Surprisingly, that paper does not mention the more satisfactory approach (Ohno-Machado 1997) of using a k-output network used on the same data set by one of its authors!)

Lapuerta et al. (1995) used for their final predictions a network with four outputs corresponding to death in one of three 40-month periods or survival for 10 years. However, during training they coped with censored data by imputing a death period for those patients lost to follow-up. This was done by training separate networks for death in periods 2 and 3. The features on a patient lost to follow-up during period 1 were input to the period 2 network; if that predicted death, death in period 2 was assigned, but if not the period 3 network was used to impute either death in period 3 or survival for 10 years.

Ravdin et al. (1992) have a variation on theme (b), in which they combine the k separate networks into one network with an additional input, the number of years for which survival is to be predicted. The training set repeats each patient for all the numbers of years for which survival or death is known. Ravdin & Clark (1992) extended this approach by attempting to ameliorate the problems of bias by randomly selecting a proportion of the deaths to match the proportion given by a classical Kaplan–Meier estimate of the survival curve. (This is not an exact procedure; if it is to be used it would be better to weight cases than to randomly choose them.)

4. Another alternative (Cox 1972) is to model the conditional probabilities

$P(\text{die in } i\text{-th interval} \mid \text{survive first } i-1 \text{ intervals}, x) = g(\eta_i),$

where g is usually the logistic function $e^x/(1 + e^x)$. Then a patient dying in the i-th interval contributes $\log\{g(\eta_i)[1 - g(\eta_{i-1})] \cdots [1 - g(\eta_1)]\}$ to the log-likelihood, and a patient lost to follow up in that interval $\log\{[1 - g(\eta_{i-1})] \cdots [1 - g(\eta_1)]\}$, and from this the log-likelihood L can be computed. The 'scores' $\eta_1, \ldots, \eta_k$ are given by the output of a neural network with k linear outputs. (This model can be regarded as a 'life-table' or discrete-time survival model (Kalbfleisch & Prentice 1980) and is sketched in those terms by Liestøl et al. (1994). It is sometimes known as a 'chain-binomial' model.)

It is possible (Efron 1988; Biganzoli et al. 1998) to fit this model using standard neural network software (although the predictions do have to be postprocessed.) We can expand the contribution to the log likelihood as a sum of $\log g(\eta_i)$ or $\log[1 - g(\eta_i)]$ over the intervals for which that patient is at risk. This is computed by having an additional input to the neural network specifying the time interval i for which $g(\eta_i)$ is required, and entering each patient into the training set for each time interval until death or the end of follow-up. Thus the training set (both inputs and outputs) is similar to that used by Ravdin et al., but patients are not entered after death and the fitted network is used in a different way. Note that although this technique is possible, special-purpose software will be substantially more efficient.

This method also has only a small bias due to censoring; it is equivalent to approach 2 but uses a different parametrization of the survival probabilities.

It may be helpful to restate the censoring problem in mathematical terms. Suppose we have $k+1$ time intervals, $[0 = t_0, t_1), [t_1, t_2), \ldots, [t_{k-1}, t_k), [t_k, \infty)$, and let $s_i = S(t_i)$ be the probability that a patient survives to time t_i, and suppose we are particularly interested in s_k. Approaches 1 and 3 estimate s_k directly. Approach 2 estimates $p_i = P(t_{i-1} \leq T < t_i)$ and then $s_k = p_{k+1} = 1 - p_1 - \cdots - p_k$. Approach 4 estimates $g_i = P(t_{i-1} \leq T < t_i \mid T > t_{i-1})$, and then $s_k = (1 - g_1) \cdots (1 - g_k)$. Approaches 2 and 4 are able to (approximately) adjust for censoring, since a patient lost to follow-up in the interval $[t_{i-1}, t_i)$ is counted as a survivor in estimating $p_1, \ldots, p_{i-1}$ or $g_1, \ldots, g_{i-1}$ rather than being ignored.

Unfortunately, the only methods that deal correctly with censoring use a different log-likelihood from that used in standard packages, and hence need software modifications or use the software inefficiently. The approaches of Lapuerta et al. (1995) and Biganzoli et al. (1998) are the most satisfactory of those using standard software.

Regression problems

Many neural network packages can tackle only regression problems; that is they are confined to fitting functions $g_j(x; \theta)$ by least squares, minimizing

$$\sum_i \sum_{j=1}^{k} [y_{ij} - g_j(x_i; \theta)]^2,$$

the first sum being over patients. This corresponds to $k \geq 1$ non-linear regressions on the explanatory variables x. The most common usage is a neural network with a single linear output (e.g. for calibration in pyrolysis mass spectrometry) or with a logistic output for a two-class classification problem. It would seem obvious to take $y = 1$ for survival and $y = 0$ for death, but as we saw in the first section, the use of least squares is not really appropriate and 'fudges' have grown up such as coding survival as $y = 0.9$ and death as $y = 0.1$. The extension to a k-class classification problem is to take $y_{ij} = 1$ for the class which occurred and $y_{ij} = 0$ for the others; then when the network is used for the prediction the class with the largest output is chosen. (Other ways to use regression methods for classification problems are discussed in Ripley (1996, Chap. 4).)

There has been a parallel development of non-linear regression methods in statistics. Additive models are of the form

$$g_j(x; \theta) = \alpha_j + \sum_{s=1}^{p} \beta_{js} g_s(x_s; \theta),$$

which allows a non-linear transformation of each of the features. The functions g_s can be chosen non-parametrically (Hastie & Tibshirani 1990) or by smoothing splines (Wahba 1990); some implementations such as multivariate adaptive regression splines (MARS) (Friedman 1991) also allow functions of more than one feature. Perhaps the most wide-ranging generalization of additive models is *projection pursuit regression* (Friedman & Stuetzle 1981) which is an additive model in linear combinations of the features. This subsumes neural networks with a single hidden layer, but the algorithms developed in the statistical literature for fitting projection pursuit regressions are less powerful than those now known for fitting neural networks.

Classification trees have a counterpart, regression trees (Breiman et al. 1984), in which once again the patients are grouped and a constant value assigned to each group; the groups are found by a tree-structured set of rules.

Great ingenuity has been shown in finding ways to apply existing regression methods and software to other problems. For example, Therneau et al. (1990) suggested applying regression trees to the residuals from a linear survival analysis to provide a non-linear survival method using existing software, and this idea could be applied equally to neural networks.

Survival analysis

The conventional set-up in survival analysis is that there is a time-to-outcome, T, which is measured continuously, plus a censoring indicator δ which indicates whether the outcome was 'death' ($\delta = 1$) or the patient was lost to follow-up ($\delta = 0$). The standard statistical procedures (Kalbfleisch & Prentice 1980; Collett 1994; Venables & Ripley 1997) relate the distribution of T to explanatory variables x via a *linear predictor* $\eta = \beta^T x$. For example, proportional hazards models have the hazard at time t (the rate of death at time t of those who are still alive)

$$h(t) = h_0(t)e^\eta, \tag{11.3}$$

where $h_0()$ is known as the baseline hazard, and an accelerated life model fits a standard distribution to $Te^{-\eta}$, so the linear predictor speeds up or slows down time for that patient. We discuss below how these models can be generalized to use neural networks.

Parametric models for survival analysis can be very useful but are often neglected. Common choices for a parametric proportional hazards model are the Weibull distribution and its special case the exponential, and for accelerated life models the Weibull (again) and the log-logistic. However, following Cox (1972), the semiparametric proportional hazard model has become extremely popular.

This assumes model (11.3), with no assumption on the baseline hazard and η is estimated by partial or marginal likelihood methods (Kalbfleisch & Prentice 1980).

Non-linear models in survival analysis are surprisingly rare in the statistical literature. There are a few references (O'Sullivan 1988; Gentleman & Crowley 1991; Gray 1992; Kooperberg et al. 1995) suggesting additive extensions of Cox models as well as a fully local approach (Gray 1996) and a modest literature (Ciampi et al. 1987; Segal 1988; Davis & Anderson 1989; LeBlanc & Crowley 1992, 1993) on tree-structured survival analysis.

The only previous attempt of which we are aware that applied neural networks directly to survival analysis is by Faraggi & Simon (1995), applied by Mariani et al. (1997). Both sets of authors considered partial-likelihood estimation of model (11.3) with $\eta = f(x; \theta)$ the output of a neural network. We have implemented this and the parametric models mentioned earlier. We should point out that there is a much easier way to fit Cox models with η given by a neural network, which is to use an iterative idea (Gentleman & Crowley 1991; LeBlanc & Crowley 1992). This alternates estimating the baseline cumulative hazard $H_0(t)$ by the Breslow estimator and choosing θ to maximize

$$\sum_i \{\delta_i \eta_i - H_0(t_i) \exp \eta_i\} \quad \eta_i = f(x_i; \theta)$$

(the sum being over patients) starting with $\eta_i \equiv 0$ or with a linear fit. Normally only a couple of iterations are required. The solution is a (local) maximum of the partial likelihood.

Fitting neural networks

Perhaps the major cause of difficulty in fitting neural networks is the ease with which it is possible to overfit, that is to tune the neural network to the peculiarities of the examples to hand rather than to extract the salient dependencies of the whole population. In a phrase borrowed from psychology, we want to fit a network to achieve good *generalization*. Why is this an especial problem for artificial neural networks? In using classical statistical methods we build up from simple models, perhaps first fitting a linear model and then allowing quadratic or interaction terms and at each stage testing for a significant improvement in fit. There is no analogue for neural networks, and there are results (Ripley 1996) that show that with enough hidden units we can make (essentially) arbitrarily complicated models.

For good generalization we do not want to use maximum likelihood fitting (or least squares fitting). We borrow the ideas of *regularization* from the numerical methods field, and penalize 'rough' functions $f(x; \theta)$. This is most conveniently done using *weight decay* in which we maximize

$$L - \lambda \sum_{\text{weights}} w_{ij}^2$$

How do we choose λ? There are some very effective guidelines (Ripley 1996) based on statistical ideas, but as with the number of hidden units it is best chosen by a validation experiment.

Not only does weight decay help to achieve good generalization, it also makes the optimization task easier and thus faster. So it is very surprising that (yet again) it is omitted from most packages, yet most experts in the field believe that it should *always* be used. Instead, most packages use the older idea of *early stopping* with an inefficient method of optimization; this will usually work but can be one or two orders of magnitude slower and is responsible for the reputation that neural networks have of being very computationally demanding. (*None* of the application studies we reviewed used weight decay nor explained how training was stopping nor how the number of hidden units were chosen. Mariani et al. (1997) are a commendable exception which appeared whilst this paper was in preparation.)

Although a neural network can handle complicated relationships, it is likely to generalize better if the problem is simplified, so as much care in preparing the data and transforming the inputs should be used for neural networks as for conventional statistical methods.

In the vast majority of neural network fitting problems there will be multiple local optima, so if the optimization is run from a different set of initial weights, different predictions will be made. Sometimes the differences between predictions at different local optima will be small, but by no means always. (Ripley (1996) has some simple examples for a medical diagnosis problem.) It is *not* a good idea to choose the best-fitting solution (that is probably the one that overfits the most); it is better to combine the predictions from the multiple solutions. The idea of averaging the probability predictions across, say, 25 fits is rather effective, and many other averaging ideas (Wolpert 1992; Perrone & Cooper 1993; Freund & Schapire 1995; Breiman 1996) have been suggested.

Several studies claimed that their neural network model outperformed a Cox regression and/or clinicians, but such findings need to be examined critically. None of the studies considered using non-linear terms nor interaction terms in the Cox regression, and this would be standard practice for a statistical expert using such models. However, the basis of the comparison is flawed. Cox models are not designed to estimate the probability of survival at a fixed time (usually the end of the study); they are intended to show the dependence of the survivor curve on the explanatory features. Even when used for prediction, they are able to predict the whole survivor curves, and it is not surprising that they are less able to predict one point on that curve than methods designed to predict just that point (e.g. logistic discrimination). Further, censoring biases in the test set will almost always favour the neural network models, which estimate the probability of survival to a fixed time *conditional* on the patient still being under follow-up, not the unconditional probability estimated by a survival analysis model or being assessed by the clinicians. The only way to ensure a fair comparison on a test set is to impute an outcome to each patient whose follow-up is for less than the fixed time. We suggest that this is best done by grouping test set patients on the basis of survival experience (perhaps using a tree-structured analysis to do the grouping), fitting a Kaplan–Meier survival curve to each group and using this to estimate the probability of survival of those patients in the group whose follow-up period is too short.

A frequent mistake is to take too small a test set; several authors have used a test set of fewer than 20 observations (Schwarzer et al. 1997). However, the size of the test set is not the whole story, as there needs to be sufficient cases that survive and sufficient that die. The study of Bottaci et al. (1997) (see also Dobson 1997) has gained considerable publicity, yet is based on the apparent success in predicting the death of just 7 out of 92 patients, and a higher accuracy (the headline measure used) would have been obtained by predicting survival for all the patients!

Examples

We tried most of the methods described here on one or both of the examples. Selecting the number of units in the neural networks and the amount of weight decay to be used was done by cross-validation (Ripley 1996), for a set of about a dozen values chosen from past experience. The measure of fit used was the *deviance*, summing minus twice the logarithms of the predicted probability of the event over all patients in the training set. (This provides a more sensitive measure of fit than the success rate, especially in the survival analysis models where the exact time of death is used.)

Breast cancer

We used a training set of size 500, and a test set of size 476 (ignoring those five patients in the full test set whose follow-up to 24 months was incomplete). All the linear methods used selection of the input variables by Akaike information criterion (AIC) (Ripley 1996); for all the methods using neural networks the number of hidden units and the amount of weight decay was chosen by 10-fold

Table 11.1. Results (%) for predictions on the test set of the breast cancer example

	Linear			Neural net		
Method	Specificity	Sensitivity	Accuracy	Specificity	Sensitivity	Accuracy
Binary classification	73	62	67	72	64	68
1-year periods	75	63	68	72	65	68
Proportional odds				72	61	66
Regression	66	68	67	63	71	67
Proportional hazards	70	62	66	71	62	66
Weibull survival	72	58	64	72	61	66
Log-logistic survival	70	66	67	68	66	67

cross-validation within the training set. Our results are summarized in Table 11.1. There *sensitivity* is the probability of correctly predicting death, *specificity* is the probability of correctly predicting survival, and the *accuracy* is the percentage of correct predictions.

There is almost nothing to choose between the methods, except that the Weibull survival models are slightly (but not significantly) poorer. This might have been expected, as Figure 11.1 shows that the overall survival distribution is not very close to Weibull. The regression methods were done with response the logarithm of survival time (using time directly gave very much worse results). This is formally equivalent to the log-normal survival analysis model, and further investigations showed that the bias towards death of the regression models is due to the exclusion of six cases with incomplete follow-up to 24 months (which were also excluded for the binary classifications).

Melanoma

This is a small data set (205 patients) with heavy censoring. We used five-fold cross-validation to assess the models: that is, we randomly divided the data set into five parts and for each fitted to the remaining four parts and predicted survival on the single part. Because there was heavy censoring, assessment on just those patients with complete follow-up to 2500 days would be seriously biased. We used a tree-based analysis to divide the data set into six groups (Figure 11.2) with homogeneous survival experience, fitted Kaplan–Meier survival curves to each group, and used these to estimate the probability that the patient would have survived from the end of observed follow-up to 2500 days. (This probability was often 1, and never less than 0.45.) These patients were then entered into the test set with both possible outcomes, weighted by the estimated probabilities.

The multiple output classification problem had classes as 0–1500, 1500–2000,

Table 11.2. Results (%) from five-fold cross-validation of the melanoma example. The second row of binary classification is using the estimated probabilities as targets for the patients with incomplete follow-up to 2500 days; these patients are completely ignored during training of the models for the first line

Method	Linear			Neural net		
	Specificity	Sensitivity	Accuracy	Specificity	Sensitivity	Accuracy
Binary classification	56.8	63.2	58.8	60.4	60.2	60.4
Full training set	87.7	27.9	69.5	88.3	26.2	69.4
4-class	89.3	23.7	69.4	92.9	15.8	69.4
Proportional odds	90.9	24.0	70.5	92.3	19.2	70.0
Proportional hazards	84.8	32.7	69.0	88.2	34.0	71.7
Weibull survival	87.7	26.4	69.0	87.6	24.7	68.5
Log-logistic survival	87.0	36.1	71.5	85.0	34.6	69.6

(a)   (b)

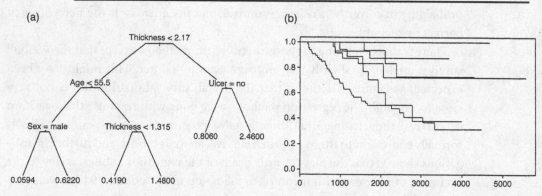

Figure 11.2. (a) Tree used to split the melanoma data into six groups. At each node the label indicates the condition to go down the left branch, and the numbers are the hazards for the groups relative to the whole dataset. (b) Kaplan–Meier plots of survival in the six groups.

2000–2500 and 2500– days, chosen by looking at the pattern of censoring times.

The results are shown in Table 11.2. Despite the use of nested cross-validation (so that evaluating each neural network method involved $5 \times 5 \times 12$ fits) the total computation time was less than an hour. Again there are generally small differences between the methods (except for the binary classifications ignoring censoring), even though the Weibull and log-logistic distributions cannot model long-term survival as shown in Figure 11.1. The large differences between sensitivity and specificity are not really surprising given that only about 28.2% of patients die within 2500 days. Thus we would achieve a higher accuracy than *all* of the methods by declaring all patients to survive. The underlying difficulty is that it is hard to find prognostic patterns and the dominance of survival leads to predicted

Table 11.3. Results for the melanoma data with differential costs of errors. The sensitivities and specificities are percentages, whereas the losses are totals over 205 patients

	Linear			Neural net		
Method	Specificity	Sensitivity	Loss	Specificity	Sensitivity	Loss
Binary classification	32.5	73.2	129.1	41.6	73.3	116.7
Full training set	69.7	57.4	96.3	69.7	62.2	90.3
4-class	64.2	57.6	103.9	77.4	47.6	97.6
Proportional odds	77.4	52.4	91.6	77.4	50.8	93.6
Proportional hazards	73.2	59.0	89.3	72.8	63.8	84.3
Weibull survival	74.6	54.2	93.4	73.2	63.8	83.3
Log-logistic survival	73.2	54.0	95.6	70.3	66.8	83.7

probabilities of death of individual patients that are above 28% but do not reach 50%. If we consider the cost of failing to spot a death as twice that of incorrectly predicting death, a different pattern emerges, shown in Table 11.3. (With this cost pattern we predict death if the probability of survival is less than 2/3.)

Under this cost pattern the methods from survival analysis show a clear superiority, and within the class the non-linear methods show a substantial advantage over the linear ones. However, as this data set is so small, only the larger differences (those between the first 'binary classification' line and the rest) are statistically significant when assessed by paired t-tests.

All the methods had been set up to predict probabilities of observed events, so it was easy to recompute the results for a different pattern of costs. There are technical arguments (Ripley 1996) that suggest we might have obtained (slightly) improved results by taking the cost pattern into account during training by weighting examples in the training set.

Acknowledgements

R.M.R. was supported by an EPSRC grant during this work. Mark Mathieson supplied the code for the proportional-odd models.

REFERENCES

Abu-Mostafa, Y. S. (1995). Machines that learn from hints. *Scientific American* **272**(4), 64–69.

Andersen, P. K., Borgan, Ø., Gill, R. D. & Keiding, N. (1993). *Statistical Models based on Counting Processes*. Springer-Verlag, New York.

Baxt, W. G. (1995). Application of artificial neural networks to clinical medicine. *Lancet* **346**, 1135–1138.

Biganzoli, E., Boracchi, P., Mariani, L. & Marubini, E. (1998). Feed forward neural networks for the analysis of censored survival data: a partial logistic regression approach. *Statistics in Medicine* **17**, 1169–1186.

Bishop, C. M. (1995). *Neural Networks for Pattern Recognition.* Clarendon Press, Oxford.

Bottaci, L., Drew, P. J., Hartley, J. E., Hadfield, M. B., Farouk, R., Lee, P. W. R., Macintyre, I. M. C., Duthie, G. S. & Monson, J. R. T. (1997). Artificial neural networks applied to outcome prediction for colorectal cancer patients in separate institutions. *Lancet* **350**, 469–472.

Breiman, L. (1996). Bagging predictors. *Machine Learning* **24**, 123–140.

Breiman, L., Friedman, J. H., Olshen, R. A. & Stone, C. J. (1984). *Classification and Regression Trees.* Wadsworth and Brooks/Cole, Monterey, CA.

Bridle, J. S. (1990a). Probabilistic interpretation of feedforward classification network outputs, with relationships to statistical pattern recognition. In F. Fogelman Soulié & J. Hérault, eds., *Neuro-computing: Algorithms, Architectures and Applications.* Springer-Verlag, Berlin, pp. 227–236.

Bridle, J. S. (1990b). Training stochastic model recognition algorithms as networks can lead to maximum mutual information estimation of parameters. In D. S. Touretzky, ed., *Advances in Neural Information Processing Systems 2.* Morgan Kaufmann, San Mateo, CA, pp. 211–217.

Bugliosi, R., Tribalto, M., Avvisati, G., Boccadoro, M., De Martinis, C., Friera, R., Mandelli, F., Pileri, A. & Papa, G. (1994). Classification of patients affected by multiple myeloma using a neural network software. *European Journal of Haematology* **52**, 182–183.

Burke, H. B., Rosen, D. B. & Goodman, P. H. (1995). Comparing the prediction accuracy of artificial neural networks and other statistical models for breast cancer survival. In G. Tesauro, D. S. Touretzky & T. K. Leen, eds., *Advances in Neural Information Processing Systems 7.* MIT Press, Cambridge, MA, pp. 1063–1067.

Cheng, B. & Titterington, D. M. (1994). Neural networks: a review from a statistical perspective. *Statistical Science* **9**, 2–54.

Ciampi, A., Chang, C.-H., Hogg, S. & McKinney, S. (1987). Recursive partitioning: a versatile method for exploratory data analysis in biostatistics. In I. B. MacNeil & G. J. Umphrey, eds., *Biostatistics.* Reidel, Dordrecht, pp. 23–50.

Collett, D. (1994). *Modelling Survival Data in Medical Research.* Chapman & Hall, London.

Cox, D. R. (1972). Regresson models and life-tables (with discussion). *Journal of the Royal Statistical Society series B* **34**, 187–220.

Davis, R. & Anderson, J. (1989). Exponential survival trees. *Statistics in Medicine* **8**, 947–961.

Dobson, R. (1997). Program predicts cancer deaths. *The Sunday Times* 28 September, 'Innovations' section.

Dybowski, R. & Gant, V. (1995). Artificial neural networks in pathology and medical laboratories. *Lancet* **346**, 1203–1207.

Efron, B. (1988). Logistic regression, survival analysis and the Kaplan–Meier curve. *Journal of the American Statistical Association* **83**, 414–425.

Faraggi, D. & Simon, R. (1995). A neural network model for survival data. *Statistics in Medicine* **14**, 73–82.

Freund, Y. & Schapire, R. E. (1995). A decision-theoretic generalization of on-line learning and an application to boosting. In *Proceedings of the 2nd European Conference on Computational Learning Theory*. Springer-Verlag, Berlin, pp. 23–37.

Friedman, J. H. (1991). Multivariate adaptive regression splines (with discussion). *Annals of Statistics* **19**, 1–141.

Friedman, J. H. & Stuetzle, W. (1981). Projection pursuit regression. *Journal of the American Statistical Association* **76**, 817–823.

Gentleman, R. & Crowley, J. (1991). Local full likelihood estimation for the proportional hazards model. *Biometrics* **47**, 1283–1296.

Gray, R. J. (1992). Flexible methods for analyzing survival data using splines, wth applications to breast cancer prognosis. *Journal of the American Statistical Association* **87**, 942–951.

Gray, R. J. (1996). Hazard rate regression using ordinary nonparametric regression smoothers. *Journal of Computational and Graphical Statistics* **5**, 190–207.

Hastie, T. J. & Tibshirani, R. J. (1990). *Generalized Additive Models*. Chapman & Hall, London.

Haykin, S. (1994). *Neural Networks. A Comprehensive Foundation*. Macmillan College Publishing, New York.

Hertz, J., Krogh, A. & Palmer, R. G. (1991). *Introduction to the Theory of Neural Computation*. Addison-Wesley, Redwood City, CA.

Kalbfleisch, J. D. & Prentice, R. L. (1980). *The Statistical Analysis of Failure Time Data*. Wiley, New York.

Kappen, H. J. & Neijt, J. P. (1993). Neural network analysis to predict treatment outcome. *Annals of Oncology* **4**, S31–S34.

Kooperberg, C., Bose, S. & Stone, C. J. (1997). Polychotomous regression. *Journal of the American Statistical Association* **92**, 117–127.

Kooperberg, C., Stone, C. J. & Truong, Y. K. (1995). Hazard regression. *Journal of the American Statistical Association* **90**, 78–94.

Lapuerta, P., Azen, S. P. & LaBree, L. (1995). Use of neural networks in predicting the risk of coronary-artery disease. *Computers and Biomedical Research* **28**, 38–52.

LeBlanc, M. & Crowley, J. (1992). Relative risk trees for censored survival data. *Biometrics* **48**, 411–425.

LeBlanc, M. & Crowley, J. (1993). Survival trees by goodness of split. *Journal of the American Statistical Association* **88**, 457–467.

Liestøl, K., Andersen, P. K. & Andersen, U. (1994). Survival analysis and neural nets. *Statistics in Medicine* **13**, 1189–1200.

Lowe, D. & Webb, A. (1990). Exploiting prior knowledge in network optimization: an illustration from medical prognosis. *Network* **1**, 299–323.

Mariani, L., Coradini, D., Biganzoli, E., Boracchi, P., Marubini, E., Pilotti, S., Salvadori, B., Silvestrini, R., Veronesi, U., Zucali, R. & Rilke, F. (1997). Prognostic factors for metachronous contralateral breast cancer: a comparison of the linear Cox regression model and its artificial neural network extension. *Breast Cancer Research and Treatment* **44**, 167–178.

Mathieson, M. J. (1996). Ordinal models for neural networks. In A.-P. N. Refenes, Y. Abu-Mostafa, J. Moody & A. Weigend, eds., *Neural Networks in Financial Engineering*. World Scientific, Singapore, pp. 523–536.

Mathieson, M. J. (1997). Ordered classes and incomplete examples in classification. In M. C. Mozer, M. J. Jordan & T. Petsche, eds., *Advances in Neural Information Processing Systems 9*. MIT Press, Cambridge, MA, pp. 550–556.

MathSoft Data Analysis Products Division (1987–97) *S-PLUS*. Seattle, WA.

Ohno-Machado, L. (1997). A comparison of Cox proportional hazards and artificial neural network models for medical prognosis. *Computers in Biology and Medicine* 27, 55–65.

Ohno-Machado, L. & Musen, M. A. (1997). Modular neural networks for medical prognosis: quantifying the benefits of combining neural networks for survival prediction. *Connection Science* 9, 71–86.

O'Sullivan, F. (1988). Nonparametric estimation of relative risk using splines and cross-validation. *SIAM Journal of Scientific and Statistical Computing* 9, 531–542.

Pardey, J., Roberts, S., Tarassenko, L. & Stradling, J. (1996). A new approach to the analysis of the human sleep/wakefulness continuum. *Journal of Sleep Research* 5, 201–210.

Perrone, M. P. & Cooper, L. N. (1993). When networks disagree: ensemble methods for hybrid neural networks. In R. J. Mammone, ed., *Artificial Neural Networks for Speech and Vision*. Chapman & Hall, London, pp. 126–142.

Ravdin, P. M. & Clark, G. M. (1992). A practical application of neural network analysis for predicting outcome of individual breast cancer patients. *Breast Cancer Research and Treatment* 22, 285–293.

Ravdin, P. M., Clark, G. M., Hilsenbeck, S. G., Owens, M. A., Vendely, P., Pandian, M. R. & McGuire, W. L. (1992). A demonstration that breast cancer recurrence can be predicted by neural network analysis. *Breast Cancer Research and Treatment* 21, 47–53.

Ripley, B. D. (1993). Statistical aspects of neural networks. In O. E. Barndorff-Nielsen, J. L. Jensen & W. S. Kendall, eds., *Networks and Chaos – Statistical and Probabilistic Aspects*. Chapman & Hall, London, pp. 40–123.

Ripley, B. D. (1994a). Flexible non-linear approaches to classification. In V. Cherkassky, J. H. Friedman & H. Wechsler, eds., *From Statistics to Neural Networks. Theory and Pattern Recognition Applications*. Springer-Verlag, Berlin, pp. 105–126.

Ripley, B. D. (1994b). Neural networks and flexible regression and discrimination. In K. V. Mardia, ed., *Statistics and Images 2*. Carfax, Abingdon, pp. 39–57.

Ripley, B. D. (1994c). Neural networks and related methods for classification. *Journal of the Royal Statistical Society series B* 56, 409–456.

Ripley, B. D. (1996). *Pattern Recognition and Neural Networks*. Cambridge University Press, Cambridge.

Ripley, R. M., Harris, A. L. & Tarassenko, L. (1998). Neural networks models for breast cancer prognosis. *Neural Computing and Applications* 7, 367–375.

Schwarzer, G. Vach, W. & Schumacher, M. (1997). On the misuses of artificial neural networks for prognosis and diagnostic classification in oncology. Technical Report. Center for Data Analysis and Model Building, University of Freiburg.

Segal, M. R. (1988). Regression trees for censored data. *Biometrics* 44, 35–47.

Tarassenko, L., Whitehouse, R., Gasparini, G. & Harris, A. L. (1996). Neural network prediction of relapse in breast cancer patients. *Neural Computing and Applications* 4, 105–113.

Theeuwen, M., Kappen, B. & Neijt, J. (1995). Neural network analysis to predict treatment outcome in patients with ovarian cancer. In F. Fogelman Soulié & G. Dreyfus, eds., *Proceedings Session 5, Medicine, International Conference on Artificial Neural Networks*. Paris, France.

Therneau, T. M., Grambsch, P. M. & Fleming, T. R. (1990). Martingale-based residuals for survival models. *Biometrika* 77, 147–160.

Titterington, D. M., Murray, G. D., Murray, L. S., Spiegelhalter, D. J., Skene, A. M., Habbema, J. D. F. & Gelpka, G. J. (1981). Comparison of discrimination techniques applied to a complex data set of head injured patients. *Journal of the Royal Statistical Society series B* 144, 145–174.

Venables, W. N. & Ripley, B. D. (1997). *Modern Applied Statistics with S-PLUS*, 2nd edn. Springer-Verlag, New York.

Wahba, G. (1990). *Spline Models for Observational Data*. SIAM, Philadelphia.

Wahba, G., Gu, C., Wang, Y. & Chappell, R. (1995). Soft classification a.k.a. risk estimation via penalized log likelihood and smoothing spline analysis of variance. In D. H. Wolpert, ed., *The Mathematics of Generalization*. Addison-Wesley, Reading, MA, pp. 331–359.

Watt, R. C., Sisemore, C. S., Kanemoto, A., Malan, T. P. & Frink, E. J. (1995). Neural networks applied to the bispectral analysis of EEG during anesthesia. *Anesthesiology* 83, A503.

Wolpert, D. H. (1992). Stacked generalization. *Neural Networks* 5, 241–259.

12

A review of techniques for extracting rules from trained artificial neural networks

Robert Andrews, Alan B. Tickle and Joachim Diederich

Introduction

Even a quick glance through the literature reveals that artificial neural networks (ANNs) have been applied across a broad spectrum of biomedical problem domains. ANNs have been used to aid in the diagnosis of cervical cancer (Mehdi et al. 1994; Mango et al. 1994) and breast cancer (Downes 1994; Feltham & Xing 1994). ANNs have also been applied to prediction tasks including the likelihood of onset of myocardial infarction (Browner 1992) and the survival rates of cancer sufferers (Burke 1994). Other application areas include interpretation of medical images (Lo et al. 1994; Silverman & Noetzel 1990), the interpretation of electrocardiograph data (Kennedy et al. 1991) and biochemical analysis. ANN architectures used in these studies include feedforward multilayer networks trained by back-propagation, recurrent networks (Blumenfeld 1990), self-organizing maps (Dorffner et al. 1993), neurofuzzy systems (Tan & Carpenter 1993) and hybrid systems (Pattichis et al. 1994).

The ANN approach has been demonstrated to have several benefits including the following:

ANNs can be trained by examples drawn from the problem domain rather than rules laboriously drawn from human experts.

ANNs are tolerant of 'noise' in the input data.

ANNs can, with a high degree of accuracy, 'generalize' over a set of unseen examples.

The use of a trained ANN eliminates issues associated with human fatigue and habituation (Eisner 1990; Boon & Kok 1993).

The use of an automated approach allows analysis of conditions and diagnosis in real time.

Somewhat surprisingly there appears to have been little effort made to understand the hows and whys of the behaviour of the trained ANN. The reporting of experimental results for cases where ANNs perform as well as, or even outperform, statistical, symbolic artificial intelligence (AI) techniques and even human experts has been sufficient encouragement for continued research into the use of ANNs for biomedical applications. However, experience has shown that an explanation capability is considered to be one of the most important functions provided by symbolic AI systems. In particular, the salutary lesson from the introduction and operation of knowledge based systems is that the ability to generate even limited explanations (in terms of being meaningful and coherent) is absolutely crucial for the user-acceptance of such systems (Davis et al. 1977). In contrast to symbolic AI systems, ANNs have no explicit declarative knowledge representation. Therefore they have considerable difficulty in generating the required explanation structures. Rule extraction provides, among other things, a means of deriving an explanation structure from a trained ANN that can give a human user insight into the decision-making processes of the trained ANN, thus allowing the user to verify that the ANN is utilizing a clinically sound basis for it decisions.

This chapter includes a discussion on the benefits that may accrue to users from including rule extraction as part of the overall use of trained ANNs, a discussion of a schema proposed by Andrews et al. (1995) for categorizing rule extraction algorithms, and a review of a set of rule extraction techniques representative of the major classes of the schema. For each technique an indication is given of whether the technique has been applied to medical domain databases. The chapter concludes with a look at current issues and directions in the field of rule extraction from trained ANNs.

The merits of including rule extraction as an adjunct to the use of a trained ANN

Andrews et al. (1995) discussed several advantages for the ANN paradigm by including rule extraction:

provision of a user explanation facility
extension of ANN systems to safety critical areas
software verification and debugging of ANN components in software systems
improving the generalization of ANN solutions
data exploration and the induction of scientific theories
knowledge acquisition for symbolic systems.

Provision of a user explanation capability

Within the field of symbolic AI the term *explanation* refers to an explicit structure that can be used internally for reasoning and learning, and externally for the explanation of results to a user. Users of symbolic AI systems benefit from an explicit declarative representation of knowledge about the problem domain, typically in the form of object hierarchies, semantic networks, frames etc. The explanation capability of symbolic AI also includes the intermediate steps of the reasoning process, for example a trace of rule firings or a proof structure, which can be used to answer 'How' questions. Further, Gallant (1988) observed that the attendant benefits of an explanation capability are that it also provides a check on the internal logic of the system as well as enabling a novice user to gain insights into the problem at hand.

While provision of an explanation capability is a significant innovation in the ongoing development of ANNs, of equal importance is the *quality* of the explanations delivered. It is here that the evolution of explanation capabilities in symbolic AI offers some valuable lessons into how this task of extracting rules from trained ANNs might be directed. For example practitioners in the field of symbolic AI have experimented with various forms of user explanation vehicles, including, in particular, rule traces. However, for some time it has been clear that explanations based on rule traces are too rigid and inflexible (Gilbert 1989; Moore 1989; Moore & Swartout 1989). Indeed one of the major criticisms of utilizing rule traces is that they always reflect the current structure of the knowledge base. Further, rule traces may have references to internal procedures (e.g. calculations), might include repetitions (e.g. if an inference was made more than once) and the granularity of the explanation is often inappropriate (Gilbert 1989). Perhaps one clear lesson from using rule traces is that the transparency of an explanation is by no means guaranteed. For example, experience has shown that an explanation based on rule traces from a poorly organized rule base with perhaps hundreds of premises per rule could not be regarded as being *transparent*.

A further example of the limitations of explanation capabilities in symbolic AI systems that should, if possible, be obviated in the extraction of rules from trained ANNs, comes from Moore & Swartout (1989). They note that the early use of *canned* text or templates as part of user explanations has been shown to be too rigid, that systems always interpret questions in the same way, and that the response strategies are inadequate. Further, although efforts have been made to take advantage of natural-language dialogues with artifices such as mixed initiatives, user-models and explicitly planned explanation strategies (Moore & Swartout 1989), there is little doubt that current systems are still too inflexible, unresponsive, incoherent, insensitive and too rigid (W. R. Swartout, unpublished data, 1989).

In summary, while the integration of an explanation capability (via rule extraction) within a trained ANN is crucial for user acceptance, such capabilities must if possible obviate the problems already encountered in symbolic AI.

Extension of ANN systems to 'safety-critical' problem domains

While the provision of a user explanation capability is one of the key benefits in extracting rules from trained ANNs, it is certainly not the only one. For example within a trained ANN the capability should also exist for the user to determine whether the ANN has an optimal structure or size. (For instance if an input dimension does not appear as the antecedent in any extracted rule the network can be pruned to remove nodes associated with this input.) A concomitant requirement is for ANN solutions not only to be transparent as discussed above but also for the internal states of the system to be both accessible and able to be interpreted unambiguously. Satisfaction of such requirements would make a significant contribution to the task of identifying and if possible excluding those ANN-based solutions that have the potential to give erroneous results without any accompanying indication as to when and why a result is suboptimal.

Such a capability is mandatory if neural network-based solutions are to be accepted into a broader range of application areas and, in particular, *safety-critical* problem domains such as air traffic control, the operation of power plants, medical diagnosis and patient monitoring. Rule extraction offers the potential for providing such a capability.

Software verification and debugging of ANN components in software systems

A requirement of increasing significance in software-based systems is that of verification of the software itself. While the task of software verification is important it is also acknowledged as being difficult, particularly for large systems. Hence if ANNs are to be integrated within larger software systems that need to be verified, then clearly this requirement must be met by the ANN as well. At their current level of development, rule extraction algorithms do not allow for the verification of trained ANNs, i.e. they do not prove that a network behaves according to some specification. However, rule extraction algorithms provide a mechanism for either partially or completely *decompiling* a trained ANN. This is seen as a promising vehicle for achieving the required goal at least indirectly by enabling a comparison to be made between the extracted rules and the software specification.

Examination of the extracted rules may allow the user to determine regions of input space where the network produces correct output, false negative or false positive outputs. This is important for ANNs trained in medical problem domains where it is important for the user to be able to attach a degree of certainty to the conclusion reached by the ANN.

Improving the generalization of ANN solutions

Where a limited or unrepresentative data set from the problem domain has been used in the ANN training process, it is difficult to determine when generalization can fail, even with evaluation methods such as cross-validation. By being able to express the knowledge embedded within the trained ANN as a set of symbolic rules, the rule extraction process may provide an experienced system user with the capability to anticipate or predict a set of circumstances under which generalization failure can occur. Alternatively the system user may be able to use the extracted rules to identify regions in input space that are not represented sufficiently in the existing ANN training set data and to supplement the data set accordingly.

Data exploration and the induction of scientific theories

Over time neural networks have proved to be extremely powerful tools for data exploration, with the capability to discover previously unknown dependencies and relationships in data sets. As Craven & Shavlik (1994) observed, 'a [learning] system may discover salient features in the input data whose importance was not previously recognized.' This is of particular interest to practitioners in the medical domain, where complex interrelationships of the various factors relevant to diagnosis and prognosis may exist in the clinical data but may not be recognized by the practitioner. However, even if a trained ANN has learned interesting and possibly non-linear relationships, these relationships are encoded incomprehensibly as weight vectors within the trained ANN and hence cannot easily serve the generation of scientific theories. Rule extraction algorithms significantly enhance the capabilities of ANNs to explore data to the benefit of the user.

Knowledge acquisition for symbolic AI systems

One of the principal reasons for introducing machine learning algorithms over the last decade was to overcome the so-called *knowledge acquisition* problem for symbolic AI systems (Saito & Nakano 1988; Sestito & Dillon 1991). Further, as Sestito & Dillon (1994, p. 156) observed, the most difficult, time-consuming, and expensive task in building an expert system is constructing and debugging its knowledge base.

The notion of using trained ANNs to assist in the knowledge acquisition task has existed for some time (Gallant 1988). An extension of these ideas is to use trained ANNs as vehicles for synthesizing the knowledge that is crucial for the success of knowledge-based systems. Alternatively, domain knowledge that is acquired by a knowledge engineering process may be used to constrain the size of the space searched during the learning phase and hence contribute to improved learning performance.

The necessary impetus for exploring these ideas could now come from two recent developments. The first is a set of recent benchmark results such as those of Thrun et al. (1991), where trained ANNs have been shown to outperform symbolic machine learning methods. The second is from developments in techniques for extracting from trained ANNs symbolic rules that could be directly added to the knowledge base.

Classification scheme for categorizing rule extraction techniques

Andrews et al. 1995; Tickle et al. 1999 presented a classification scheme for categorizing and describing rule extraction techniques. The scheme is based on:

the expressive power of the extracted rules

the *translucency* of the view taken by the rule extraction algorithm of the underlying ANN

the use of a specialized training regime or network architecture

the quality of the extracted rules

the algorithmic complexity of the rule extraction technique.

Expressive power of the extracted rules

Expressive power is taken to describe the form of the extracted rules. Most commonly rule extraction techniques use either conventional two-valued Boolean logic *if . . . then . . . else* rules or fuzzy rules that use the concept of membership functions to represent *partial* truths and can include probabilistic certainty factors in the rule conclusion. While methods that extract propositional rules form the bulk of the rule extraction techniques described to date, there are a variety of methods that extract rules in other formats. A small set of techniques extract so-called *M-of-N* rules first described by Towell & Shavlik (1993). *M-of-N* rules are of the form *if* M *of the following* N *antecedent conditions are true then the rule consequent is true.* The use of *M-of-N* rules was extended by Craven (1996) to a technique that extracts decision trees from any learned model where *M-of-N* rules are used in the nodes of the decision tree. Saito & Nakano (1996) described a technique that extracts scientific laws in which the power values are not restricted to integers. Nayak et al. (1997) described a technique where propositional rules are extracted from a feedforward network and used to generate a knowledge base of generic predicates, rules and facts for a connectionist knowledge representation system that is capable of dynamically binding variables to values.

The translucency of the view taken by the rule extraction algorithm of the underlying ANN

Andrews et al. 1995; Tickle et al. 1999 used translucency to describe the degree to which a rule extraction algorithm makes use of knowledge of the network weights and architecture in extracting rules. At one end of the translucency continuum are the *decompositional* algorithms that extract rules at the level of individual hidden and output units. The rules extracted from each unit are then aggregated to form the composite rule base extracted from the network as a whole. A basic requirement of decompositional algorithms is that the computed output of the ANN node under consideration must be mapped into a binary (*yes/no*) output that corresponds to the notion of a rule consequent. Hence each hidden or output unit can be interpreted as a *step* function or a Boolean rule that reduces the rule extraction problem to one of determining the situations in which the rule is *true*, i.e. when a subset of the incoming links has a summed value that exceeds the unit's bias regardless of the values of the other incoming links. *Pedagogical* rule extraction techniques, on the other hand, assume no knowledge of network architecture and treat the network as a 'black box'. In general, pedagogical techniques use the trained network to attach a class label to a set of examples/cases that are either drawn from the training data or generated/sampled from the entire input space. These labelled examples then are noise free and contain no conflicts. A symbolic learning method is then employed to generate rules that map inputs directly to outputs. Between decompositional and pedagogical techniques are the so-called *eclectic* techniques that utilize knowledge of the network weights and architecture to complement a symbolic learning algorithm.

The use of a specialized training regime

This aspect of the rule extraction algorithm is important because it provides a measure of the portability of the technique. Rule extraction techniques that are tightly coupled to the architecture of a particular ANN are not portable and cannot be applied immediately to any in situ trained network. Instead, for the particular rule extraction technique to be applicable, the associated network must first be trained on the problem domain with the possibility that this network may not give optimum performance.

The quality of the extracted rules

Towell & Shavlik (1993) proposed criteria by which the quality of the extracted sets could be assessed. These criteria were revised by Andrews et al. (1995) and include (a) the accuracy, (b) the fidelity, (c) the consistency, and (d) the comprehensibility of the extracted rule sets.

In this context a rule set is considered to be *accurate* if it can correctly classify previously unseen examples. (Accuracy is calculated as the percentage of correctly classified patterns in the test set data.) Similarly a rule set is considered to display a high level of *fidelity* if it can mimic the behaviour of the ANN from which it was extracted by capturing all of the information embodied in the ANN. (Fidelity here is calculated as the percentage agreement between the generalization performance of the ANN on the test set and the generalization performance of the extracted rule set on the test set data.) A rule extraction algorithm is deemed to be *consistent* if, under different runs of the algorithm on the same trained ANN and test set the algorithm generates the same rule set. Finally the *comprehensibility* of a rule set is determined by measuring the size of the rule set (in terms of the number of rules) and the number of antecedents per rule.

The algorithmic complexity of the rule extraction technique

The inclusion of this dimension of the classification scheme reflects the necessity for any rule extraction technique to be as efficient as possible. Many of the algorithms that are discussed in this chapter require the use of either a *search and test* strategy through weight space (decompositional algorithms) or a *generate and test* strategy through input space (pedagogical techniques). Clearly the efficiency of the algorithm is dependent on the size of the weight space to be searched or the number of cases that must be generated to adequately 'cover' the input space. Algorithms that rely on an exhaustive search of weight/input space to generate all possible rules are inefficient because the size of the space to be searched grows exponentially with the number of input dimensions. Algorithms that employ heuristics to limit the search space reduce algorithmic complexity but increase the likelihood of overlooking potentially important rules that are represented by only a small number of examples in the search space. The goal then is to find heuristics that make the algorithm tractable without adversely affecting rule quality.

It should be observed at this point that it may not be possible, or even desirable, to simultaneously optimize all of the above-mentioned evaluation criteria. For example, in safety-critical applications such as patient monitoring systems or automated diagnostic systems a high premium should be placed on accuracy and fidelity at the possible expense of rule comprehensibility.

Decompositional rule extraction techniques

The earliest decompositional algorithm is the KT approach described by Fu (1991, 1994). The KT algorithm extracts Boolean rules at the level of individual hidden and output units within a multilayer, feedforward network that has been trained by back-propagation. The algorithm searches for sets of weights containing a single positively weighted link, $link_n$, sufficient to exceed the bias of the unit under consideration regardless of the weights of the other incoming links. If such a link is found, a rule of the form *if input$_n$, then the concept represented by the unit is true* is written where $input_n$ is the input node connected to the unit under consideration by $link_n$. KT maps the output from each unit into a Boolean function via the simple artifice of *if $0 \leq output \leq threshold\_1 \Rightarrow no$*, and *if $threshold\_1 \leq output \leq threshold\_2 \Rightarrow yes$*, where $threshold\_1 \leq threshold\_2$. The search then proceeds to look for subsets of two incoming links etc. At the completion of the process, the rules extracted from the individual units are aggregated to form the composite rule base for the ANN as a whole.

A more recent example of this style of approach is the Subset algorithm of Towell & Shavlik (1993). For Subset the network is constructed in such a way that the output of each unit is either *near* a value of 1 (i.e. maximally active), or *near* a

Table 12.1. The Subset algorithm

For each hidden and output unit:

    extract up to S_p subsets of the positively weighted incoming links for which the summed weight is greater than the bias on the unit;

    For each element p of the S_p subsets:

    – search for a set S_N of a set of negative attributes so that the summed weights of p plus the summed weights of $N-n$ (where N is the set of all negative attributes and n is an element of S_N) exceed the threshold on the unit;

    – with each element n of the set S_N form a rule: 'if p and NOT n then the concept designated by the unit'

value of 0 (inactive). Hence each link carries a signal equal to its weight or no signal at all. The Subset algorithm is given in Table 12.1.

While Fu (1991, 1994) reported initial success with KT in the problem domain of detecting wind shears by infrared sensors and Towell & Shavlik (1993) showed that their algorithm is capable of delivering a set of rules that are at least potentially tractable and 'smaller than many handcrafted expert systems' (Towell & Shavlik 1993), both analyses suffer the same problem, i.e. the solution time for finding all possible subsets of suitable incoming links is a function of the size of the power set of links to each unit – the algorithm is exponential.

To make the algorithm more tractable Fu (1991, 1994) restricted the search space by placing a limit on the maximum number of antecedents per rule. Saito & Nakano (1988) restricted the search space by placing a limit on the depth of the search. Both these heuristics have the potential for adverse rule quality outcomes as the method could overlook some important rules.

Maire (1997), Krishnan (1996) and Nayak et al. (1997) all suggested methods based on weight ordering to limit the search space without overlooking important rules. The method suggested by Maire (1997) is similar to the COMBO algorithm (Krishnan 1996). COMBO is applicable to feedforward networks with Boolean inputs. COMBO first sorts the incoming weights of a particular node in descending magnitude then forms a 'combination tree' of the sorted weights. The combination tree for a unit with four incoming weights (already sorted) is shown in Figure 12.1. The premise is that judicious pruning of the combination tree can reduce the search space while at the same time preserving all important rules. Pruning can occur:

1. *At the same level in the tree.* If any combination at any level fails then all other combinations at this level can be pruned away. This is because all the combinations at the same level have the same length, and, because of the ordering of the

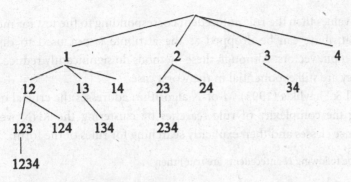

Figure 12.1. A combination tree.

weights, if a combination at a level fails, then all other combinations at the same level will also fail as their weighted sum will be less than the weighted sum of the combination that failed. Hence they need not be considered in the search for rules.

2. *At deeper levels of the tree.* If a combination at a level succeeds in forming a rule then all combinations in the subtree of which it is a root can be pruned away. Although these combinations will also succeed in forming a rule, these rules will be less general than the rule formed from the root of the subtree.

The LAP technique described by Nayak et al. (1997) is suitable for application to feedforward networks with Boolean inputs and extracts all possible rules from each hidden and output node of the network. LAP assumes an N-dimensional input such that any input vector x_i has N corresponding attributes $A_1, A_2, \ldots A_N$ and any attribute A_j has $\| A_j \| > 1$ associated possible values that correspond to network inputs, which is sparse coded to a k-dimensional input space in $\{0, 1\}^k$ where $k = \Sigma_{j=1}^{N} \| A_j \|$. Sets of weights corresponding to each attribute are formed and then ordered. A sum is formed from the largest weight from each set and this sum is tested against the bias to see whether the unit will have a high output. A procedure that recursively drops weights and tests the sum of the maximum weights of those remaining in the sets against the network bias is employed to find a set of inputs in each dimension such that dropping any of them will cause the unit not to fire. The resulting set can be expressed as a rule of the form:

IF x_i value for attribute $1 \in \{$subset of attribute 1 values$\}$
AND x_i value for attribute $2 \in \{$subset of attribute 2 values$\}$
. . .
AND x_i value for attribute $N \in \{$subset of attribute N values$\}$
THEN   perceptron will fire

where x_i is some input vector. If any subset of values for an attribute contains all possible values then the rule antecedent corresponding to the test for membership for the attribute can be dropped as the attribute is not used to discriminate between input vectors. Although these methods do significantly reduce the search space they are still exponential in the worst case.

Towell & Shavlik's (1993) M-of-N algorithm addresses the crucial question of reducing the complexity of rule searches by clustering the ANN weights into equivalence classes and then explicitly searching for rules of the form:

If (M of the following N antecedents are true) then . . .

For example, with reference to the unit shown below:

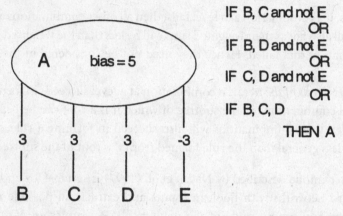

the four extracted rules could be written as the single rule

If 3 of (B,C,D, not E) then A.

Towell & Shavlik (1993) cited as one of the main attractions of the M-of-N approach a natural affinity between M-of-N rules and the *inductive bias* of ANNs. Towell & Shavlik used two dimensions, namely (a) 'the rules must accurately categorize examples that were not seen during training', and (b) 'the extracted rules must capture the information contained' in the knowledge-based ANN (KNN), for assessing the quality of rules extracted both from their own algorithm and from the set of algorithms they use for the purposes of comparison. In their view the M-of-N idea inherently yields a more compact rule representation than conventional conjunctive rules produced by algorithms such as Subset. In addition the M-of-N algorithm outperformed a subset of published symbolic learning algorithms in terms of the accuracy and fidelity of the rule set extracted from a cross-section of problem domains including two from the field of molecular biology, namely the *gene promoter recognition* problem and the *splice-junction determination* problem. The phases of M-of-N algorithm are shown in Table 12.2.

Techniques that can directly decompile network weights to rules obviate the

Table 12.2. The M-of-N technique

---

1. Generate an artificial neural network using the KBANN system and train using back-propagation. With each hidden and output unit, form groups of similarly weighted links.
2. Set link weights of all group members to the average of the group.
3. Eliminate any groups that do not significantly affect whether the unit will be active or inactive.
4. Holding all link weights constant, optimize biases of all hidden and output units using the back-propagation algorithm.
5. Form a single rule for each hidden and output unit; the rule consists of a threshold given by the bias and weighted antecedents specified by the remaining links.
6. Where possible, simplify rules to eliminate superfluous weights and thresholds.

KBANN, knowledge-based artificial neural network.

need to involve exhaustive search-and-test strategies in the rule extraction algorithm and thus make the algorithm computationally efficient. In order that direct decompilation be possible, a meaning relevant to the problem domain must be able to be ascribed to each:

1. hidden and output unit of the ANN; and
2. each weight of each hidden and output unit.

Local function networks such as radial basis function (RBF) networks with a single hidden layer of basis function units perform function approximation and classification by mapping a local region of input space (hypercube or hyperellipsoid) directly to an output. Conditions (1) and (2) above can be met by either constraining the network such that at most one hidden unit exhibits appreciable activation in response to an input pattern, or by including in the extracted rule a 'belief value' or 'certainty factor' that indicates the degree to which the individual unit contributed to the output.

Under these circumstances individual hidden units can be decompiled to form a rule of the form:

IF   the input lies in the hypercube represented by the hidden unit
THEN   consequent represented by the hidden unit output is TRUE.

Examples of rule extraction by direct decompilation of weights to rules include the method described by Tresp et al. (1993), the RULEX algorithm of Andrews & Geva (1995, 1996a,b, 1997) and the technique described by Berthold & Huber (1995a,b). (A more complete description of RULEX and the method described by Tresp et al. can be found under Rule refinement, p. 277, below.)

Berthold & Huber (1995a,b) structure their rectangular basis function (RecBF) networks in such a way that there is a one-to-one correspondence between hidden

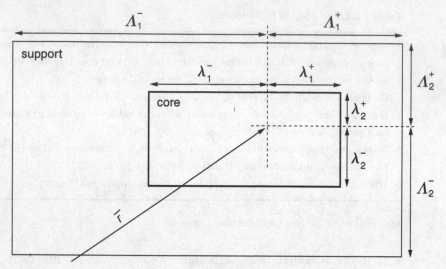

Figure 12.2. A RecBF unit. For explanation of symbols, see the text.

units and rules. RecBF networks consist of an input layer, a hidden layer of RecBF units, and an output layer with each unit in the output layer representing a class. The hidden units of RecBF networks are constructed as *hyper-rectangles* with their training algorithm derived from that used to train RBF networks.

The hyper-rectangles are parameterized by a reference vector, *r*, which gives the centre of the rectangle, and two sets of radii, $\lambda_i^{+,-}$, which defines the *core*-rectangle, and $\Lambda_i^{+,-}$, which describes the *support* rectangle (see Figure 12.2).

The core rectangle includes data points that definitely belong to the class and the boundary of the support rectangle excludes data points that definitely *do not* belong to the class, i.e. the support rectangle is simply an area where there are no data points.

$R(\cdot)$, the activation function for a RecBF unit is:

$$R(\boldsymbol{x}) = \min_{1 \leq i \leq n} A(\boldsymbol{x}_i, \boldsymbol{r}_i, \lambda_i^-, \lambda_i^+), \tag{12.1}$$

where *x* represents the input vector, *r* represents the reference vector of the unit, *σ* (see below) is a vector representing individual radii in each dimension and $A(\cdot)$ is the Signum activation function:

$$A(\boldsymbol{x}_i, \boldsymbol{r}_i, \boldsymbol{\sigma}_i) = \begin{cases} 1: r - \lambda_i^- \leq x_i \leq r_i + \lambda_i^+ \\ 0: \text{else} \end{cases}. \tag{12.2}$$

Training the RecBF network is by the dynamic decay algorithm (DDA) (Berthold & Huber 1995a). This algorithm is based on three steps:

Covered: a new training point lies inside the support rectangle of an existing RecBF. Extend the core rectangle of the RecBF to cover the new point.

Commit: a new pattern is *not* covered by a RecBF of the correct class. Add a new RecBF with centre the same as the training instance and widths as large as possible to avoid overlapping any existing RecBF.

Shrink: a new pattern is incorrectly classified by an existing RecBF. The RecBF's widths are shrunk so that the conflict is resolved.

Because RecBF hyper-rectangles have finite radii in each input dimension a straightforward conversion from RecBF weights to rules can be performed resulting in rules of the form:

IF $\qquad 1 \le i \le n : x_i \in [r_i - \lambda_i^-, r_i - \lambda_i^+] \subset (r_i - \Lambda_i^-, r_i - \Lambda_i^+)$
THEN   Class c.

Here $[r_i - \lambda_i^-, r_i - \lambda_i^+]$ represents the core rectangle region of the RecBF unit and $(r_i - \Lambda_i^-, r_i - \Lambda_i^+)$ represents the support rectangle region of the RecBF unit.

Rules of this form have a condition clause for each of the n dimensions of the problem domain. This reduces the comprehensibility of the extracted rule set by including rules that contain antecedents for *don't care* dimensions i.e. dimensions that the network does not use to discriminate between input patterns. *Don't care* dimensions are those where $r_i - \lambda_i^- \le x_{i\min}$ and $r_i - \lambda_i^+ \ge x_{i\max}$ where $x_{i\min}$ is the smallest possible allowable value of the i-th input dimension and $x_{i\max}$ is the largest possible allowable value of the i-th input dimension. Using the above scheme condition clauses for *don't care* dimensions are removed from the rules extracted from RecBF networks.

Saito & Nakano's (1996) RF5 (rule extraction from facts version 5) algorithm extracts scientific laws of the form:

$$y_t = c_0 + \sum_{i=1}^{h} c_i x_{t1}^{w_{i1}} \ldots x_{tn}^{w_{in}},$$

where each parameter c_i or w_{ij} is an unknown real number and h is an unknown integer. The technique is based on an ANN that uses *product units* (Durbin & Rumelhart 1989) in the hidden layer. Product units calculate a weighted product of input values, where each input value is raised to a power determined by a variable weight. Saito & Nakano (1996) developed their own second-order learning algorithm called BPQ. After training, each product unit represents a term in the above expression. Because it is not possible to determine a priori the optimum number of hidden layer product units, several networks with different numbers of hidden layer units are trained and then a technique called minimum description length (MDL) criterion (Rissanen 1989) is utilized to select the best-law candidate

Table 12.3. The VIA algorithm

1. Assign arbitrary intervals to all (or a subset of all) units in the ANN. These intervals constitute constraints on the values for the inputs and the activations of the output.
2. Refine the intervals by iteratively detecting and excluding activation values that are provably inconsistent with the weights and biases of the network.
3. The result of step (2) is a set of intervals that are either consistent or inconsistent with the weights and biases of the network. (In this context an interval is defined as being inconsistent if there is no activation pattern whatsoever that can satisfy the constraints imposed by the initial validity intervals.)

from among the trained networks. The technique has been applied to artificial data with both integer and real-valued exponents and to real-world data including discover-ing Hagen–Ruben's law, Kepler's third law and Boyle's law. Experiments showed that RF5 successfully discovered the underlying laws even if the data contained a small amount of noise.

Pedagogical rule extraction techniques

One of the earliest published *pedagogical* approaches to rule extraction is that of Saito & Nakano (1988). In this implementation the underlying ANN is treated as a 'black box', with rules from a medical diagnostic problem domain being extracted from changes in the levels of the input and output units. Saito & Nakano also deal with the problem of constraining the size of the solution space to be searched by avoiding meaningless combinations of inputs (i.e. medical symptoms in this problem domain) and restricting the maximum number of coincident symptoms to be considered. Even with these heuristics in place, the number of rules extracted on a relatively simple problem domain was exceedingly large. This result high-lights one of the major concerns with rule extraction techniques, namely that the end-product is explanation and not obfuscation.

The validity interval analysis (VIA) technique developed by Thrun (1994) is the epitome of a pedagogical approach in that it extracts rules that map inputs directly into outputs. The algorithm uses a generate-and-test procedure to extract symbolic rules from standard back-propagation ANNs which have not been specifically constructed to facilitate rule extraction. The basic steps in the procedure are shown in Table 12.3.

Thrun (1994) likens the approach to sensitivity analysis in that it characterizes the output of the trained ANN by systematic variations in the input patterns and examining the changes in the network classification. The technique is fundamentally different from other techniques that analyse the activations of individual

Table 12.4. The rule-extraction-as-learning technique

```
/* initialize rules for each class */
  for each class c
    R_c := 0
  repeat
    e := Examples()
    c := Classify(e)
    if e not covered by R_c then
      /* learn a new rule */
      r := conjunctive rule formed from e
      for each antecedent r_i of r
        ŕ := r but with r_i dropped
        if Subset(c, ŕ) = true then r := ŕ
      R_c := R_c ∪ r
  until stopping criterion met
```

units within a trained ANN in that focus is on what are termed *validity intervals*. A validity interval of a unit specifies a maximum range for its activation value. The resultant technique provides a generic tool for checking the consistency of rules within a trained ANN. The VIA algorithm is designed as a *general purpose* rule extraction procedure. Thrun uses a number of examples to illustrate the efficacy of his VIA technique including (1) the XOR problem, (2) the 'Three Monks' problem(s), and (3) a robot arm kinematics (i.e. continuously valued domain) problem. While the VIA technique does not appear to be limited to any specific class of problem domains Thrun (1994) reported that VIA failed to generate a complete set of rules in a relatively complex problem domain involving the task of training a network to read aloud (*NETtalk*).

The *Rule-extraction-as-learning* approach of Craven & Shavlik (1994) is another significant development in rule extraction techniques utilizing the pedagogical approach. The core idea is to 'view rule extraction as a learning task where the target concept is the function computed by the network and the input features are simply the network's input features'. A schematic outline of the overall algorithm is shown in Table 12.4.

The role of the *Examples* function is to provide training examples for the rule-learning algorithm. The options used are (1) select members of the set used for training the ANN, (2) random sampling, or (3) random creation of examples of a specified class (see Table 12.5).

Craven & Shavlik use a function which they call *Subset* which is different from the Subset algorithm proposed by Towell & Shavlik (1993) to determine whether

Table 12.5. Option 3 of Examples algorithm in rule-extraction-as-learning

---

/* create a random example */

for each feature e_i with possible values $v_{i1}, \ldots, v_{in}$

$e_i := $ randomly-select$(v_{i1}, \ldots, v_{in})$.

calculate the total input s to output unit (which has a threshold value θ)

if $s \geq \theta$ then return e

impose random order on all feature values

/* consider the values in order */

for each value v_{ij}

   if changing feature e_i's value to v_{ij} increases s

     $e_i := v_{ij}$

   if $s \geq \theta$ then return e

---

the modified rule still agrees with the network, i.e. whether all instances that are covered by the rule are members of the given class.

A salient characteristic of this technique is that, depending on the particular implementation used, the rule-extraction-as-learning approach can be classified either as pedagogical or *decompositional*. The key is in the procedure used to establish if a given rule agrees with the network. This procedure accepts a class label c and a rule r, and returns *true* if all instances covered by r are classified as members of class c by the network. If, for example, Thrun's (1994) VIA algorithm (as discussed previously) is used for this procedure then the approach is pedagogical, whereas if an implementation such as that of Fu (1991) is used the classification of the technique is decompositional.

The algorithm is designed as a general purpose rule extraction procedure and its applicability does not appear to be limited to any specific class of problem domains. Craven and Shavlik illustrate the efficacy of their technique on the prokaryotic promoter recognition problem from the field of molecular biology.

One of the stated aims of the authors is to reduce the amount of computation to achieve the same degree of rule fidelity as the decompositional (or search-based) algorithms. One of the crucial differences between this algorithm and search-based extraction methods is that it explores the space of rules from the bottom up as distinct from the conventional top down approach.

As with the VIA technique discussed earlier, the rule-extraction-as-learning technique does not require a special training regime for the network. The authors suggest two *stopping criteria* for controlling the rule extraction algorithm: (1) estimating whether the extracted rule set is a sufficiently accurate model of the ANN from which the rules have been extracted; or (2) terminating after a certain number of iterations have resulted in no new rules (i.e. a *patience* criterion).

Craven's (1996) TREPAN (see Table 12.6) is a general purpose algorithm for

Table 12.6. The TREPAN algorithm

TREPAN (training_examples, features)

  Queue := 0;   /* sorted queue of nodes to expand */

  for each example $E \in$ training_examples   /*use trained ANN to label examples*/

    class label for E := ORACLE(E)

  initialize the root of the tree, T, as a leaf node

  put $\langle T$, training_examples, $\{\}\rangle$ into Queue

  while Queue is not empty and size(T) < tree_limit_size   /*expand a node*/

    remove node N from head of Queue

    examples$_N$:= examples of set stored with N

    constraints$_N$:= constraint set stored with N

    use features to build a set of candidate splits

    use examples$_N$ and calls to ORACLE(constraints$_N$) to evaluate splits

    S := best binary split

    search for best M-of-N split, S', using S as a seed

    make N an internal node with spit S'

    for each outcome s, of S' /*make children nodes*/

    make C, a new child node of N

    constraints$_C$:= constraints$_N \cup \{S' = s\}$

    use calls to ORACLE(constraints$_C$) to determine whether C should remain a leaf, otherwise

      examples$_C$:= members of examples$_N$ with outcome s on split S' put $\langle C$, examples$_C$,

      constraints$_C\rangle$ into Queue

---

extracting a decision tree from any learned model (ANN or symbolic). TREPAN uses queries to induce a decision tree that approximates the concept acquired by a given inductive learning method.

TREPAN has been evaluated on the Cleveland Heart Disease database from the University of California at Irvine machine learning repository, a variation of the gene promoter recognition problem used by Towell & Shavlik (1993), and a problem in which the task was to recognize protein-coding regions in DNA (Craven & Shavlik 1993). Analysis of results showed that TREPAN exhibits high fidelity with the model from which its trees are derived, high predictive accuracy and is comparable in complexity with other decision trees trained on the same problem, for example C4.5 (Quinlan 1993) and ID2-of-3 (Murphy & Pazzani 1991). Craven & Shavlik (1993) pointed out that another significant advantage of this model over other rule extraction techniques is that it scales well to problems of higher dimensionality.

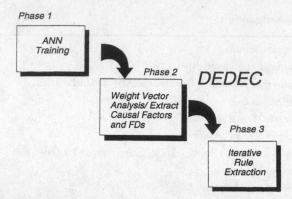

Figure 12.3. Schematic outline of the three basic phases of the DEDEC approach. FD, functional dependency.

Eclectic rule extraction technique

In addition to the two main categories of rule extraction techniques (decompositional and pedagogical), Andrews et al. (1995) also proposed a third category, which they labelled *eclectic*. This category was designed to accommodate those rule extraction techniques which incorporate elements of both the decompositional and pedagogical approaches. In reality the eclectic category is a somewhat diffuse group. This can be illustrated by the fact that one prominent example of an eclectic technique is the variant of the rule-extraction-as-learning technique of Craven & Shavlik (1994), which utilizes the (decompositional) KT algorithm of Fu (1991, 1994) in the role of determining whether a given rule is consistent with the underlying ANN network.

Another example of the eclectic approach to ANN knowledge elicitation is the DEDEC (Decision Detection) approach of Tickle et al. (1994, 1996). Essentially, DEDEC extends into the domain of knowledge elicitation from trained ANNs the work on identifying ANN causal factors (Garson 1991), reducts (Pawlak 1991) and functional dependencies (Geva & Orlowski 1996) as a precursor to rule extraction.

Figure 12.3 shows an overall schematic outline of the three basic phases of the DEDEC approach. DEDEC is designed to be applicable across a broad class of multilayer feedforward ANNs trained using the back-propagation technique and the starting point is Phase 1, in which an ANN solution to a given problem domain is synthesized. The intermediate phase (Phase 2) is where the task of identifying a set of causal factors and functional dependencies is performed. Hence it is this phase that distinguishes DEDEC from other pedagogically based rule extraction techniques and which provides the basis for assigning DEDEC to the eclectic rule extraction category.

To date, two different weight vector analysis techniques have been developed and applied in DEDEC Phase 2. The first of these utilizes an existing algorithm (Garson 1991) for determining causal factors in a trained ANN based on calculating the relative weight shares of the ANN inputs. Within DEDEC Phase 2 this basic algorithm has been adapted and extended for use in a broad range of ANN architectures including cascade correlation (Fahlman & Lebiere 1991) and an implementation of a local response ANN network (Geva & Sitte 1993). In addition to the weight sharing technique, DEDEC also incorporates a coefficient reduction approach to identifying causal factors and functional dependencies in a trained ANN using an adaptation of an algorithm originally designed to be used in conjunction with linear programming problems.

For the DEDEC approach, the final phase (Phase 3) is essentially the learning or pedagogical phase. It comprises a set of basic algorithms and techniques for eliciting the requisite sets of symbolic rules by learning from a selected set of cases generated by the trained ANN using the causal factor/functional dependency information extracted at Phase 2.

Techniques for the extraction of fuzzy rules

Parallel to the development of techniques for extracting Boolean rules from trained ANNs has been the synthesis of corresponding techniques for extracting fuzzy rules – the so-called *neurofuzzy* systems. Analogous to the techniques discussed previously for conventional Boolean logic systems, typically, neurofuzzy systems comprise three distinct elements. The first is a set of mechanisms/procedures to insert existing expert knowledge in the form of fuzzy rules into an ANN structure (i.e. a knowledge initialization phase). The essential difference here is that this step involves the generation of representations of the corresponding membership functions. The second element is the process of training the ANN, which, in this case, focuses on tuning the membership functions according to the patterns in the training data. The third element in the process is the analysis and extraction of the refined knowledge embedded in the form of a set of modified membership functions. Horikawa et al. (1992) observed that the identification of the initial set of fuzzy inference rules to be modelled has proved to be a difficult task as have attempts at simultaneously undertaking the tasks of rule identification and membership tuning.

One of the earliest works in this area was that of Masuoka et al. (1990), who used a decompositional approach to refine an initial set of fuzzy rules extracted from experts in the problem domain. The technique incorporates a specialized three-phase ANN architecture. In the input phase a three-layer ANN comprising an input unit, one or two hidden units, and an output unit was used to represent the membership function of each rule antecedent (i.e. the input variables). The fuzzy operations on the input variables (e.g. AND, OR, etc.) are represented by a second distinct phase labelled as the rule net (RN) phase and the membership functions that constitute the rule consequents are represented in a third (output) phase using the same motif as for the input phase. In this technique the problem of eliciting a compact set of rules as the output is tackled by pruning at the RN phase those connections in the network which are less than a threshold value.

In a similar vein, Berenji (1991) demonstrated the use of a specialized ANN to refine an approximately correct knowledge base of fuzzy rules used as part of a controller. (The problem domain selected in this case was a cart-pole balancing application.) The salient characteristic of this technique is that the set of rules governing the operation of the controller are known and the ANN is used to modify the membership functions both for the rule preconditions and the rule conclusions.

Horikawa et al. (1992) developed three types of fuzzy neural networks that can automatically identify the underlying fuzzy rules and tune the corresponding membership functions by modifying the connection weights of the ANNs using the back-propagation algorithm. In this approach, the initial rule base is created either by using expert knowledge or by selectively iterating through possible combinations of the input variables and the number of membership functions. The fuzzy neural network model *FuNe I* developed by Halgamuge & Glesner (1994) generalizes this work by using a (rule based) process to initially identify 'rule relevant nodes for conjunctive and disjunctive rules for each output'. Halgamuge & Glesner reported on the successful application of the FuNe I technique to a benchmark problem involving the classification of iris species as well as three real-world problems involving the classification of solder joint images, underwater sonar image recognition, and handwritten digit recognition.

Both the FNES (*fuzzy neural expert system*) of Hayashi (1990) and the *fuzzy-MLP* model of Mitra (1994) specifically address the problem of providing the end-user with an explanation (justification) as to how a particular conclusion has been reached. In both techniques the set of rule antecedents is determined by analysing and ranking the weight vectors in the trained ANN to determine their relative influence (impact) on a given output (class). However, whereas FNES relies on the involvement of an expert at the input phase to convert the input data into the required format, in the fuzzy-MLP procedure, this process has been automated. Both the FNES and fuzzy-MLP models have been applied to the medical problem domain of diagnosing hepatobiliary disorders, the latter showing an improved set of results (in terms of rule accuracy) over the former. In part this improvement is attributable to the more complex ANN architecture used in fuzzy-MLP, namely three hidden layers vs. one hidden layer in FNES. (The FNES architecture also includes direct connections between the input and output layers.)

Okada et al. (1993) incorporated elements of knowledge initialization, rule refinement (via the tuning of membership functions), and rule extraction in a fuzzy inference system incorporating a seven-layer structured ANN. In this implementation, two layers of the model are used to provide representations of the membership functions for the input variables (presented in a separate input layer) and another layer is used to represent membership functions for the rule consequents. Separate layers are also used to construct the rule antecedents (incorporating mechanisms for supporting fuzzy logical operations) and rule consequents. The authors report a significant improvement in prediction accuracy of the model in comparison with a conventional three-layer neural network in the application problem domain of financial bond rating.

Fuzzy ARTMAP developed by Tan & Carpenter 1993; Carpenter & Tan, 1995 is another example of a situation in which a highly effective rule extraction algorithm has been designed to work in conjunction with a specific supervised learning ANN, i.e. the fuzzy ARTMAP system. The algorithm is decompositional because a characteristic feature of the Fuzzy ARTMAP system is that each (category) node roughly corresponds to a rule. Furthermore, the weight vector associated with each node can be directly translated into a verbal or algorithmic description of the rule antecedents. This is in contrast to a 'conventional' back-propagation network where the role of hidden and output units in the total classification process is not usually as explicit. Fuzzy ARTMAP has been applied to the problem of diagnosing diabetes in Pima Indians according to World Health Organization criteria, with a resulting 76% prediction accuracy from six extracted fuzzy rules. Extracted rules are of the form:

IF   number of times pregnant is medium to very high,
AND   plasma glucose concentration is medium to high,
AND   diastolic blood pressure is medium to very high,
AND   triceps skin fold thickness is very low to medium,
AND   2-hour serum insulin is below medium,
AND   body mass index is not very high,
AND   diabetes pedigree function is below medium,
AND   age is not extreme,
THEN   diabetes is very likely.

Rule refinement

A problem ancillary to that of rule extraction from trained ANNs is that of using the ANN for the *refinement* of existing rules within symbolic knowledge bases. Whereas the rule extraction process normally commences with an empty symbolic

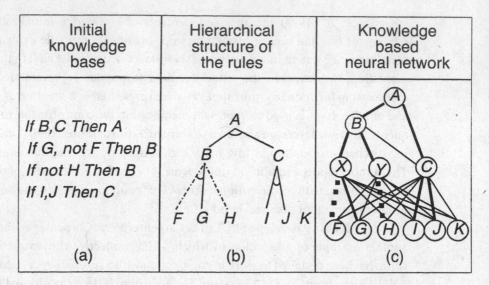

Initial knowledge base	Hierarchical structure of the rules	Knowledge based neural network
If B,C Then A *If G, not F Then B* *If not H Then B* *If I,J Then C*		
(a)	(b)	(c)

Figure 12.4. Construction of a KNN by the KBANN algorithm.

rule base, the starting point for the rule refinement process is some initial knowledge about the problem domain expressible in the form of symbolic rules. A crucial point, however, is that the initial set of rules may not necessarily be complete or even correct (Giles & Omlin 1993a,b). Irrespective of the quality of the initial rule base, the goal in rule refinement is to use a combination of ANN learning and rule extraction techniques to produce a *better* (i.e. a *refined*) set of symbolic rules that can then be applied back in the original problem domain. In the rule refinement process, the initial rule base (i.e. what may be termed *prior knowledge*) is inserted into an ANN by programming some of the weights. (In this context, prior knowledge refers to all of the production rules known prior to commencement of the ANN training phase.) The rule refinement process then proceeds in the same way as normal rule extraction, namely (a) train the network on the available data set(s) and (b) extract (in this case the refined) rules – with the proviso that the rule refinement process may involve a number of iterations of the training phase rather than a single pass.

The first successful method for prestructuring an ANN such that the classification behaviour of the network was consistent with a given set of propositional rules was Towell & Shavlik's (1993) KBANN algorithm. KBANN is in essence a domain theory refinement system. An initial approximately correct domain theory is provided as a propositional rule base, the KBANN network is created from the rules and then trained with examples drawn from the problem domain. Finally a refined set of M-of-N rules are extracted from the trained network. Figure 12.4 shows the process of converting a rule-based knowledge base (a) to the corresponding hierarchical representation of the knowledge base (b) to a knowledge-based neural network (KNN) (c) that represents the rule base.

In Figure 12.4b the solid and dotted lines represent necessary and prohibitory dependencies, respectively. The KNN shown in Figure 12.4c results from the translation of the knowledge base. Units X and Y in Figure 12.4c are introduced to handle the disjunction in the rule set. Otherwise each unit in the KNN corresponds to a consequent or an antecedent in the knowledge base. The thick lines in part c represent heavily weighted links in the KNN that correspond to dependencies in the knowledge base. The thin lines in part c represent links added to the network to allow refinement of the knowledge base.

The core requirements of the KBANN/M-of-N approach are: (a) the requirement for either a rule set to initialize the ANN or a special training algorithm that uses a *soft-weight sharing* algorithm to cluster weights; (b) the requirement for a special network training regime; (c) the requirement for hidden units to be approximated as threshold units (this is achieved by setting the parameter s in the activation function $1/[1 + e^{-sx}]$ to be greater than a value of 5.0); and (d) the requirement that the extracted rules use an intermediate term to represent each hidden unit. This gives rise to the concern that the approach may not enable a sufficiently accurate description of the network to be extracted (Towell & Shavlik 1993). It is also worth noting that one of the basic tenets of the KBANN approach is that the meaning of a hidden unit in the ANN, generated as part of the initialization process, does not change during the training process. Given that KBANN is essentially a rule refinement system this may be true in general and, in fact, Towell & Shavlik (1993) reported empirical confirmation from trained ANNs in their study. However, in the case where the meaning of a unit *does* change during training, the comprehensibility of the extracted rules may be significantly degraded. Opitz & Shavlik (1995) described the TopGen algorithm that significantly enhances the utility of KBANN by allowing the addition of semantically meaningful nodes to the network during training. The facility to add such nodes reduces the dependency on having the initial domain theory nearly complete and correct.

Local function networks (such as RBF networks) are inherently suitable for rule refinement because there is a one-to-one correspondence between rules and basis function units. (The conversion from basis function unit to rule and vice versa is achieved by describing the area of response of the unit in terms of a reference vector that represents the centre of the unit and a set of radii that determine the effective range of the unit in each input dimension. The rule associated with the unit has antecedents formed by the conjunct of these effective ranges in each dimension and consequent given by the concept represented by the unit.) This means that

initial rules can be readily converted to hidden layer basis function units during
the network initialization phase;

new units that have a meaning directly related to the problem domain can be
added during training to supplement an initial weak domain theory;

the initialized 'meaning' of a hidden layer unit can alter during the training and
the rule extracted from the unit after training has been completed will still have
a valid meaning within the problem domain;

each hidden layer basis function can be easily and directly decompiled to a rule
after training has been completed.

Tresp et al. (1993) described a technique for refining rules using RBF networks. An
ANN $y = NN(x)$, which makes a prediction about the state of y given the state of its
input x, can be instantiated as a set of basis functions, $b_i(x)$, where each basis
function describes the premise of the rule that results in prediction y. The degree
of certainty of the rule premise is given by the value of $b_i(x)$, which varies
continuously between 0 and 1. The rule conclusion is given by $w_i(x)$ and the
network architecture is given as:

$$y = NN(x) = \frac{\sum_i w_i(x) b_i(x)}{\sum_j b_j(x)}. \tag{12.3}$$

If the w_i values are constants and the basis functions chosen are multivariate
Gaussians (i.e. individual variances in each dimension), Eq. (12.3) reduces to the
network described by Moody & Darken (1989).

They show how the basis functions can be parameterized by encoding simple
logical if–then expressions as multivariate Gaussians, thus facilitating both rule
initialization and extraction. For instance the rule

IF $[(x_1 \approx a)$ AND $(x_4 \approx b)]$ OR $(x_2 \approx c)$ THEN $y = dx^2$

is encoded as

premise: $b_i(x) = \exp\left(-\frac{1}{2} \frac{(x_1 - a)^2 + (x_4 - b)^2}{\sigma^2}\right) + \exp\left(-\frac{1}{2} \frac{(x_2 - c)^2}{\sigma^2}\right)$

conclusion_i: $w_i(x) = dx^2.$

The initial knowledge base can be refined by allowing network training to proceed
in any of four modes including:

1. *Forget,* where training data is used to adapt NN^{init} by gradient descent (i.e. the
   sooner training stops, the more initial knowledge is preserved);
2. *Freeze,* where the initial configuration is frozen (i.e. if a discrepancy between
   prediction and data occurs, a new basis function is added);

3. *Correct* where a parameter is penalized if it deviates from its initial value; and
4. *Internal Teacher* where the penalty is formulated in terms of the mapping rather than in terms of the parameters.

Classification is performed by applying Bayesian probability and rule extraction is performed by directly decompiling the Gaussian (*centre:* μ_{ij}, *width:* δ_{ij}) pairs to form the rule premise and attaching a certainty factor, w_i to the rule.

After training is complete, a *pruning* strategy is employed to arrive at a solution that has the minimum number of basis functions (rules), and the minimum number of conjuncts for each rule.

The RULEIN/RULEX rule refinement algorithm of Andrews & Geva (1995, 1996a,b, 1997) is based on the RBF network (Geva & Sitte 1994), which consists of an input layer, a hidden layer of local basis function units, and an output layer and performs function approximation and classification in a manner similar to RBF networks. The hidden layer basis function units are constructed using pairs of sigmoids; one pair forms each input dimension. An incremental, constructive training algorithm is used, with training that involves adjusting, by gradient descent, the centre c_i, breadth b_i and edge steepness k_i parameters of the sigmoids that define the local basis function units. During training for classification problems, the output weight, w, is held constant at a value such that the hidden units are prevented from 'overlapping', i.e. no more than one unit contributes appreciably to the network output. This measure facilitates rule extraction by allowing individual hidden units to be interpreted as rules in isolation of all other units.

RULEX extracts a rule set from the network solution by interpreting each hidden unit as a single if–then rule. The antecedents for the rule associated with a hidden unit are formed from the conditions that cause the hidden unit to produce appreciable output, i.e. an input pattern lies wholly within the hypercube represented by the responsive area of the hidden unit (each component x_i of the input vector x lies within the active range of the basis function in the i-th input dimension). The rule describing the behaviour of the hidden unit will then be of the form:

IF $1 \leq i \leq n: x_i \in [x_{i\text{lower}}, x_{i\text{upper}}]$
THEN   pattern belongs to the target class,

where $x_{i\text{lower}}$ represents the lower limit of activation of the unit in the i-th input dimension and $x_{i\text{upper}}$ represents the upper limit of activation of the unit in the i-th input dimension and n is the dimensionality of the input.

The range of input values, $[x_{i\text{lower}}, x_{i\text{upper}}]$, in the i-th input dimension that will produce appreciable output from the hidden units corresponding to the i-th ridge can be calculated directly from the network equations without the need for employing a search-and-test strategy, thus making RULEX computationally efficient.

RULEIN converts a propositional if–then rule into the parameters that define a local basis function unit by determining from the rule the active range in each dimension for the unit to be configured. RULEIN sets the upper and lower bounds of the active range, $[x_{i_{lower}}, x_{i_{upper}}]$, and then calculates the centre, breadth, and steepness parameters (c_i, b_i, k_i) for each of the sigmoid pairs used to construct the local basis function that will represent the rule.

Setting $x_{i_{lower}}$ and $x_{i_{upper}}$, appropriately involves choosing values such that they 'cut off' the range of antecedent clause values. For discriminating ranges, i.e. those ranges that represent input pattern attributes that are used by the unit in classifying input patterns, these required values will be those that are mentioned in the antecedent of the rule to be encoded. For non-discriminating ranges, the active range can be set to include all possible input values in the corresponding input dimension. (Non-discriminating ranges will be those that correspond to input pattern attributes that do not appear as antecedent clauses of the rule to be encoded.) After the network has been initialized hidden units that represent rules that are known to be accurate or deemed to be important can be 'frozen' so that they will not be altered during network training. RULEIN/RULEX has been evaluated on the Cleveland Heart Disease database and the Hypothyroid database from the University of California at Irvine machine learning repository. Results indicate that RULEIN/RULEX can extract accurate, comprehensible rules that show high fidelity with the underlying trained RBF network.

Work in the area of rule refinement and recurrent networks has centred on the ability of recurrent networks to learn the rules underlying a regular language (where a regular language is the smallest class of formal languages in the Chomsky hierarchy; Hopcroft & Ullman 1979). Giles & Omlin (1993a,b, 1996) stated that a regular language is defined by a grammar $G = \langle S, N, T, P \rangle$ where S is the start symbol, N is the non-terminal symbol, T is the terminal symbol; and $P =$ is a production of the form $A \rightarrow a$ or $A \rightarrow aB$ where $AB \in N$, and $a \in T$.

The regular language generated by G is denoted $L(G)$.

Giles & Omlin (1993a,b, 1996) also discussed the equivalence between the regular language L and the deterministic finite-state automata (DFA) M, which acts as an *acceptor* for the language $L(G)$, i.e. DFA M accepts only strings that are members of $L(G)$. They formally define a DFA as a quintuple $M = \langle \Sigma, Q, R, F, \delta \rangle$ where:

$\Sigma = \{a_1, \ldots, a_m\}$ is the alphabet of the language L;
$Q = \{q_1, \ldots, q_n\}$ is a set of states;
$R \in Q$ is a start state;

Table 12.7. Giles & Omlin's (1993a,b) method for extracting DFA from recurrent networks

1. Divide the output of each of the N state neurons into q intervals (quantization levels). This results in q^N partitions of the hidden state unit space.
2. Starting in a defined initial network state generate a search tree with the initial state as its root and the number of successors of each node equal to the number of symbols in the input alphabet. (Links between nodes correspond to transitions between DFA states.)
3. Perform (breadth first) search of the tree by presenting all strings up to a certain length in alphabetical order starting with length 1. Make a path from one partition to another. When:
   (a) A previously visited partition is reached; then only the new transition is defined between the previous and the current partition, i.e. no new DFA state is created and the search tree is pruned at that node.
   (b) An input causes a transition immediately to the same partition; then a loop is created and the search tree is pruned at that node.
4. Terminate the search when no new DFA states are created from the string set initially chosen and all possible transitions from all DFA states have been extracted.
5. For each resulting path, if the output of the response neuron is greater than 0.5 the DFA state is accepting; otherwise the DFA state is rejecting.

DFA, deterministic finite-state automata.

$F \subseteq Q$ is a set of accepting states; and
$\delta: Q \times \Sigma \to Q$ defines state transitions in M.

Acceptance of a string x by the DFA M is defined as the DFA M reaching an accepting state after being read by M. Acceptance of the string x by the DFA M implies that x is a member of the regular language $L(M)$, (and hence also by the regular language $L(G)$).

Cleeremans et. al. (1989), Williams & Zipser (1989) and Elman (1990) showed that recurrent networks were capable of being trained such that the behaviour of the trained network emulated a given DFA. Cleeremans et al. (1989) concluded that the hidden unit activations represented past histories and that clusters of these activations represented the states of the generating automaton. Giles et al. (1992) extended the work of Cleeremans and described a technique for extracting complete from second-order, dynamically driven recurrent networks and is described in Table 12.7.

The networks used by Giles & Omlin (1993a,b) have N recurrent hidden units labelled S_j, K special non-recurrent input units labelled I_k, and $N^2 \times K$ real-valued weights labelled W_{ijk}. The values of the hidden neurons are referred to collectively as state vectors $\mathbf{S}$ in the finite N-dimensional space $[0, 1]^N$. (Second order is taken to mean that the weights W_{ijk} modify a *product* of the hidden (S_j) and input (I_k)

neurons, which allows a direct mapping of {state, input} ⇒ {next state} and means the network has the representational potential of at least finite-state automata; Giles & Omlin 1993a,b.)

The extracted DFA depends on:

1. the quantization level, q, chosen. Different DFAs will be extracted for different values of q;
2. the order in which strings are presented (which leads to different successors of a node visited by the search tree).

Giles & Omlin (1993a,b) stated that these distinctions are usually not significant as they employ a minimization strategy (Hopcroft & Ullman 1979), which guarantees a unique, minimal representation for any extracted DFA. Thus DFAs extracted under different initial conditions may collapse into equivalence classes (Giles et al. 1992).

Rule insertion for known DFA transitions is achieved by programming some of the initial weights of a second-order recurrent network with N state neurons. The rule insertion algorithm assumes $N > N_s$, where N represents the number of neurons in the network and N_s is the number of states in the DFA to be represented.

In the recurrent networks used by Giles & Omlin (1993a,b), the network changes state S at time $t+1$ according to the equations:

$$S_i^{(t+1)} = g(\Xi_i), \tag{12.4}$$

$$\Xi_i = \sum_{j,k} W_{ijk} S_j^{(t)} I_k^{(t)}, \tag{12.5}$$

where g is a sigmoid discriminant function.

To encode a known transition $\delta(s_j, a_k) = s_i$ Giles & Omlin (1993a,b) arbitrarily identified DFA states s_j and s_i with state neurons S_j and S_i, respectively. This transition can be represented by having S_i have a high output (≈ 1), and S_j have a low output (≈ 0), after the input symbol a_k has entered the network via input neuron I_k.

Setting W_{ijk} to a large positive value will ensure that $s_i^{(t+1)}$ will be high, and setting W_{ijk} to a large negative value will ensure that $s_j^{(t+1)}$ will be low. All other weights are set at small random values.

To program the response neuron to indicate whether the resulting DFA state is an accepting or rejecting state the weight W_{0ie} is set large and positive if s_i is an accepting state, and large and negative if s_i is a rejecting state. (Where e is a special symbol that marks the end of an input string.)

Network training proceeds after all known transitions are inserted into the network by encoding the weights according to the above method. After training, the refined rule/DFA is extracted using the method described above. Giles & Omlin (1993a,b) concluded that network initialization reduces training time and improves generalization with the example problems studied.

Current issues in rule extraction/refinement

The field of rule extraction from trained ANNs has achieved a degree of maturity. Researchers have moved beyond merely describing new techniques and reporting empirical results to formulating benchmark standards and developing a consistent theoretical base. The following is a discussion of some of the issues raised by recent theoretical work.

Limitations imposed by inherent algorithmic complexity

The survey paper of Andrews et al. (1995) used algorithmic complexity of the rule extraction algorithm as one of their criteria for categorizing rule extraction processes. This criterion was introduced due to the observations of several authors notably Fu (1991, 1994), Towell & Shavlik (1993), Thrun (1994) and more recently Viktor et al. (1995) that for certain *real-world* problem domains there exist potential problems due to the algorithmic complexity of various implementations of the rule extraction process. Typically these problems relate to the algorithm either requiring a long time to find the maximally general solution or producing a large number of rules (with a consequent loss of comprehensibility). Further such authors have usually shown how a variety of heuristics may be employed to achieve a balance between solution time/effort, fidelity (degree to which the rule set mimics the underlying ANN) and accuracy (measure of the ability of the rule set to classify previously unseen examples from the problem domain) of the rule set, and comprehensibility of the rule set.

Golea (1996) identified issues relating to the intrinsic complexity of the rule extraction problem. The three key results were that, in the worst case, extracting:

1. the minimum disjunctive normal form (DNF) expression from a trained (feedforward) ANN; and
2. the best monomial rule from a single perceptron within a trained ANN; and
3. the best M-of-N rule from a single perceptron within a trained ANN

are all NP-hard problems.

Limitations on achieving simultaneously high accuracy, high fidelity and high comprehensibility

Recently, rule extraction techniques have been applied in an increasingly diverse range of problem domains. This increased exposure has also brought to light a

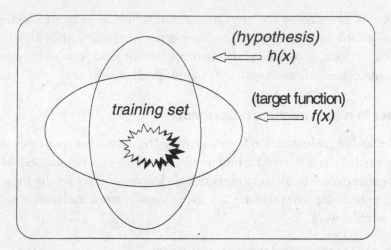

Figure 12.5. Training set, target function (f) and ANN solution (h). Bold area, input space.

potential conflict in attempting to maximize simultaneously the fidelity, accuracy and comprehensibility criteria for evaluating the quality of the rules extracted from a trained ANN. The general nature of this problem was described by Golea (1996) and is illustrated as in Figure 12.5. (Recall that rule *accuracy* is a measure of the capability of the extracted rules to classify correctly a set of previously unseen examples from the problem domain. Rule *fidelity* is a measure of the extent to which the extracted rules mimic the behaviour of the ANN from which they were drawn whereas rule *comprehensibility* is assessed in terms of the size of the extracted rule set and the number of antecedents per rule.)

Let I be the complete input space for a given problem domain and let D be a distribution defined on I where $D(x)$ represents the probability of seeing a given x in I. Let $f(x)$ be the function that actually maps or classifies a set of training cases drawn from the problem domain (i.e. the function that is the 'target' for the ANN training). In addition let $h(x)$ be the functional representation of the ANN solution and let R be the set of rules extracted from the ANN.

On the basis of the definitions presented above, the set of extracted rules R exhibits a high level of fidelity with respect to the ANN solution h if R can act as a surrogate for h (i.e. R and h can be used interchangeably). Hence a set of extracted rules R with a high level of fidelity will be as accurate as the ANN itself in classifying previously unseen examples from the problem domain. (In passing it should also be noted that a number of authors, e.g. Towell & Shavlik (1993) and Andrews & Geva (1997), have reported situations in which the extracted rule set exhibits a better generalization performance than the trained ANN from which the rule set was extracted.)

A standard measure of the accuracy of the ANN solution (h) (which results from the ANN training process involving the given training set) is given by the generalization error (ε) in using h (i.e. the ANN solution) as a surrogate for the target function f, namely

$$\varepsilon = \text{probability}\{x \in D \mid h(x) \neq f(x)\}. \tag{12.6}$$

Hence, if the generalization error ε is small, a set of extracted rules R, with a high level of fidelity, will simultaneously exhibit a high level of rule accuracy (as defined above). Moreover, R can therefore act as a surrogate for the original target function f.

However, if the distribution D is localized in some region of the input space I then it is possible to synthesize an ANN solution h for which the generalization error ε, is small but for which h is neither equal to nor perhaps even close to f. Importantly, if the function h is significantly more complex than f, then the extracted rule set R will exhibit high levels of accuracy and fidelity but a correspondingly lower level of comprehensibility than the set of rules extracted, for example by applying a symbolic induction algorithm directly to the data in the original training set.

The survey paper of Andrews et al. (1995) listed one of the important benefits in extracting rules from a trained ANN as being the ability to identify situations in which certain regions of an input space were not represented sufficiently by data in an ANN training set. The view expressed in the survey was that this would enable the data set to be supplemented accordingly. The preceding discussion has highlighted the importance of this observation.

Rule extraction and the quality of ANN solution

In most ANN architectures the initial values for the weight vectors that ultimately characterize an ANN solution are randomly assigned within the ANN training algorithm. Consequently the result of each separate instance of the ANN training is normally a unique ANN solution. After training the ANN solution is assessed in terms of:

1. the size of the residual error on the training set;
2. the size of the generalization error on the test or validation set; and
3. the number of hidden units required in the trained ANN.

Some trade-off between these three measures is often required, particularly in situations involving noise in the training set. However, in most cases the implicit or in some cases explicit goal of the training phase is to arrive at an ANN solution with the minimum number of hidden units consistent with satisfying certain threshold criteria for the residual/generalization errors.

An issue that was not expanded upon in the survey paper of Andrews et al. (1995) is the extent of the dependence of the efficacy of rule extraction techniques on the quality of the ANN solution (and by extension, the algorithm used in the ANN training phase). For example, because of their algorithmic complexity, the tractability of most decompositional approaches to rule extraction (and specifically those that involve some form of search process to find possible rule sets) is heavily dependent on the ANN having as close as practical to the minimum number of hidden units in the final configuration. More importantly, such decompositional techniques are critically dependent on each (hidden and output) unit possessing a separate and distinct *meaning* or representing a single concept or feature within the context of the problem domain.

A recent result by Bartlett (1996) raises certain problems in this regard. In particular Bartlett (1996) has shown that the generalization error ε of a trained ANN can be expressed in the form:

$$\varepsilon \propto A^2/n, \tag{12.7}$$

where n is the number of cases in the training set; and $\Sigma |w| \le A$ i.e. the sum of the absolute values of the weights w for each (hidden and output) unit in the trained ANN is bounded by some positive constant A.

This result shows that an ANN solution may be found that exhibits good generalization behaviour (i.e. has acceptable low generalization error ε) whilst being suboptimal in terms of having the minimum number of hidden units. Moreover an important corollary is that an ANN solution could be found with good generalization capability in problems involving binary classifications but in which some or all of the hidden units do not possess a separate and distinct meaning or represent a single concept or feature within the context of the problem domain. As such the result has important implications for all rule extraction techniques and in particular for those decompositional rule extraction techniques for which this is a prerequisite.

Functional dependencies, causal factors and rule extraction

To date almost the entire focus of the discussion regarding knowledge elicitation from trained ANNs has centred on the task of extracting as efficiently as possible a set of (symbolic) rules that explain the behaviour of the trained ANN. However, as was pointed out at the beginning of this chapter another reason for performing rule extraction is to discover previously unknown dependencies and relationships in data sets. In particular, a useful interim result from an end-user's point of view might simply be one that identifies which attributes, or combination of attributes, from the problem domain that are the most significant (or alternatively the least significant) determinants of the decision/classification. Moreover Holte (1993)

Table 12.8. Case attributes and functional dependencies

Case/attribute	A	B	C	D
t_1	a_1	b_1	c_1	d_1
t_2	a_1	b_2	c_1	d_2
t_3	a_2	b_2	c_2	d_2
t_4	a_2	b_3	c_2	d_3
t_5	a_3	b_3	c_2	d_4

showed that for a broad range of data sets involving in some situations a large number of attributes, it is frequently possible to classify cases from the problem domain to an acceptable level of accuracy based on two or fewer dominant attributes.

A numerous and diverse range of techniques has been developed that is designed to enable the dominant attributes in a problem domain to be isolated. This range includes statistical techniques such as multiple regression analysis, discriminant analysis, and principal component analysis. Within the context of knowledge elicitation from trained ANNs, Garson (1991) focused on the task of determining the relative importance of input factors used by the ANN to arrive at its conclusions. Garson (1991) termed these *causal factors* between ANN inputs and outputs. In a similar vein Tickle et al. (1996) identified certain parallels between the processes for identifying *keys, superkeys,* and in particular *functional dependencies* (Korth & Silberschatz 1991), within the realm of relational database design. Specifically, for a given problem domain and a set of cases drawn from the problem domain (where each case comprises a set of attribute/value pairs), then in essence a *functional dependency* (FD) $X \rightarrow Y$ (read X determines Y) exists if the value of the attribute Y can be uniquely determined from the values of the attributes belonging to set X. More precisely the functional dependency $X \rightarrow Y$ is satisfied if for each pair of cases t_1 and t_2 in a given problem domain such that $t_1[X] = t_2[X]$ (i.e. the set of attributes X for cases t_1 and t_2 are equivalent) it follows that $t_1[Y] = t_2[Y]$.

By way of illustration of the concept of functional dependencies consider the set of cases $T = \{t_1 \ldots t_5\}$ involving attributes A, B, C and D shown in Table 12.8. (Korth & Silberschatz 1991). In this example the functional dependency $A \rightarrow C$ is satisfied because each case that has the same value of attribute A has the same value for attribute C. However, the functional dependency $C \rightarrow A$ is *not* satisfied because the cases t_4 and t_5 both have the value c_2 for attribute C (i.e. $t_4[C] = t_5[C]$ but $t_4[A] \neq t_5[A]$). In a similar way it can be shown that the functional dependency $AB \rightarrow D$ is satisfied.

Both the notion of a causal factor as introduced by Garson (1991) and the concept of a functional dependency as has been previously discussed can be viewed as one in which a conceptual relationship is established between the domain attributes and the decision attribute(s). However, a functional dependency relies on having discrete values for the attributes whereas a causal factor as described by Garson (1991) can embrace both discrete and continuous valued attributes. Moreover the notion of a rule can be viewed as an extension of the functional dependency concept to the point of expressing a relationship between specific values of the domain attributes and the decision attribute(s) (Geva & Orlowski 1996).

In any given problem domain there could exist numerous functional dependencies. Hence in a relational database context attention is focused primarily on determining only what are termed *left-reduced functional dependencies*, i.e. those that possess the property that while the functional dependency $X \to Y$ is satisfied, any proper subset $X \subset Y$ is not sufficient to determine Y. Applying these concepts in the realm of ANNs it is expected that a trained ANN would not necessarily reflect all of the possible functional dependencies in a given data set. This is because the intrinsic nature of the training process is to give prominence to those attribute/values or combination of attribute/values that lead to global error minimization.

In both the relational database context and also in the context of applying the functional dependency concept to knowledge elicitation from trained ANNs, the identification of the set of left-reduced functional dependencies is important because the goal is to identify and eliminate superfluous/insignificant attributes. In addition, eliminating such attributes augurs well for ultimately determining a set of rules with the minimum number of antecedents (Geva & Orlowski 1996).

As indicated previously in certain applications, the identification of causal factors and/or functional dependencies may of themselves provide considerable insight into the problem domain for the end-user. However, this may not be the only benefit. In the context of rule extraction from trained ANNs, one of the issues upon which comment has already been made is the complexity of the various rule extraction algorithms. In particular, algorithms such as KT and Subset are exponential in the number of ANN inputs. Hence reducing the number of attributes by eliminating those that are irrelevant in determining the decision has the potential of making a direct impact on the tractability of such algorithms by significantly reducing the search space. In addition this has the potential to obviate one of the key problems in both the VIA and the rule-extraction-as-learning (Craven & Shavlik 1994) algorithms, namely finding an initial set of specific cases that can then be used to synthesize more general rules.

One impediment to the use of functional dependencies to preprocess the training set data is that the determination of all functional dependencies is in itself exponential in the number of domain attributes. Geva & Orlowski (1996) sugges- ted some heuristics by which the process of discovering and enumerating all functional dependencies may be made more tractable.

Conclusions

As evidenced by the diversity of real-world application problem domains in which rule extraction techniques have been applied, there appears to be a strong and continuing demand for the end-product of the rule extraction process, namely a comprehensible explanation as to how and why the trained ANN arrived at a given result or conclusion. This demand appears to fall broadly within two groups: (a) ANN solutions that have already been implemented and where ipso facto the user is interested in identifying and possibly exploiting the potentially rich source of information that already exists within the trained ANN; and (b) a green-field situation where a user has a data set from a problem domain and is interested in what relationships exist within the data given and what general conclusions can be drawn.

The first group requires the development of rule extraction techniques that can be applied to existing ANNs. At this stage it would appear that, notwithstanding the initial success of decompositional approaches such as that of the KT algorithm of Fu (1991, 1994) the pedagogical approach is well placed to serve this set. Similarly it could be argued that the second group might well become the province of those rule extraction techniques that use specialized ANN training regimes, given the reported success of, for example, KBANN/M-of-N, BRAINNE, RULEX, etc. However, it also clear that no single rule extraction/rule refinement technique or method is currently in a dominant position to the exclusion of all others.

A pressing problem then is the formulation of a set of criteria for matching the set of techniques to the requirements of a given problem domain. For example, at a practical level, what has not yet emerged is a means of determining which rule extraction technique is optimal for application problem domains involving real valued data as distinct from discrete data. Further it is also uncertain as to whether the reported improvement in performance of ANN/rule extraction techniques vis-à-vis other induction techniques for extracting rules from data, applies in all problem domains. Hence a pressing requirement is for a set of comparative benchmark results across a range of problem domains similar to that undertaken with the original Three Monks problem proposed by Thrun et al. (1991).

A related issue is that in an increasing number of applications there are reports of situations in which the extracted rule set has shown better generalization performance than the trained ANN from which the rule set was extracted (Towell

& Shavlik 1993; Andrews & Geva 1997). Similar observations have also been made in the area of extracting symbolic grammatical rules from recurrent ANNs (Giles et al. 1992; Omlin et al. 1992; Giles & Omlin 1993a,b). However, Giles & Omlin (1993a,b) also reported that larger networks tend to show a poorer generalization performance. While these results are significant, what is not clear at this stage is the extent to which this superior performance can be ascribed to the elimination of the remaining error over the output unit(s) after the ANN training has been completed (i.e. the *rest* error). Hence an important research topic is also to identify the set of conditions under which an extracted rule set shows better generalization than the original network.

This chapter has described the reasons for the emergence of the fields of rule extraction and rule refinement from ANNs and described a taxonomy for classifying rule extraction algorithms. A selection of published rule extraction/refinement techniques was discussed to illustrate the taxonomy. The chapter also highlighted a variety of important issues relevant to the field that deserve the attention of researchers in the field. Rule extraction can have an important role in medical AI systems when used in conjunction with trained ANNs for the reasons given at the beginning of the chapter, namely: the ability to provide a human comprehensible explanation facility through extracting rules from the trained ANN; the ability to be able to use the extracted rules to gain an insight into the regions of input space where the ANN produces correct, false positive and false negative decisions; the possible explicitation of previously unrecognized relationships between clinical factors important for diagnosis and prognosis; and finally by rule refinement making possible the use of symbolic knowledge with connectionist inductive learning techniques for the refinement of existing domain knowledge by network training and subsequent rule extraction.

REFERENCES

Andrews, R. & Geva, S. (1995). RULEX & CEBP networks as the basis for a rule refinement system. In J. Hallam, ed., *Hybrid Problems, Hybrid Solutions*. 10th Biennial Conference on AI and Cognitive Sciences. IOS Press, Amsterdam, pp. 1–12.

Andrews, R. & Geva, S. (1996a). Rules and local function networks. In R. Andrews & J. Diederich, eds., Rules and Networks. Queensland University of Technology, Brisbane, pp. 1–15.

Andrews, R. & Geva, S. (1996b). Rule refinement and local function networks. In M. J. Jordan, M. J. Kearns & S. A. Solla, eds., *Proceedings of the NIPS *96 Rule Extraction From Trained Artificial Neural Networks Workshop*. Queensland University of Technology, Brisbane, pp. 1–12.

Andrews, R. & Geva, S. (1997). Using expert knowledge with an artificial neural network. In N.

Kasabov, R. Kozma, K. Ko, R. O'Shea, G. Coghill & T. Gedeon, eds., *Proceedings of the International Conference on Neural Information Processing (ICONIP '97)*, vol. 2. IEEE Press, New York, pp. 847–850.

Andrews, R., Diederich, J. & Tickle, A. B. (1995). A survey and critique of techniques for extracting rules from trained artificial neural networks. *Knowledge Based Systems*, **8**, 373–389.

Bartlett, P. L. (1996). For valid generalization the size of the weights is more important than the size of the network. In M. Mozer, M. Jordan & T. Petsche, eds., *Advances in Neural Information Processing (NIPS *96)*, Denver, CO. MIT Press, Cambridge, MA, pp. 134–140.

Berenji, H. R. (1991). Refinement of approximate reasoning-based controllers by reinforcement learning. In L. A. Birnbaum & G. C. Collins, eds., *Proceedings of the Eighth International Machine Learning Workshop*, Evanston, IL. Morgan Kaufmann, San Mateo, CA, pp. 475–479.

Berthold, M. & Huber, K. (1995a). From radial to rectangular basis functions: a new approach for rule learning from large databases. Technical Report 15-95, University of Karlsruhe.

Berthold, M. & Huber, K. (1995b). Building precise classifiers with automatic rule extraction. In F. Fogelman-Soulié & P. Gallinari, eds., *Proceedings of the IEEE International Conference on Neural Networks*. Perth, Western Australia **3**. EC2, Nanterre, pp. 1263–1268.

Blumenfeld, B. (1990). A connectionist approach to the processing of time dependent medical parameters. In M. Caudill, ed., *Proceedings of the 1990 International Joint Conference on Neural Networks, (IJCNN '90)*, Washington, DC, vol. 2. IEEE Service Center, pp. 575–578.

Boon, M. E. & Kok L. P. (1993). Neural network processing can provide means to catch errors that slip through human screening of pap smears. *Diagnostic Cytopathology*, **9**, 411–416.

Browner, W. S. (1992). Myocardial infarction prediction by artificial neural networks. *Annals of Internal Medicine*, **116**, 701–702.

Burke, H. (1994). A computerized prediction system for cancer survival that uses an artificial neural network. In *First World Congress on Computational Medicine, Public Health and BioTechnology*, Austin TX.

Carpenter, G. & Tan, A. H. (1995). Rule extraction: from neural architecture to symbolic representation. *Connection Science* **7**, 3–27.

Cleeremans, A., Servan-Schreiber, D. & McClelland, J. L. (1989). Finite state automata and simple recurrent networks. *Neural Computation* **1**, 372–381.

Craven, M. (1996). Extracting comprehensible models from trained neural networks. PhD thesis, University of Wisconsin, Madison.

Craven, M. W. & Shavlik, J. W. (1993). Learning to predict reading frames in *E. coli* sequences. In *Proceedings of the 26th Hawaii International Conference on System Sciences*, Wailea, HI. IEEE Press, New York.

Craven, M. W. & Shavlik, J. W. (1994). Using sampling and queries to extract rules from trained neural networks, In W. W. Cohen & H. Hirsh, eds., *Machine Learning: Proceedings of the 11th International Conference*, New Brunswick. Morgan-Kaufmann, San Mateo, CA, pp. 73–80.

Davis, R., Buchanan, B. G. & Shortliffe, E. (1977). Production rules as a representation for a knowledge-based consultation program. *Artificial Intelligence* **8**, 15–45.

Dorffner, G., Rappelsberger, P. & Flexer, A. (1993). Using selforganizing feature maps to classify EEG coherence maps. In B. Kappen & S. Gielen, eds., *International Conference on Artificial Neural Networks (ICANN '93)*. Springer-Verlag, Berlin, pp. 882–887.

Downes, P. T. (1994). Neural network recognition of multiple mammographic lesions. *World Congress on Neural Networks*, San Diego, CA. INNS Press/Lawrence Erlbaum Associates, New York, pp. 133–137.

Durbin, R. & Rumelhart, D. (1989). Product units: a computationally powerful and biologically plausible extension. *Neural Computation* 1, 133–166.

Eisner, R. (1990). Help for the weary: an automated pap smear screening system. *Diagnostic Clinical Testing* 28, 10.

Elman, J. L. (1990). Finding structure in time. *Cognitive Science* 14, 179–211.

Fahlman, S. & Lebiere, C. (1991). The Cascade-correlation learning architecture. In D. S. Touretzky, ed., *Advances in Neural Information Processing Systems*, vol. 2. Morgan Kaufmann, San Mateo, CA, pp. 524–532.

Feltham, R. & Xing, G. (1994). Pyramidal neural networking for mammogram tumour pattern recognition. In *Proceedings of the International Conference on Neural Networks (ICNN '94)*, Orlando FL. IEEE Press, New York, pp. 3546–3551.

Fu, L.M. (1991). Rule learning by searching on adapted nets. In K. Dean & T. L. McKeown, eds., *Proceedings of the 9th International Conference on Artificial Intelligence*, Anaheim, CA. MIT Press/AAAI Press, Cambridge, MA, pp. 590–595.

Fu, L. M. (1994). Rule generation from neural networks. *IEEE Transactions on Systems, Man and Cybernetics* 28, 1114–1124.

Gallant, S. (1988). Connectionist expert systems. *Communications of the ACM* 31, 152–169.

Garson, D. G. (1991). Interpreting neural-network connection weights. *AI Expert*, pp. 47–51.

Geva, S. & Orlowski, M. (1996). Simplifying the identification of decision rules with functional dependencies processing. Technical Report. Queensland University of Technology, Brisbane.

Geva, S. & Sitte, J. (1993). Local response neural networks and fuzzy logic for control. In *Proceedings of the 2nd IEEE International Workshop on Emerging Technologies and Factory Automation (EFTA '93)*, Cairns. IEEE Press, New York, pp. 51–57.

Geva, S. & Sitte, J. (1994). Constrained gradient descent. In *Proceedings of the 5th Australian Conference on Neural Computing*, Brisbane. Dept. of Electrical Engineering and Computing Science, University of Queensland, Brisbane.

Gilbert, N. (1989). Explanation and dialogue. *The Knowledge Engineering Review* 4, 235–247.

Giles, C. L. & Omlin, C. W. (1993a). Rule refinement with recurrent neural networks. In H. R. Berenji, E. Sanchez & S. Usui, eds., *Proceedings of the IEEE International Conference on Neural Networks*, San Francisco, CA. IEEE Press, New York, pp. 801–806.

Giles, C. L. & Omlin, C. W. (1993b). Extraction, insertion, and refinement of symbolic rules in dynamically driven recurrent networks. *Connection Science* 5, 307–328.

Giles, L. & Omlin C. (1996). Rule revision with recurrent networks. *IEEE Transactions on Knowledge and Data Engineering* 8, 183–188.

Giles, C. L., Miller, C. B., Chen, D., Chen, H., Sun G. Z. & Lee, Y. C. (1992). Learning and extracting finite state automata with second-order recurrent neural networks. *Neural Computation* 4, 393–405.

Golea, M. (1996). On the complexity of rule extraction from neural networks and network querying. In R. Andrews & J. Diederich, eds., *Rules and Networks*. Queensland University of Technology, Brisbane, pp. 51–59.

Halgamuge, S. K. & Glesner, M. (1994). Neural networks in designing fuzzy systems for real world applications. *Fuzzy Sets and Systems* **65**, 1–12.

Hayashi, Y. (1990). A neural expert system with automated extraction of fuzzy if–then rules. In R. P. Lippmann, J. E. Moody & D. S. Touretzky, eds., *Advances in Neural Information Processing Systems* (*NIPS *90*), vol. 3. Morgan Kaufmann, San Mateo, CA, pp. 578–584.

Holte, R. C. (1993). Very simple classification rules perform well on most commonly used datasets. *Machine Learning* **11**, 63–91.

Hopcroft, J. & Ullman, J. (1979). *Introduction to Automata Theory, Languages, and Computation*. Addison-Wesley Publishing Company Inc., Reading, MA.

Horikawa, S., Furuhashi, T. & Uchikawa, Y. (1992). On fuzzy modeling using fuzzy neural networks with the back-propagation algorithm. *IEEE Transactions on Neural Networks* **3**, 801–806.

Kennedy, R. L., Harrison, R. F., Marshall, S. J. & Hardisty, C. A. (1991). Analysis of clinical and electrocardiographic data from patients with acute chest pain using a neurocomputer. *Quarterly Journal of Medicine* **80**, 788–789.

Korth, H. F. & Silberschatz, A. (1991). *Database Systems Concepts*. McGraw-Hill, New York.

Krishnan, R. (1996). A systematic method for decompositional rule extraction from neural networks. In R. Andrews & J. Diederich, eds., *Proceedings of the NIPS *96 Rule Extraction From Trained Artificial Neural Networks Workshop*. Queensland University of Technology, Brisbane, pp. 38–45.

Lo, S., Lin, J., Freedman, M. & Mun, S. (1994). Application of artificial neural networks to medical image pattern recognition. In *Proceedings of the World Congress on Neural Networks* (*WCNN '94*), vol. 1. Lawrence Erlbaum Associates, New York, pp. 37–42.

Maire, F. (1997). A partial order for the M-of-N rule extraction algorithm. *IEEE Transactions on Neural Networks* **8**, 1542–1544.

Mango, L., Tjon, R. & Herriman, J. (1994). Computer assisted pap smear screening using neural networks. In *Proceedings of the World Congress on Neural Networks* (*WCNN '94*), vol. 1. Lawrence Erlbaum Associates, New York, pp. 84–89.

Masuoka, R., Watanabe, N., Kawamura, A., Owada, Y. & Asakawa, K. (1990). Neurofuzzy systems – fuzzy inference using a structured neural network. In *Proceedings of the International Conference on Fuzzy Logic and Neural Networks*, Iizuka, Japan, pp. 173–177.

Mehdi, B., Stacey, D. & Harauz, G. (1994). A hierarchical neural network assembly for classification of cervical cells in automated screening. *Analytical Cellular Pathology* **7**, 171–180.

Mitra, S. (1994). Fuzzy MLP based expert system for medical diagnosis. *Fuzzy Sets and Systems* **65**, 285–296.

Moody, J. & Darken, C.J. (1989). Fast learning in networks of locally-tuned processing units. *Neural Computation* **1**, 281–294.

Moore, J. D. (1989). A reactive approach to explanation in expert and advice-giving systems. Ph.D. thesis, University of California, Los Angeles.

Moore, J. D. & Swartout, W. R. (1989). A reactive approach to explanation. In N. S. Sridharan, ed., *International Joint Conference on Artificial Intelligence*, vol. 2. Morgan Kaufmann, San Mateo, CA, pp. 1504–1510.

Murphy, P. M. & Pazzani, M. J. (1991). ID2-of–3: constructive induction of M-of-N concepts for discriminators in decision trees. In L. Birnbaum & G. Collins, eds., *Proceedings of the 8th International Machine Learning Workshop*, Evanston, IL. Morgan-Kaufmann, San Mateo, CA, pp. 183–187.

Nayak, R., Hayward, R. & Diederich, J. (1997). Connectionist knowledge base representation by generic rules from trained feed-forward networks. In F. Maire, R. Hayward & J. Diederich, eds., *Connectionist Systems for Knowledge Representation and Deduction*, Queensland. University of Technology Publication, Brisbane, pp. 87–98.

Okada, H., Masuoka, R. & Kawamura, A. (1993). Knowledge based neural network – using fuzzy logic to initialise a multilayered neural network and interpret postlearning results. *Fujitsu Scientific and Technical Journal FAL* **29**, 217–226.

Omlin, C. W., Giles. C. L. & Miller, C. B. (1992). Heuristics for the extraction of rules from discrete time recurrent neural networks. In *Proceedings of the International Joint Conference on Neural Networks (IJCNN '92)*, Baltimore, MD. IEEE Press, New York, pp. I-33–I-38.

Optiz, D. W. & Shavlik, J. W. (1995). Dynamically adding symbolically meaningful nodes to knowledge-based neural networks. *Knowledge-based Systems* **8**, 301–311.

Pattichis, C. S., Schizas, C. N., Sergiou, A. & Schnorrenberg, F. (1994). A hybrid neural network electromyographic system: incorporating the WISARD net. In *Proceedings of the World Congress on Computational Intelligence*, Orlando, FL. IEEE Press, New York, pp. 3478–3483.

Pawlak, Z. (1991). *Rough Sets – Theoretical Aspects of Reasoning About Data*. Kluwer Academic Publishers, Dordrecht.

Quinlan, R. (1993). *C4.5: Programs for Machine Learning*. Morgan-Kaufmann, San Mateo, CA.

Rissanen, J. (1989). *Stochastic Complexity in Statistical Inquiry*. World Scientific, Singapore.

Saito, K. & Nakano, R. (1988). Medical diagnostic expert system based on PDP model. In *Proceedings of IEEE International Conference on Neural Networks*, vol. 1. IEEE, New York, pp. 255–262.

Saito, K. & Nakano, R. (1996). Law discovery using neural networks. In R. Andrews & J. Diederich, eds., *Proceedings of the NIPS *96 Rule Extraction From Trained Artificial Neural Networks Workshop*. Queensland University of Technology, Brisbane, pp. 62–69.

Sestito, S. & Dillon, T. (1991). The use of sub-symbolic methods for the automation of knowledge acquisition for expert systems. In J. C. Rault, ed., *Proceedings of the 11th International Conference on Expert Systems and their Applications (AVIGNON '91)*, Avignon, France. EC2, Nanterre, pp. 317–328.

Sestito, S. & Dillon, T. (1994). *Automated Knowledge Acquisition*. Prentice Hall, Englewood Cliffs, NJ.

Silverman, R. H. & Noetzel, A. S. (1990). Image processing and pattern recognition in ultrasonograms by backpropagation. *Neural Networks* **3**, 593–603.

Tan, A. & Carpenter, G. (1993). Rule extraction, fuzzy ARTMAP and medical databases. In *Proceedings of the World Congress on Neural Networks (WCNN '93)*, Portland, OR, vol. 1. Lawrence Erlbaum Associates, New York, pp. 501–506.

Thrun, S. B. (1994). Extracting provably correct rules from artificial neural networks, Technical Report IAI-TR-93-5. Institut für Informatik III Universität, Bonn.

Thrun, S. B., Bala, J., Bloedorn, E., Bratko, I., Cestnik, B., Cheng, J., De Jong, K., Dzeroski, S.,

Fahlman, S. E., Fisher, D., Hamann, R., Kaufman, K., Keller, S., Kononenko, I., Kreuziger, J., Michalski, R. S., Mitchell, T., Pachowicz, P., Reich, Y., Vafaie, H., Van de Welde, K., Wenzel, W., Wnek, J. & Zhang, J. (1991). The MONK's problems: a performance comparison of different learning algorithms. Technical Report CMU-CS-91-197. Carnegie Mellon University, Pittsburgh, PA.

Tickle, A. B., Orlowski, M. & Diederich, J. (1994). DEDEC: decision detection by rule extraction from neural networks. Technical Report QUTNRC-95-01. Queensland University of Technology, Neurocomputing Research Centre, Brisbane.

Tickle, A. B., Orlowski, M. & Diederich, J. (1996). DEDEC: a methodology for extracting rules from trained artificial neural networks. In R. Andrews & J. Diederich, eds., *Rules and Networks*. Queensland University of Technology, Brisbane, pp. 90–102.

Tickle, A. B., Andrews, R., Golea, M. & Diederich, J. (1999). The truth will come to light: directions and challenges in extracting the knowledge embedded within trained artificial neural networks. *IEEE Transactions on Neural Networks* **9**, 1057–1068.

Towell, G. & Shavlik, J. (1993). The extraction of refined rules from knowledge based neural networks. *Machine Learning* **131**, 71–101.

Tresp, V., Hollatz, J. & Ahmad, S. (1993). Network structuring and training using rule-based knowledge. In S. Hanson, J. Cowan & C. L. Giles, eds., *Advances in Neural Information Processing Systems (NIPS '93)*. Morgan Kaufmann, San Mateo, CA, pp. 871–878.

Viktor, H. L., Engelbrecht, A. P. & Cloete, I. (1995). Reduction of symbolic rules from artificial neural networks using sensitivity analysis. In *Proceedings of the IEEE International Conference on Neural Networks*, Perth, WA, vol. 3. IEEE Press, New York, pp. 1788–1793.

Williams, R. J. & Zipser, D. (1989). A learning algorithm for continually running fully recurrent neural networks. *Neural Computation* **1**, 270–280.

13

Confidence intervals and prediction intervals for feedforward neural networks

Richard Dybowski and Stephen J. Roberts

Artificial neural networks have been used as predictive systems for a variety of medical domains, but none of the systems encountered by Baxt (1995) and Dybowski & Gant (1995) in their reviews of the literature provided any measure of confidence in the predictions made by those systems. In a medical setting, measures of confidence are of paramount importance (Holst et al. 1998), and we introduce the reader to a number of methods that have been proposed for estimating the uncertainty associated with a value predicted by a feedforward neural network.

The chapter opens with an introduction to regression and its implementation within the maximum likelihood framework. This is followed by a general introduction to classical confidence intervals and prediction intervals. We set the scene by first considering confidence and prediction intervals based on univariate samples, and then we progress to regarding these intervals in the context of linear regression and logistic regression. Since a feedforward neural network is a type of regression model, the concepts of confidence and prediction intervals are applicable to these networks, and we look at several techniques for doing this via maximum likelihood estimation. An alternative to the maximum likelihood framework is Bayesian statistics, and we examine the notions of Bayesian confidence and prediction intervals as applied to feedforward networks. This includes a critique on Bayesian confidence intervals and classification.

Regression

Regression analysis is a common statistical technique for modelling the relationship between a *response* (or *dependent*) *variable* y and a set x of regressors $x_1, \ldots, x_d$ (also known as *independent* or *explanatory variables*). For example, the relationship could be between whether a patient has a malignant breast tumour (the response variable) and the patient's age and level of serum albumin (the regressors). When an article includes a discussion of artificial neural networks, it is customary to refer to response variables as *targets* and regressors as *inputs*.

Furthermore, the ordered set $\{x_1, \ldots, x_d\}$ is sometimes referred to as an *input vector*. We will adopt this practice for the remainder of this chapter.

Regression assumes that target y is related to input vector x by stochastic and deterministic components. The stochastic component is the random fluctuation of y about its mean $\mu_y(x)$; for example, one possibility is

$$y = \mu_y(x) + \varepsilon,$$

where *noise* ε, with zero mean, has a Gaussian distribution. The deterministic component is the functional relationship between $\mu_y(x)$ and x.

If the 'true' functional relationship between $\mu_y(x)$ and x is given by

$$\mu_y(x) = f(x; w_{\text{true}}), \tag{13.1}$$

where w is a set of parameters, regression attempts to estimate this relationship from a finite data set (a *derivation* or *training set*) by estimating the parameter values from the data. This is done by adjusting the values of w, under the assumption that f is the true function, to give

$$\hat{\mu}_y(x; \hat{w}) = f(x; \hat{w}), \tag{13.2}$$

where a hat denotes an estimated value. The function $f(x; \hat{w})$ will be referred to as a *regression function*,[1] and it will be used interchangeably with $\hat{\mu}_y(x; \hat{w})$. The best-known example of Eq. (13.2) is the *simple linear regression function*,

$$\hat{\mu}_y(x; \hat{w}) = \hat{w}_0 + \sum_{i=1}^{d} \hat{w}_i x_i, \tag{13.3}$$

where $\hat{w}_0, \hat{w}_1, \ldots, \hat{w}_d$ are the regression coefficients.

The maximum likelihood framework

Suppose we have a dataset $\{x^{(1)}, y^{(1)}, \ldots, x^{(N)}, y^{(N)}\}$, where $y^{(n)}$ is the target value associated with the n-th input vector $x^{(n)}$, and we wish to fit a regression function $f(x; \hat{w})$ to this data. How do we select $\hat{w}$?

Maximum likelihood estimation (MLE) is based on the intuitive idea that the best estimate of $\hat{w}$ for $f(x; \hat{w})$ is that set of parameter values $\hat{w}_{\text{MLE}}$ for which the observed data have the highest probability of arising. More formally,

$$\hat{w}_{\text{MLE}} = \arg \max_{\hat{w}} p(y^{(1)}, \ldots, y^{(N)} \mid x^{(1)}, \ldots, x^{(N)}, \hat{w}), \tag{13.4}$$

$p(\cdot \mid \cdot \cdot)$ denoting a probability function.[2]

Let the distribution of y about $\mu_y(x)$ be defined by a conditional probability distribution $p(y \mid x)$. For regression function $f(x; \hat{w})$, this distribution is approximated by $\hat{p}(y \mid x, \hat{w})$ with mean $\hat{\mu}_y(x; \hat{w})$; therefore, if the cases of dataset $\{x^{(1)}, y^{(1)}, \ldots, x^{(N)}, y^{(N)}\}$ are sampled independently from the same population, Eq. (13.4) can be simplified to

$$\hat{w}_{\text{MLE}} = \underset{\hat{w}}{\arg\min} \left[-\sum_{n=1}^{N} \ln \hat{p}(y^{(n)} \mid x^{(n)}, \hat{w}) \right]. \tag{13.5}$$

If the distribution of y about $\mu_y(x)$ is assumed to be Gaussian,

$$\hat{p}(y \mid x, w) = \frac{1}{\sqrt{2\pi}\sigma_y} \exp\left\{ \frac{-[\hat{\mu}_y(x; w) - y]^2}{\sigma_y^2} \right\}, \tag{13.6}$$

substitution of Eq. (13.6) into the negative sum of Eq. (13.5) (and ignoring constant terms) gives

$$\hat{w}_{\text{MLE}} = \underset{w}{\arg\min} \, Err(w), \tag{13.7}$$

where

$$Err(w) = \frac{1}{2} \sum_{n=1}^{N} [\hat{\mu}_y(x^{(n)}; w) - y^{(n)}]^2, \tag{13.8}$$

$Err(\cdot)$ denoting an *error function*.

If a feedforward neural network (FNN) $f(x; \hat{w})$ is trained on data set $\{x^{(1)}, y^{(1)}, \ldots, x^{(N)}, y^{(N)}\}$ by minimizing $Err(w)$, where w are the network weights, it can be shown that the resulting network approximates the mean value for y conditioned on x (Bishop 1995, pp. 201–203),

$$f(x; \hat{w}_{\text{MLE}}) \approx \mu_y(x), \tag{13.9}$$

the approximation becoming equality if N goes to infinity and $f(x; \hat{w})$ has unlimited flexibility. Thus, from Eq. (13.2), an FNN trained via $Err(w)$ can be regarded as a regression function.

Sources of uncertainty

There are two types of prediction that we may want from a regression function for a given input x: one is the mean $\mu_y(x)$; the other is the target value y associated with x.

Even if we are fortunate to have a regression function equal to the true model, so that $\hat{\mu}_y(x; \hat{w})$ is equal to $\mu_y(x)$ for all x, y cannot be determined with certainty. This is due to the intrinsic random fluctuation of y about its mean $\mu_y(x)$ (*target noise*).

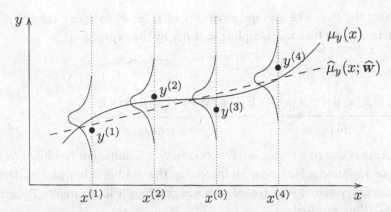

Figure 13.1. An illustration of a regression function. The 'true' model consists of a probability function $p(y|x)$ for y, with a mean $\mu_y(x)$ (bold curve) which is dependent on x. Data set $\{(x^{(1)}, y^{(1)}), (x^{(2)}, y^{(2)}), (x^{(3)}, y^{(3)}), (x^{(4)}, y^{(4)})\}$ can be regarded as having been obtained by first randomly sampling $\{x^{(1)}, x^{(2)}, x^{(3)}, x^{(4)}\}$ from a population and then randomly sampling $y^{(1)}$ from $p(y|x^{(1)})$, $y^{(2)}$ from $p(y|x^{(2)})$, $y^{(3)}$ from $p(y|x^{(3)})$, and $y^{(4)}$ from $p(y|x^{(4)})$. Given the resulting data set $\{(x^{(1)}, y^{(1)}), (x^{(2)}, y^{(2)}), (x^{(3)}, y^{(3)}), (x^{(4)}, y^{(4)})\}$, a regression function $\hat{\mu}_y(x; \hat{w})$ (dashed line) attempts to estimate $\mu_y(x)$ by adjustment of a set of model parameters w.

When y is continuously valued, the best one can do is establish a predictive probability density on y or a region where y is most likely to occur – a prediction interval. We will return to the concept of prediction intervals in the next section, our attention here being focused on $\hat{\mu}_y(x; \hat{w})$.

The acquisition of a training set $\{x^{(1)}, y^{(1)}, \ldots, x^{(N)}, y^{(N)}\}$ is prone to *sampling variation*. There are two reasons for this. Firstly, there is variability in the random sampling of $x^{(1)}, \ldots, x^{(N)}$ from the associated population. Secondly, for each selected $x^{(n)}$, there is a random fluctuation in the value of y about the mean $\mu_y(x)$, as defined by $p(y|x)$ (Figure 13.1 illustrates the univariate case). Consequently, the training set used for an FNN is only one of a large (possibly infinite) number of possibilities. Since each possible training set can give rise to a different set of network weights $\hat{w}$, it follows that there is a distribution of $\hat{\mu}_y(x; \hat{w})$ values for a given input x.

If we randomly sample (with replacement) an infinite number of data sets $\mathscr{D}$, the resulting $\hat{\mu}_y(x; \hat{w})$ values will be distributed about the mean (or *expected value*) $\mathsf{E}_{\mathscr{D}}[\hat{\mu}_y(x; \hat{w})]$ with *sampling variance*

$$\mathsf{E}_{\mathscr{D}}[\{\hat{\mu}_y(x; \hat{w}) - \mathsf{E}_{\mathscr{D}}[\hat{\mu}_y(x; \hat{w})]\}^2]$$

but $\mathsf{E}_{\mathscr{D}}[\hat{\mu}_y(x; \hat{w})]$ is not necessarily equal to $\mu_y(x)$, the difference

$$\mathsf{E}_{\mathscr{D}}[\hat{\mu}_y(x; \hat{w})] - \mu_y(x)$$

being the *bias*. The average proximity of $\hat{\mu}_y(x; \hat{w})$ to $\mu_y(x)$, taken over all $\mathscr{D}$, is related to the bias and sampling variance by the expression

$$E_{\mathscr{D}}[\{\hat{\mu}_y(x; \hat{w}) - \mu_y(x)\}^2] =$$

$$\underbrace{\{E_{\mathscr{D}}[\hat{\mu}_y(x; \hat{w})] - \mu_y(x)\}^2}_{\{bias\}^2} + \underbrace{E_{\mathscr{D}}[\{\hat{\mu}_y(x; \hat{w}) - E_{\mathscr{D}}[\hat{\mu}_y(x; \hat{w})]\}^2]}_{variance}. \tag{13.10}$$

Bias is due to a regression function having insufficient flexibility to model the data adequately. However, on increasing the flexibility in order to decrease bias, sampling variance is increased (this was graphically illustrated by Bishop (1995, p. 336); thus, optimal

$$E_{\mathscr{D}}[\{\hat{\mu}_y(x; \hat{w}) - \mu_y(x)\}^2]$$

requires a trade-off between bias and variance (Gemen et al. 1992). The standard method for achieving this trade-off with FNNs is to augment the error function with a term that penalizes against overfitting (a regularization term), such as the weight decay procedure (Hinton 1989).

When a regression function is an FNN, there are additional sources of error in $\hat{w}$ (Penny & Roberts 1997). One is due to the fact that an error function can have many local minima resulting in a number of possible $\hat{w}$. Another potential error in $\hat{w}$ arises from suboptimal training, for example by premature termination of a training algorithm.

In the above discussion, uncertainty in $\hat{\mu}_y(x; \hat{w})$ has been attributed to uncertainty in $\hat{w}$, but there are two sources of uncertainty not originating from $\hat{w}$, namely uncertainty in the input values (*input noise*, see p. 322) and uncertainty in the structure of the regression model (*model uncertainty*). As regards the latter, the regression model consists of two parts: an assumed structure for the model and a set of parameters w whose meaning is specific to the choice of model structure; therefore, uncertainty in $\hat{\mu}_y(x; \hat{w})$ should reflect the uncertainty in model structure as well as the uncertainty in $\hat{w}$. An approach to this problem has been suggested by Draper (1995), in which a range of structural alternatives are considered, but we are not aware of an application of this method to FNNs.

Classical confidence intervals and prediction intervals

There is uncertainty in the values of $\hat{\mu}_y(x; \hat{w})$ and y due to their respective distributions about the true mean $\mu_y(x)$. Such uncertainties can, in principle, be quantified by confidence and prediction intervals. We will define these terms and consider their application to regression, and thus to FNNs.

Let μ_v be the mean of a population of values v. The mean $\bar{v}$ of a sample S drawn randomly from the population is a point estimate of μ_v but, given that $\bar{v}$ is unlikely to be exactly equal to μ_v, how reliable a measure of μ_v is $\bar{v}$? A response to this question is to derive a lower limit $\lambda_L(S)$ and an upper limit $\lambda_U(S)$ from S such that there is a 95% probability that interval $[\lambda_L(S), \lambda_U(S)]$ will contain μ_v. By this we mean that, if an infinite number of samples $S_1, S_2, \ldots$ of equal size are drawn randomly (with replacement) from the population, 95% of the intervals

$$[\lambda_L(S_1), \lambda_U(S_1)], [\lambda_L(S_2), \lambda_U(S_2)], \cdots$$

associated with these samples will overlap μ_v, which is fixed. Such an interval is referred to as a (*classical*) 95% *confidence interval* for μ_v.[3]

If sample S consists of univariate values $v^{(1)}, \ldots, v^{(N)}$, one can also consider an interval $[\psi_L(S), \psi_U(S)]$ such that there is a 95% probability that a new value $v^{(N+1)}$ drawn randomly from the population will occur within the interval. Such an interval is referred to as a 95% *prediction interval* for $v^{(N+1)}$. Whereas a confidence interval is for a population parameter, a prediction interval is for a single value randomly drawn from the population.

As an example, for sample $v^{(1)}, \ldots, v^{(N)}$, where v is continuously valued, the 95% prediction interval for $v^{(N+1)}$ is given by (Geisser 1993, pp. 6–9)

$$\bar{v} \pm t_{0.025[N-1]} \left(s \sqrt{\frac{1}{N} + 1} \right),$$

where $t_{0.025[N-1]}$ is the required critical value of Student's t-distribution ($N-1$ degrees of freedom), and s is the standard deviation of the sample. This interval is wider than the 95% confidence interval for μ_v,

$$\bar{v} \pm t_{0.025[N-1]} \left(s \sqrt{\frac{1}{N}} \right),$$

because $v^{(N+1)}$ is variable whereas μ_v is constant.

When v is binary valued, μ_v is equivalent to $p(v=1)$, but the construction of a confidence interval for $p(v=1)$ is complicated by the fact that $\bar{v}$ is discrete (Dudewicz & Mishra 1988, pp. 561–566). The discrete nature of $\bar{v}$ results in a confidence interval $[\lambda_L(S), \lambda_U(S)]$ with *at least a* 95% probability of containing $p(v=1)$. However, for large N, $\bar{v}$ can be assumed to have a normal distribution (Hogg & Craig 1995; pp. 272–273). Given that v is either 0 or 1 when it is binary valued, and nothing in between, there is no prediction interval for $v^{(N+1)}$ as such.[4] For the remainder of this chapter, confidence and prediction intervals will be understood to be of the classical type, unless stated otherwise.

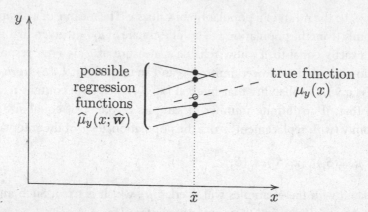

Figure 13.2. True function (dashed line) and several regression functions (solid lines) in the vicinity of x_0. The different regression functions are caused by variation in $\hat{w}$ due to sampling variation. Each black dot is a possible value for $\hat{\mu}_y(x_0; \hat{w})$, the open circle representing the correct value $\mu_y(x_0)$. (After Wonnacott & Wonnacott 1981.)

Confidence and prediction intervals for simple linear regression

Confidence and prediction intervals can also be applied to regression, where they are collectively referred to as *error bars* by some authors. Variation in a finite sample S leads to variation in $\hat{w}$ and thus variation in $\hat{\mu}_y(x; \hat{w})$. Consequently, there is a distribution of possible values for $\hat{\mu}_y(x_0; \hat{w})$ about $\mu_y(x_0)$, where x_0 is a particular value for x. This is illustrated in Figure 13.2. Above, we described the idea of attaching an interval $[\lambda_L(S), \lambda_U(S)]$ to $\bar{v}$ such that the interval has a 95% probability of overlapping with μ_v. In an analogous manner, we can conceptualize the existence of a 95% confidence interval $[\lambda_L(S, x_0), \lambda_U(S, x_0)]$ for $\mu_y(x_0)$ attached to each $\hat{\mu}_y(x_0; \hat{w})$ by defining it in a manner analogous to the probabilistic interpretation given to confidence interval $[\lambda_L(S), \lambda_U(S)]$ above, namely that $[\lambda_L(S, x_0), \lambda_U(S, x_0)]$ has a 95% probability of overlapping $\mu_y(x_0)$, which is fixed. A conceptual representation of this idea is given in Figure 13.3. Furthermore, motivated by the above definition of prediction interval $[\psi_L(S), \psi_U(S)]$, one can also conceptualize the existence of a 95% prediction interval $[\psi_L(S, x_0), \psi_U(S, x_0)]$ for the unknown value of y associated with x_0. For example, if we linearly regress y on x using $\{x^{(1)}, y^{(1)}, \ldots, x^{(N)}, y^{(N)}\}$ as the sample S, the 95% confidence interval for $\mu_y(x_0)$ is

$$\hat{\mu}_y(x_0; \hat{w}) \pm t_{0.025[N-2]}\left(s\sqrt{\frac{1}{N} + \frac{(x_0 - \bar{x})^2}{\sum_{n=1}^{N}(x^{(n)} - \bar{x})^2}}\right), \tag{13.11}$$

and the 95% prediction interval for y at x_0 is

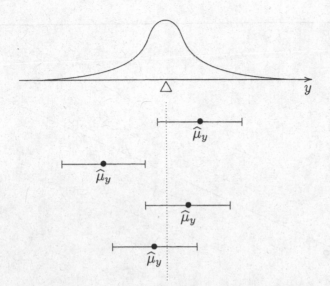

Figure 13.3. An illustration of classical confidence intervals. Variation in $\hat{w}$ due to sampling variation results in a distribution of possible $\hat{\mu}_y(x_o; \hat{w})$ values (Figure 13.2). This distribution is defined by a probability distribution $p(\hat{\mu}_y(x_o; \hat{w}))$ (the Gaussian curve). Four possible values of $\hat{\mu}_y(x_o; \hat{w})$ randomly sampled from $p(\hat{\mu}_y(x_o; \hat{w}))$ are shown (black dots). Also shown are the 95% confidence intervals associated with these four values. The triangle indicates the position of $\hat{\mu}_y(x_o)$. Ninety-five per cent of all values sampled from $p(\hat{\mu}_y(x_o; \hat{w}))$ will have their intervals correctly bracketing $\mu_y(x_o)$ if $\hat{\mu}_y(x_o; \hat{w})$ is not biased. If $\hat{\mu}_y(x_o; \hat{w})$ is biased, then the mean of $p(\hat{\mu}_y(x_o; \hat{w}))$ will not coincide with $\mu_y(x_o)$. (After Wonnacott & Wonnacott 1985.)

$$\hat{\mu}_y(x_o; \hat{w}) \pm t_{0.025[N-2]}\left(s\sqrt{\frac{1}{N}+\frac{(x_o-\bar{x})^2}{\sum\limits_{n=1}^{N}(x^{(n)}-\bar{x})^2}+1}\right),\tag{13.12}$$

where s is the standard deviation for $y^{(1)}, \ldots, y^{(N)}$ and $\bar{x}$ is the mean of $x^{(1)}, \ldots, x^{(N)}$ (Figure 13.4). Wonnacott & Wonnacott (1981, pp. 42–47) gave a derivation of these intervals in the context of simple linear regression, and Penny & Roberts (1997) have reviewed prediction intervals associated with other forms of linear regression.

A set of confidence intervals constructed continuously over an input x produces a two-dimensional *confidence band*. In a similar manner, a continuous set of prediction intervals over x produces a *prediction band*.

Confidence intervals for logistic regression

Logistic regression is the most popular technique for modelling a binary target y as a function of input vector x (Hosmer & Lemeshow 1989; Collett 1991).[5] This is

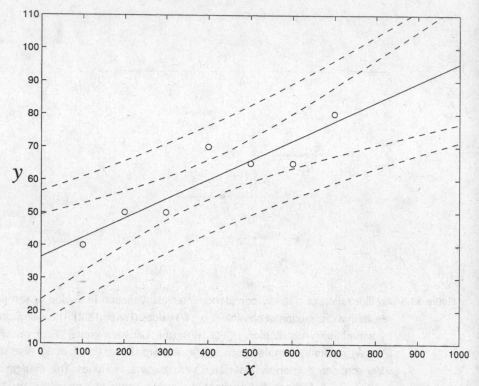

Figure 13.4. Linear regression function (solid line) with a 95% confidence band for $\mu_y(x)$ (region bounded by the inner dashed lines) and a 95% prediction band for y (region bounded by the outer dashed lines) based on intervals (13.11) and (13.12), respectively. Each open circle represents a data point.

done by assuming that probability $p(y=1\,|\,x)$ is related to x by a logistic function,

$$p(y=1\,|\,x) = \left\{ 1 + \exp\left[-\left(w_0 + \sum_{i=1}^{d} w_i x_i \right) \right] \right\}^{-1}. \tag{13.13}$$

When y is binary, $\mu_y(x)$ is equivalent to $p(y=1\,|\,x)$, therefore, Eq. (13.13) can be estimated as a regression function

$$\hat{p}(y=1\,|\,x;\hat{w}) = \left\{ 1 + \exp\left[-\left(\hat{w}_0 + \sum_{i=1}^{d} \hat{w}_i x_i \right) \right] \right\}^{-1}. \tag{13.14}$$

In the context of maximum likelihood, Eq. (13.5) still applies but the binary nature of y implies a binomial distribution for y,

$$p(y\,|\,x) = p(y=1\,|\,x)^y [1 - p(y=1\,|\,x)]^{(1-y)}.$$

It follows that the error function for Eq. (13.7), which is the negative logarithm of the relevant probability density, becomes

$$Err(w) = -\sum_{n=1}^{N} \{y^{(n)}\hat{p}(y=1\,|\,x^{(n)};\,w) + [1-y^{(n)}][1-\hat{p}(y=1\,|\,x^{(n)};\,w)]\}. \tag{13.15}$$

As with any regression modelling, logistic regression is susceptible to sampling variation; consequently, the regression parameters, and thus the logistic regression function, are subject to variation. A representation of this variation is obtained from Figure 13.2 by replacing $\mu_y(x_o)$ with $p(y=1\,|\,x_o)$ and $\hat{\mu}_y(x_o;\,\hat{w})$ with $\hat{p}(y=1\,|\,x_o;\,\hat{w})$, respectively. Just as with linear regression, the variation of $\hat{p}(y=1\,|\,x_o;\,\hat{w})$ about $p(y=1\,|\,x_o)$ due to variation in $\hat{w}$ leads to the concept of a confidence interval $[\lambda_L(S,x_o),\ \lambda_U(S,\ x_o)]$ for $p(y=1\,|\,x_o)$. This interval has been derived analytically by Hauck (1983). If sample size N is large ($N > 100$), that 95% confidence interval for $p(y=1\,|\,x)$ is approximated by the logistic transform of

$$\text{logit } \hat{p}(y=1\,|\,x;\,\hat{w}) \pm \sqrt{\chi^2_{\alpha[d+1]}x^T\hat{\Sigma}x/N}, \tag{13.16}$$

where x is a $d+1$ dimensional vector $(1, x_1, \ldots, x_d)^T$, $\hat{\Sigma}$ is the covariance matrix for $\hat{w}$, and $\chi^2_{\alpha[d+1]}$ is the χ^2 critical value for the $100(1-\alpha)$ percentage point for $d+1$ degree of freedom (Figure 13.5).[6] See Santner & Duffy (1989, pp. 238–239) for further discussion.

Confidence intervals for feedforward neural networks

So far, we have looked at linear and logistic regression, but if we have $\hat{\mu}_y(x;\,\hat{w})$ from an FNN, how can we obtain a confidence interval for $\mu_y(x)$? We start with two approaches: the delta method and the bootstrap method.

The delta method

If a variable v has a Gaussian distribution with variance $\text{Var}(v)$, a 95% confidence interval for the mean of v is given by

$$v \pm z_{0.025}\sqrt{\text{Var}(v)},$$

where $z_{0.025}$ is the critical point of the standard normal distribution. The delta method provides an estimate of this variance via the Taylor series.

If $\mu_{\hat{w}}$ is the mean vector for $\hat{w}$, the first-order Taylor expansion of $\hat{\mu}_y(x;\,\hat{w})$ around $\mu_{\hat{w}}$ gives the approximation

$$\hat{\mu}_y(x;\,\hat{w}) \approx \hat{\mu}_y(x;\,\mu_{\hat{w}}) + g(x)(\hat{w}-\mu_{\hat{w}}), \tag{13.17}$$

where the i-th element of vector $g(x)$ is the partial derivative $\partial\hat{\mu}_y(x;\,\hat{w})/\partial\hat{w}_i$ evaluated at $\hat{w}=\mu_{\hat{w}}$. According to the *delta method* (Efron & Tibshirani 1993, pp.

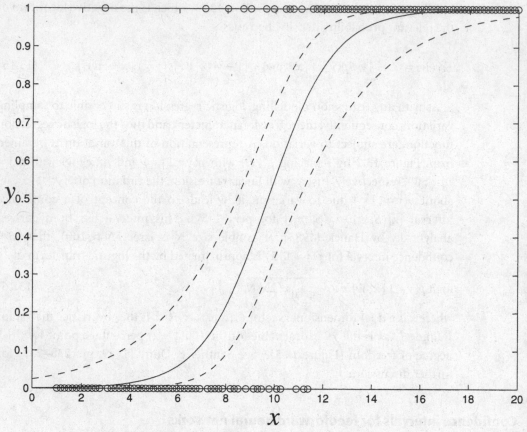

Figure 13.5. Logistic regression function (solid line) with a 95% confidence band for $p(y=1\,|\,x)$ (region bounded by the dashed lines) according to Hauck's method (i.e. interval (13.16)).

313–315), it follows from Eq. (13.17) that the variance for $\hat{\mu}_y(x; \hat{w})$ over all possible samples is approximated by

$$\widehat{\mathrm{Var}}(\hat{\mu}_y(x; \hat{w})) = g^T(x)\, \Sigma g(x),\qquad\qquad (13.18)$$

where Σ is the covariance matrix for $\hat{w}$.

The elements of a Hessian matrix H are second-order partial derivatives[7]

$$H_{i,j} = \frac{\partial^2 Err(w)}{\partial w_i \partial w_j},$$

evaluated at $w = \hat{w}$, where $Err(w)$ is the relevant error function. Covariance matrix Σ is related to the Hessian (Press et al. 1992, pp. 672–673, 685), and if the error function is defined as in Eq. (13.8) and noise variance σ_ε^2 is independent of x then Eq. (13.18) can be replaced by[8]

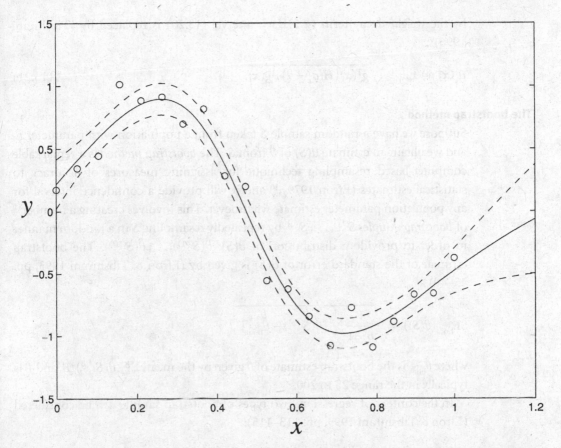

Figure 13.6. Regression function (solid line) obtained from a feedforward network with a 95% confidence band for $\mu_y(x)$ (region bounded by dashed lines) based on the delta method (i.e. interval (13.20)).

$$\widehat{\mathrm{Var}}(\hat{\mu}_y(x; \hat{w})) = \sigma_\varepsilon^2 g^T(x) H^{-1} g(x). \tag{13.19}$$

Tibshirani (1996) estimates σ_ε^2 using

$$\sigma_\varepsilon^2 = \sum_{i=1}^{N} [y^{(i)} - \hat{\mu}_y(x^{(i)}; \hat{w})]^2/N.$$

From Eq. (13.19), and assuming a Gaussian target noise distribution, we have the approximate 95% confidence interval for $\mu_y(x)$ (Figure 13.6)

$$\hat{\mu}_y(x; \hat{w}) \pm z_{0.025} \sqrt{\sigma_\varepsilon^2 g^T(x) H^{-1} g(x)}. \tag{13.20}$$

Regularization is the inclusion of a penalty term in an error function to discourage overfitting of the network to the training data. This improves the ability of the network to generalize from the data. If regularization is implemented by the weight-decay term $(\alpha/2)\Sigma_i w_i^2$, interval (13.20) is replaced by (Tibshirani 1996)[9]

$$\hat{\mu}_y(\boldsymbol{x}; \hat{\boldsymbol{w}}) \pm z_{0.025}\sqrt{\boldsymbol{g}^T(\boldsymbol{x})(\boldsymbol{H}/\sigma_\varepsilon^2 - \alpha)^{-1}\boldsymbol{g}(\boldsymbol{x})}. \tag{13.21}$$

The bootstrap method

Suppose we have a random sample S taken from a population with parameter θ, and we obtain an estimate $\hat{\theta}(S)$ of θ from S. The *bootstrap method* is a remarkable computer-based resampling technique for assigning measures of accuracy to statistical estimates (Efron 1979),[10] and it will provide a confidence interval for any population parameter estimate whatsoever. This involves creating a number[11] of *bootstrap samples* $S^{(*1)}, \ldots, S^{(*B)}$ by repeatedly resampling S in a random manner in order to provide a distribution of $\hat{\theta}(S)$: $\hat{\theta}(S^{(*1)}), \ldots, \hat{\theta}(S^{(*B)})$. The bootstrap estimate of the standard error of $\hat{\theta}(S)$ is given by (Efron & Tibshirani 1993, pp. 45–49)

$$\widehat{SE}_{boot}(\hat{\theta}(S)) = \sqrt{\frac{1}{B-1}\sum_{b=1}^{B}[\hat{\theta}(S^{(*b)}) - \hat{\theta}_{boot}]^2},$$

where $\hat{\theta}_{boot}$ is the bootstrap estimate of $\hat{\theta}$ given by the mean $\Sigma_{b=1}^{B}\hat{\theta}(S^{(*b)})/B$, and B is typically in the range 25 to 200.

In the context of regression, two types of bootstrap sample can be considered (Efron & Tibshirani 1993, pp. 113–115):

pairs sampling in which regression is based on the bootstrap sample

$$\{\boldsymbol{x}^{(*i,1)}, y^{(*i,1)}, \ldots, \boldsymbol{x}^{(*i,N)}, y^{(*i,N)}\}$$

taken from the true sample $\{\boldsymbol{x}^{(1)}, y^{(1)}, \ldots, \boldsymbol{x}^{(N)}, y^{(N)}\}$, where $(*i, 1), \ldots, (*i, N)$ is the i-th random sample with replacement of the integers $1, \ldots, N$;

residual sampling in which regression is based on the bootstrap sample

$$\{\boldsymbol{x}^{(1)}, \hat{\mu}_y(\boldsymbol{x}^{(1)}; \hat{\boldsymbol{w}}) + r^{(*i,1)}, \ldots, \boldsymbol{x}^{(N)}, \hat{\mu}_y(\boldsymbol{x}^{(N)}; \hat{\boldsymbol{w}}) + r^{(*i,N)}\},$$

where $r^{(*i,1)}, \ldots, r^{(*i,N)}$ is a random sample of the N residuals associated with $\hat{\mu}_y(\boldsymbol{x}^{(1)}; \hat{\boldsymbol{w}}), \ldots, \hat{\mu}_y(\boldsymbol{x}^{(N)}; \hat{\boldsymbol{w}})$, respectively.

Residual sampling has the advantage that it limits inferences to the set of input values $\boldsymbol{x}^{(1)}, \ldots, \boldsymbol{x}^{(N)}$ actually observed (Baxt & White 1995), but, unlike pairs sampling, it uses the strong assumption that residuals are independent of the inputs. Furthermore, the $\boldsymbol{x}$ values are assumed to be random in pairs sampling but fixed in residual sampling. The algorithms for pairs sampling and residual sampling are as follows.

Algorithm 1. (*Bootstrap pairs sampling*)
begin
> let $\{(x^{(1)}, y^{(1)}), \ldots, (x^{(N)}, y^{(N)})\}$ be the true sample S;
> **for** $b = 1$ **to** B **do**
>> randomly sample (with replacement) N (x, y)-pairs from S;
>> let $\{(x^{(*b,1)}, y^{(*b,1)}), \ldots, (x^{(*b,N)}, y^{(*b,N)})\}$ be the random sample;
>> derive regression function $\hat{\mu}_y(x; \hat{w}^{(*b)})$ from training set
>> $\{(x^{(*b,1)}, y^{(*b,1)}), \ldots, (x^{(*b,N)}, y^{(*b,N)})\}$;
> **endfor**
end

Algorithm 2. (*Bootstrap residual sampling*)
begin
> let $\{(x^{(1)}, y^{(1)}), \ldots, (x^{(N)}, y^{(N)})\}$ be the true sample S;
> derive regression function $\hat{\mu}_y(x; \hat{w})$ from S;
> let R be the set of *residuals* $\{r^{(1)}, \ldots, r^{(N)}\}$, where $r^{(n)} = y^{(n)} - \hat{\mu}_y(x^{(n)}; \hat{w})$;
> **for** $b = 1$ **to** B **do**
>> randomly sample (with replacement) N residuals from R;
>> let $\{r^{(*b,1)}, \ldots, r^{(*b,N)}\}$ be the random sample;
>> derive regression function $\hat{\mu}_y(x; \hat{w}^{(*b)})$ from training set
>> $\{(x^{(1)}, \hat{\mu}_y(x^{(1)}; \hat{w}) + r^{(*b,1)}), \ldots, (x^{(N)}, \hat{\mu}_y(x^{(N)}; \hat{w}) + r^{(*b,N)})\}$;
> **endfor**
end

For both the pairs-sampling and residual-sampling approaches, the bootstrap estimate of $\hat{\mu}_y(x)$ is given by the mean provided by the ensemble of regression functions $\hat{\mu}_y(x; \hat{w}^{(*1)}), \ldots, \hat{\mu}_y(x; \hat{w}^{(*B)})$:

$$\hat{\mu}_{y,\text{boot}}(x) = \frac{1}{B} \sum_{b=1}^{B} \hat{\mu}_y(x; \hat{w}^{(*b)}). \tag{13.22}$$

Furthermore, the bootstrap estimate of the standard error of $\hat{\mu}_y(x; \hat{w})$, which is a function of x, is given by

$$\widehat{\text{SE}}_{\text{boot}}(\hat{\mu}_y(x; \cdot)) = \sqrt{\frac{1}{B-1} \sum_{b=1}^{B} [\hat{\mu}_y(x; \hat{w}^{(*b)}) - \hat{\mu}_{y,\text{boot}}(x)]^2}, \tag{13.23}$$

with $\hat{\mu}_{y,\text{boot}}(x)$ defined as in Eq. (13.22). Assuming a normal distribution for $\hat{\mu}_y(x; \hat{w})$ over the space of all possible $\hat{w}$, we have

$$\hat{\mu}_{y,\text{boot}}(x) \pm t_{0.025[B]} \widehat{\text{SE}}_{\text{boot}}(\hat{\mu}_y(x; \cdot))$$

as the 95% bootstrap confidence interval for $\mu_y(x)$ (Heskes 1997).

As stated earlier, logistic regression provides a regression function that estimates the conditional probability $p(y=1 \,|\, x)$. By using a logistic transfer function for the output node, and the cross-entropy error function (Eq. 13.15), $p(y=1 \,|\, x)$ can also be estimated by an FNN trained with binary target values. Furthermore, the bootstrap estimate $\hat{\mu}_{y,\text{boot}}(x)$ provides a mean conditional probability with the advantages of a *bagged* predictor (Breiman 1996). The concept of a confidence interval for $p(y=1 \,|\, x)$, as used for logistic regression, can also be applied to an FNN; however, we have not found a published description of a bootstrap confidence interval for $p(y=1 \,|\, x)$ via an FNN.

A disadvantage of the bootstrap method is that the computational cost could be high when data sets or networks are large; however, Tibshirani (1996) found that the bootstrap approach provided more accurate confidence intervals than did the delta method. A contribution to this success is that bootstrap sampling takes into account the variability of FNNs due to different initial network weights. Another factor in favour of the bootstrap method is the fact that the delta method requires computation of derivatives and Hessian matrix inversion, the latter being a potential source of failure.

Prediction intervals for feedforward neural networks

If y has a Gaussian distribution with mean $E[y \,|\, x]$ and variance $\text{Var}(y \,|\, x)$, a 95% prediction interval for y is given by

$$E[y \,|\, x] \pm z_{0.025}\sqrt{\text{Var}(y \,|\, x)}.$$

This is the basis for an approximate prediction interval, as follows.

The variance of y conditioned on x is defined by

$$\text{Var}(y \,|\, x) = E[(E[y \,|\, x] - y)^2 \,|\, x].$$

Recall that an FNN $\hat{\mu}_y(x^{(n)}; \hat{w})$ trained with respect to error function

$$\frac{1}{2}\sum_{n=1}^{N}[\hat{\mu}_y(x^{(n)}; w) - y^{(n)}]^2, \tag{13.24}$$

can approximate $E[y \,|\, x]$. This suggests that, in order to obtain $E[(E[y \,|\, x] - y)^2 \,|\, x]$ in place of $E[y \,|\, x]$ by means of an FNN $\hat{\sigma}_y^2(x; \hat{u})$, we should replace y in error function (13.24) with $(E[y \,|\, x] - y)^2$. Therefore, if $\hat{\mu}_y(x; \hat{w})$ is assumed to be equal to $E[y \,|\, x]$, an FNN $\hat{\sigma}_y^2(x; \hat{u})$ for the estimation of $\text{Var}(y \,|\, x)$ can be derived by using

$$\frac{1}{2}\sum_{n=1}^{N}[\hat{\sigma}_y^2(x; u) - [\hat{\mu}_y(x^{(n)}; \hat{w}) - y^{(n)}]^2]^2 \tag{13.25}$$

as the error function. This leads to the approximate 95% prediction interval

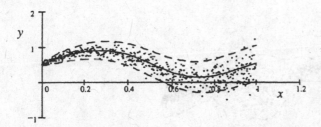

Figure 13.7. Data with increasing variance. The regression function (solid line) was estimated by a feedforward network. Another feedforward network was used to estimate the input-dependent variance from which a 95% prediction band (region bounded by dashed lines) was obtained by interval (13.26).

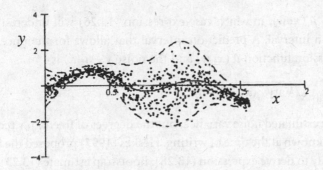

Figure 13.8. Both the regression function (solid line) and its associated 95% prediction band (region bounded by dashed lines) were obtained from a Nix–Weigend network.

$$\hat{\mu}_y(x; \hat{w}) \pm z_{0.025}\sqrt{\hat{\sigma}_y^2(x; \hat{u})}. \tag{13.26}$$

A 95% prediction band resulting from this interval is shown in Figure 13.7.

Rather than using two separate networks, Nix & Weigend (1995) proposed a single network with one output for $\hat{\mu}_y(x; \hat{w})$ and another for $\hat{\sigma}_y^2(x; \hat{u})$, using

$$\frac{1}{2}\sum_{n=1}^{N}\left[\frac{[\hat{\mu}_y(x^{(n)}; w) - y^{(n)}]^2}{\hat{\sigma}_y^2(x; u)} + \ln \hat{\sigma}_y^2(x; u)\right]^2 \tag{13.27}$$

as the error function. This approach can produce improved prediction intervals for y compared with the previous approach as a result of it acting as a form of weighted regression (weighted in favour of low noise regions) (Figure 13.8). The simpler approach based on expression (13.25) tries to fit around high noise regions, possibly distorting the low noise regions (Figure 13.9), whereas weighted regression is not influenced by regions of high fluctuation.

An underlying assumption in using either expression (13.25) or (13.27) is that $\hat{\mu}_y(x; \hat{w})$ is equal to $E[y|x]$, but, when this assumption is false, there will be

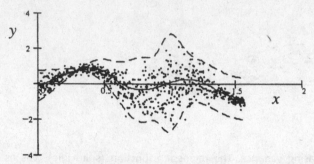

Figure 13.9. Same data as that in Figure 13.8 but, instead of using a Nix–Weigend network, a separate feedforward network estimated the variance. This resulted in a decrease in the accuracy of the 95% prediction band (region bounded by dashed lines).

uncertainty in $\hat\mu_y(x; \hat w)$, in which case expression (13.26) will underestimate the 95% prediction interval. A prediction interval that allows for the uncertainty in both the regression function $\hat\mu_y(x; \hat w)$ and the noise $y - \mu_y(x)$ is

$$\hat\mu_y(x; \hat w) \pm t_{0.025[\nu]}\sqrt{\widehat{\mathrm{Var}}(\hat\mu_y(x; \hat w)) + \hat\sigma_\varepsilon^2}, \tag{13.28}$$

where $\hat\sigma_\varepsilon^2$ is the estimated noise variance, but the degrees of freedom ν required for an FNN is not known at the time of writing. Heskes (1997) proposed the bootstrap method as a way to derive expression (13.28). Bootstrap estimate (13.23) was used for $\widehat{\mathrm{Var}}(\hat\mu_y(x; \hat w))$, and an auxiliary FNN, trained on the unused portions of the bootstrap samples, was used to estimate $\hat\sigma_\varepsilon^2$. Although Heskes obtained more realistic prediction intervals than those provided by the Nix & Weigend (1995) method, we feel that his technique requires further analysis.

The methods used in this section are based on maximum likelihood estimation, but variances estimated by MLE are biased:

$$E[\widehat{\mathrm{Var}}_{\mathrm{MLE}}(y\,|\,x)] < \mathrm{Var}(y\,|\,x).$$

This is caused by a tendency of an interpolant to try to fit to the data, thereby underestimating $\mathrm{Var}(y\,|\,x)$. Consequently, if interval (13.26) or (13.28) is used as the 95% prediction interval for y, the length of the interval will be underestimated.

The Bayesian framework

The primary purpose of statistics is to make an inference about a population on the basis of a sample taken from the population. In classical statistics, the inference is based solely on the data constituting the sample, whereas, in *Bayesian statistics*, the inference is based on a combination of prior belief and sample data (Lee 1997). In order to make a Bayesian inference about a random variable θ, prior belief about θ in the form of a *prior (probability) distribution* $p(\theta)$, is combined with a sample S of values in order to produce a *posterior (probability) distribution* $p(\theta \mid S)$ for θ.

Confidence and prediction intervals are also defined within the Bayesian framework. Let μ_v be the mean of a population of values v, and let S be an observed sample of values drawn from the population. If μ_v is regarded as a random variable with posterior distribution $p(\mu_v \mid S)$, $[\lambda_L(S), \lambda_U(S)]$ is a 95% *Bayesian confidence interval* for μ_v if, according to $p(\mu_v \mid S)$, there is a 95% probability that μ_v will fall within $[\lambda_L(S), \lambda_U(S)]$ (Barnett 1982, pp. 198–202). Note the difference between a classical confidence interval and a Bayesian confidence interval: in the classical approach, μ_v is fixed and $[\lambda_L(S), \lambda_U(S)]$ varies with S; in the Bayesian approach, μ_v is a random variable and $[\lambda_L(S), \lambda_U(S)]$ is fixed once S is available (Lee 1997, pp. 49–50).

If sample S consists of univariate values $v^{(1)}, \ldots, v^{(N)}$, and $p(v^{(N+1)} \mid S)$ is the posterior distribution for $v^{(N+1)}$, $[\psi_L(S), \psi_U(S)]$ is a 95% *Bayesian prediction interval* for $v^{(N+1)}$ if, according to $p(v^{(N+1)} \mid S)$, there is a 95% probability that $[\psi_L(S), \psi_U(S)]$ will contain $v^{(N+1)}$ (Barnett 1982, pp. 204–205).

Bayesian intervals for regression

Bayesian statistics provides a very different approach to the problem of unknown model parameters such as network weights. Instead of considering just a single value for a model parameter, as done by maximum likelihood estimation, Bayesian inference expresses the uncertainty of parameters in terms of probability distributions and integrates them out of the distribution of interest. For example, by expressing the uncertainty in weight vector w as the posterior probability distribution $p(w \mid S)$, where S is the observed sample, we have

$$p(y \mid x, S) = \int_w p(y \mid x, w) p(w \mid S) dw \tag{13.29}$$

$$\propto \int_w p(y \mid x, w) p(S \mid w) p(w) dw. \tag{13.30}$$

The integral of Eq. (13.30) can be solved analytically with approximations (MacKay 1991). If the distribution of the noise and the prior weight distribution $p(w)$ are assumed to be Gaussian, a Gaussian posterior distribution $p(y \mid x, w_{MP})$ for y can be derived in which

$$\hat{E}[y \mid x] = \hat{\mu}_y(x; w_{MP}), \tag{13.31}$$

where w_{MP} is w at the maximum of the posterior weight distribution $p(w \mid S)$ (where subscript MP denotes 'most probable'), and

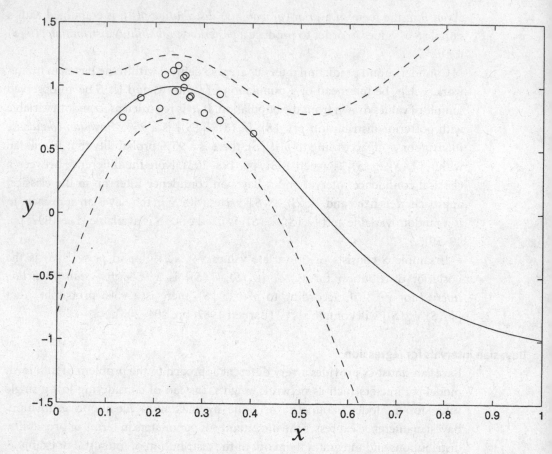

Figure 13.10. A 95% Bayesian prediction band for y (region bounded by dashed lines) based on interval (13.34). The regression function (solid line) is from a feedforward network.

$$\widehat{\mathrm{Var}}(y\,|\,\boldsymbol{x}) = \beta^{-1} + \boldsymbol{g}^T(\boldsymbol{x})\boldsymbol{A}^{-1}\boldsymbol{g}(\boldsymbol{x}), \qquad (13.32)$$

where the elements of matrix $\boldsymbol{A}$ are the second-order partial derivatives (with respect to $\boldsymbol{w}$) of the regularized error function

$$\frac{\beta}{2}\sum_{n=1}^{N}[\hat{\mu}_y(\boldsymbol{x}^{(n)};\boldsymbol{w}) - y^{(n)}]^2 + \frac{\alpha}{2}\sum_i w_i^2 \qquad (13.33)$$

evaluated at $\boldsymbol{w} = \boldsymbol{w}_{\mathrm{MP}}$. The second term in expression (13.33) (the regularization term) results from the assumption that $p(\boldsymbol{w})$ in Eq. (13.30) is Gaussian. This leads to the approximate 95% Bayesian prediction interval for y (Figure 13.10)

$$\hat{\mu}_y(\boldsymbol{x};\boldsymbol{w}_{\mathrm{MP}}) \pm z_{0.025}\sqrt{\beta^{-1} + \boldsymbol{g}^T(\boldsymbol{x})\boldsymbol{A}^{-1}\boldsymbol{g}(\boldsymbol{x})}. \qquad (13.34)$$

Note that MLE has been avoided through the use of Eq. (13.29).

The Bayesian analysis resulting in expression (13.32) demonstrates that the variance for $p(y|x, S)$ has contributions from the intrinsic noise variance β^{-1} and from the weight uncertainty. Qazaz et al. (1996) discussed how, in the context of generalized linear regression, this is affected by the distribution of data points.

Instead of using a constant value for noise variance β^{-1}, Bishop & Qazaz (1995) allowed it to be dependent on x. From 100 artificially generated data sets, each consisting of 10 data points, they demonstrated that the Bayesian approach can give an improved estimate of noise variance compared with a more biased estimate obtained from the same data using MLE.

Bayesian intervals for regression-based classification

We consider, as before, a feedforward system that estimates class-conditional posterior probabilities. For class C_i, say, given datum x, this is denoted as $p(C_i|x) = p(y_i = 1|x)$. The K outputs $\hat{p}(y_1 = |x; w), \ldots, \hat{p}(y_K = 1|x; w)$ of such a classifier, hence, must lie in the interval $[0, 1]$ and sum to unity. This may be simply achieved via the *softmax* (or generalized sigmoid) mapping of a set of latent variables, $r_1, \ldots, r_K$, such that

$$\hat{p}(y_i = 1|x; w) = \frac{\exp(r_i)}{\sum_{j=1}^{K} \exp(r_j)}. \tag{13.35}$$

For a two-class problem, we need consider only one output, $\hat{p}(y = 1|x; w)$, and Eq. (13.35) reduces to the well-known logistic sigmoid,

$$\hat{p}(y = 1|x; w) = g(r(x; w)) = \{1 + \exp[-r(x; w)]\}^{-1}.$$

For ease of notation we will consider, henceforth, the two-class case, with a single output estimating $p(C_1|x)$ (which may also be denoted $p(y = 1|x)$).

MacKay (1992b) suggested approximating the variation of r with w by a linear (first-order) expansion, and the density over w, $p(w|S)$, by a unimodal normal distribution. This enables $p(r|x; w, S)$ to be evaluated easily from $p(w|S)$. If we make a Laplace approximation to the latter (de Bruijn 1970) then $p(r|x; w, S)$ will also be approximated by a Gaussian (normal) distribution with mean (and mode) at

$$r_{\text{MP}}(x) = r(x; w_{\text{MP}}).$$

The variance of $p(r|x; w, S)$ is given as (e.g. Bishop 1995, p. 405)

$$\widehat{\text{Var}}(r|x; w, S) = h^T(x)B^{-1}h(x), \tag{13.36}$$

where $h(x)$ is the partial derivative $\partial r(x; w)/\partial w_i$ evaluated at $w = w_{\text{MP}}$ and the elements of the Hessian matrix, B, are the second-order partial derivatives of the error function with respect to w, evaluated at $w = w_{MP}$,

$$B_{i,j} = \frac{\partial^2 Err(w)}{\partial w_i \partial w_j}.$$

The error function is normally a cross-entropy measure (Eq. (13.15)) with an additive regularization term.

We may consider the location of the mode (most probable value) of the latent distribution, $r_{MP}(x)$, as propagating through the sigmoidal non-linearity, $g(.)$, to form a MLE for the posterior,

$$\hat{p}(y = 1 \mid x; w, S) = g(r_{MP}(x)).$$

The monotonicity of $g(.)$ means that the upper and lower bounds of a confidence interval on the latent distribution $p(r \mid x; w, S)$ could be mapped to equivalent points in the posterior space. This is supported by advocates of set-based (or interval-based) probability (e.g. Kyburg & Pittarelli 1996).

From the viewpoint of Bayesian decision theory, however, the notion of a confidence interval on posterior probabilities in a classification setting is redundant as uncertainty (confidence) is uniquely taken into account under a Bayesian derivation of the single-valued posteriors. We consider an optimal classifier, which probably operates by assigning an unknown datum x to class C_{k^*} if and only if

$$p(C_{k^*} \mid x) = \max_k \{p(C_k \mid x)\},$$

in other words, in a two-class setting for which $p(C_1 \mid x) = p(y = 1 \mid x)$, x is classified to class C_1 if $p(y = 1 \mid x) > 1 - p(y = 1 \mid x)$. A strict measure of the loss or uncertainty associated with a decision to C_{k^*} is $1 - p(C_{k^*} \mid x)$. Our inherent confidence in a decision is given by this quantity. Note that, if equal penalties are accrued for misclassification from all classes (i.e. the so-called *loss matrix* is isotropic) the same *decision* will be made, in a two-class case, for $p(C_{k^*} \mid x) = 0.51$ or 0.99, but our confidence in the decision is dramatically different. Indeed, it is common practice to include a 'reject' class such that x is rejected if $p(C_{k^*} \mid x) < 1 - d$, where $d \in [1/2, 1]$ is a measure of the cost associated with falsely rejecting the sample x. How then is uncertainty incorporated in the Bayesian derivation of the posteriors?

Consider the measure $p(y = 1 \mid x; w, S)$ (the posterior for class C_1) explicitly dependent upon the input x and implicitly on the 'training' data set S and the set of unknown parameters, w, which code the analysis model. The MLE framework considers only the most probable parameter set, w_{MP}, which is used to estimate $p(y=1 \mid x; w, S)$. This results in $p(y=1 \mid x; w_{MP}, S)$.

In contrast, the Bayesian paradigm integrates over the unknown parameters,

$$\bar{p}(y=1 \mid x; S) = \int_w p(y=1 \mid x; S, w)p(w \mid S)dw.$$

If we consider our analysis model in which $p(y=1 \mid x; w, S)$ is obtained via a monotone mapping $g(.)$ (the logistic sigmoid) from a continuous-valued latent variable r, i.e. $p(y=1 \mid x; w, S) = g(r; x, w, S)$, then we may rewrite the above as

$$\bar{p}(y=1 \mid x; S) = \int_r g(r; x, w, S)p(r \mid x; w, S)dr,$$

where $p(r \mid x; w, S)$ is the distribution in r induced by the distribution in the weights w upon which r is dependent. The above integral, however, is typically analytically intractable but may be easily evaluated using numerical techniques. MacKay (1992a) popularized some approximations (originally considered by Spiegelhalter & Lauritzen (1990)) that not only avoid this process but also highlight intuitively the way in which uncertainty in w, which propagates as an uncertainty in r (i.e. $p(r \mid x; w, S)$ is wide), changes the posterior probability. This change in the posterior is known as *moderation* and typically results in improved cross-entropy errors (MacKay 1992a). This approximation considers a modification to the sigmoid equation of the form

$$\bar{p}(y=1 \mid x, S) \approx g\{\kappa[\sigma_r^2(x)]r_{MP}(x)\}, \tag{13.37}$$

in which

$$\kappa[\sigma_r^2(x)] = \left(1 + \frac{\pi\sigma_r^2(x)}{8}\right)^{-1/2}$$

and $\sigma_r^2(x)$ is the variance of the latent variable distribution, as defined in Eq. (13.36). Figure 13.11 depicts the effect changes in the latent variance (uncertainty) have on the classification probability, $\bar{p}(y=1 \mid x, S) = p(C_1 \mid x, S)$. Consider, for example, $r_{MP}(x) = 2$. Note that the resultant estimated posterior probability goes down towards 1/2 as the uncertainty in r increases. The uncertainty in a decision is the distance from unity of the largest posterior, which is worst when the posterior equals the class prior (1/2 in this two-class problem). In a principled way, therefore, uncertainty (high variance) in the latent distribution is automatically represented as a lower certainty of decision.

The tacit assumption has been made in the above analysis that the density over

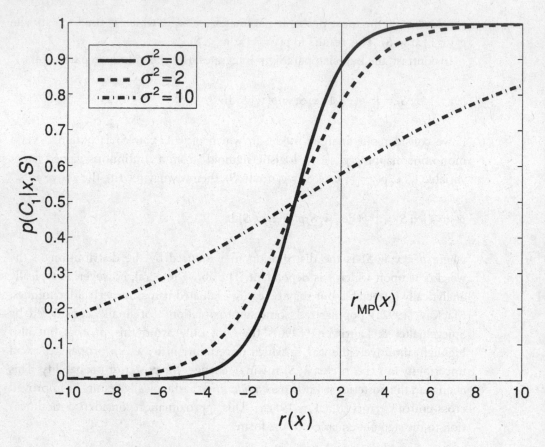

Figure 13.11. Changes in slope of the sigmoid due to latent variable uncertainty.

the weights, $p(w \mid S)$, is unimodal. For the vast majority of analysis systems, however, there are many non-equivalent local maxima in the density which would be taken into account if the requisite marginal integral was indeed over all w space. We may assume, however, that most probability mass is concentrated in the regions of w space associated with peaks in $p(w \mid S)$. Integration over all w space may hence be approximated by integration over a (finite) number of regions, $\mathcal{R}_i$, each of which contains a peak in $p(w \mid S)$. Hence

$$p(r \mid x; S) \approx \sum_i p(\mathcal{R}_i \mid S) \int_{w \in \mathcal{R}_i} p(r \mid x; w, S, \mathcal{R}_i) p(w \mid S, \mathcal{R}_i) dw$$

which may be written as

$$p(r \mid x; S) = \sum_i \gamma_i p(r \mid x; S, \mathcal{R}_i).$$

The latter equation represents a weighted average (with weightings given by γ_i) of latent densities from a *committee* of classifiers. Each latent distribution in the summation may, for example, be approximated as a Gaussian, as may the resultant committee distribution. The latter has mean

$$r_{MP}^{comm}(x) = \sum_i \gamma_i r_{MP,i}(x),$$

where $r_{MP,i}(x)$ are the modes (and means) of $p(r \mid x; S, \mathcal{R}_i)$, and a variance of

$$\sigma_{comm}^2(x) = \sum_i \gamma_i \sigma_{r,i}^2(x) + \sum_i \gamma_i (r_{MP,i}(x) - r_{MP}^{comm}(x))^2. \tag{13.38}$$

This variance may thence be used, for example, with Eq. (13.37) to provide a moderated posterior probability that takes into account uncertainty due to imprecision in the parameters of each constituent member of the committee (the first term in Eq. (13.38)) and also uncertainty due to disagreement between committee members (the second term in Eq. (13.38)). It is noted that committees are probably better in performance than the average performance of their members (Bishop 1995, pp. 364–369).

Markov chain Monte Carlo sampling

Determination of the integral in Eq. (13.29) can, in principle, be achieved numerically using

$$p(y \mid x, S) \approx \frac{1}{L} \sum_{i=1}^{L} p(y \mid x, w^{(i)}). \tag{13.39}$$

This avoids the Gaussian approximation adopted on p. 315 and elsewhere.

The set $\{w^{(1)}, \ldots, w^{(L)}\}$ of weight vectors used for approximation (13.39) is sampled from $p(w \mid S)$ by means of *Markov chain Monte Carlo* (MCMC) sampling (Gilks et al. 1996). In the two standard versions of MCMC sampling (the Metropolis method and Gibbs sampling), the space of possible w values (state-space) is explored by random walk; however, sampling through a random walk can perform poorly when the state-space has a large number of dimensions. In such a situation, Neal (1996) advocates the *hybrid Monte Carlo method* in which state-space is replaced by a phase-space consisting of (w, p) pairs in which 'position' vector w is augmented with a 'momentum' vector p. Unlike Metropolis and Gibbs sampling, this exploits the gradient information contained in a back-propagation-trained network.

An example of the application of MCMC is its use by Goldberg et al. (1998) to model input-dependent variance, which they did using a Gaussian process (Williams 1999).

The assumption that $p(y|x, w)$ is Gaussian whenever y is continuous-valued will not always be appropriate in the real world as it is possible for $p(y|x, w)$ to be skewed or multimodal due to the noise being non-Gaussian. Distribution $p(y|x, w)$ can take on non-Gaussian forms by setting it equal to a *mixture model* composed of a sum of Gaussian kernel functions (Everitt & Hand 1981). The input-dependent mean and variance of the distribution can be derived from the mixture model by MLE (Bishop 1994) and by MCMC (Dybowski 1997), but there is then the problem of defining an interval when a distribution is asymmetric or multimodal.

Input noise

As mentioned on p. 302, one source of uncertainty in the output of an FNN is uncertainty in the input values. Some methods for estimating errors due to input noise have been reviewed by Press et al. (1992, pp. 666–670), Tresp et al. (1994) and Townsend & Tarassenko (1997).

Wright (1999) has taken a Bayesian approach to the problem in which the true but unobserved input x is perturbed by noise to give a noisy, observed input z. If z_0 denotes a new observed input, and y_0 is the associated target value, the predictive distribution $p(y_0|z_0, S)$ can be expressed by integrating over the unknown x_0:

$$p(y_0|z_0, S) = \int_{x_0} p(y_0|x_0, S)p(x_0|z_0)dx_0. \tag{13.40}$$

If there is a small level of Gaussian noise on the true input, Eq. (13.40) leads to the following expression for the variance of y_0:

$$\widehat{Var}(y_0|z_0) = \beta^{-1} + \sigma_x^2 h^T(z_0)h(z_0) + g^T(z_0)A^{-1}g(z_0), \tag{13.41}$$

which is similar to Eq. (13.32) but with an additional term due to the introduction of noise to x. The extra term consists of the variance σ_x^2 of x multiplied by the squared partial derivative $\partial \hat{\mu}_y(x; w)/\partial x_i$ evaluated at $x = z_0$.

If the assumptions leading to Eq. (13.41) do not hold then $p(y_0|z_0, S)$ is evaluated numerically, with MCMC used to estimate the inner integral in

$$p(y_0|z_0, S) = \int_{x_0} p(x_0|z_0)\left[\int_{x,w} p(y_0|x_0, w)p(x, w|S)dxdw\right]dx_0,$$

but a limitation of this approach is that $p(x_0|z_0)$ is required.

Conclusion

A neural network correctly trained with binary target values can estimate conditional class probabilities and, although it is possible to define a Bayesian confidence interval for a posterior probability, the section on Bayesian intervals for regression-based classification described why, from the viewpoint of Bayesian decision theory, such an interval is unnecessary. Furthermore, for the case when target values are real-valued, Bishop & Qazaz (1995) have demonstrated that variances estimated within the Bayesian framework can be less biased than those estimated by MLE; consequently, the Bayesian approach is preferred to MLE.

A problem with the Bayesian approach (whether by hybrid MCMC or via Gaussian approximations) is that implementing it tends to be more troublesome than with MLE. These difficulties are restricted to neural networks and are due to the approximations used to obtain the mathematical formalism. When generalized linear models are used, the implementation becomes easy and straightforward because the approximations become exact. The accounting for parameter uncertainty in Bayesian methods works only if the computations are done reasonably exactly, and not by gross approximations. In contrast, MLE is easier to implement in terms of both stability of the algorithm and speed of convergence (as measured by central processing unit time). Of the MLE-based methods, the bootstrap method has been reported to provide more accurate confidence intervals than the delta method and more accurate prediction intervals than the Nix–Weigend method. Nevertheless, the advantages of the Bayesian framework suggest that efforts should be made towards developing stable techniques in this area so that Bayesian prediction and confidence intervals can be obtained reliably.

Acknowledgements

We thank Cazhaow Qazaz and Brian Ripley for their constructive comments during the writing of this chapter.

NOTES

1. We have used the expression *regression function* instead of *regression model* as the former refers to an estimated relationship between $\mu_y(x)$ and x (Robbins & Munro 1951), whereas the latter refers to a family of possible relationships.
2. Symbol p will be used both for probability density functions and probability mass functions, the correct meaning being understood from the context in which it is used. For those readers unfamiliar with probability theory, we recommend Wonnacott & Wonnacott (1985, pp. 52–150) followed by Ross (1988).
3. Although confidence intervals with equal tails are the most common form, there are other possibilities (Barnett 1982, pp. 172–176).
4. The predictive distribution for $v^{(N+1)}$ is given by

$$p(v^{(N+1)} = 1 \mid \bar{v}, N) = (\bar{v}N + 1)/(N + 1).$$

5. Both linear and logistic regression models belong to the class of models called *generalized linear models* (Dobson 1990). These have the general form

$$g(\mu_y(\boldsymbol{x}; \boldsymbol{w})) = w_0 + \sum_{i=1}^{d} w_i x_i,$$

where g is the *link function*. In simple linear regression, $g(a) = a$, whereas in logistic regression, $g(a) = \text{logit}(a)$.

6. A clear account of vectors and matrices is provided by Anton (1984).

7. The Hessian matrix and calculation of its inverse H^{-1} are discussed by Bishop (1995, pp. 150–160).

8. If noise variance σ_ε^2 is *not* independent of $\boldsymbol{x}$ then H/σ_ε^2 in Eq. (13.18) is replaced by a matrix G defined by (Penny & Roberts 1997)

$$G_{k,l} = \sum_{i=1}^{N} \frac{1}{\sigma_\varepsilon^2(\boldsymbol{x}^{(i)})} \left\{ \frac{\partial \hat{\mu}_y(\boldsymbol{x}^{(i)}; \hat{\boldsymbol{w}})}{\partial \hat{w}_k} \frac{\partial \hat{\mu}_y(\boldsymbol{x}^{(i)}; \hat{\boldsymbol{w}})}{\partial \hat{w}_l} + [y^{(i)} - \hat{\mu}_y(\boldsymbol{x}^{(i)}; \hat{\boldsymbol{w}})] \frac{\partial^2 \hat{\mu}_y(\boldsymbol{x}^{(i)}; \hat{\boldsymbol{w}})}{\partial \hat{w}_k \partial \hat{w}_l} \right\}.$$

9. Maximum likelihood is referred to as *maximum penalized likelihood* if the error function is regularized.

10. The *bootstrap* method should not be confused with the *jack-knife* or *cross-validation* (Efron & Gong 1983).

11. The number of bootstrap samples needed for reliable estimates depends on the type of statistics we are after. In the case of estimating the mean of a random variable, a relatively small number of samples are required, whilst for estimating variance, a larger number is needed, since the estimate of the variance is more sensitive to noise.

REFERENCES

Anton, H. (1984). *Elementary Linear Algebra*, 4th edn. John Wiley, New York.

Barnett, V. (1982). *Comparative Statistical Inference*, 2nd edn. Wiley, Chichester.

Baxt, W. G. (1995). Application of artificial neural networks to clinical medicine. *Lancet* **346**, 1135–1138.

Baxt, W. G. & White, H. (1995). Bootstrapping confidence intervals for clinical input variable effects in a network trained to identify the presence of acute myocardial infarction. *Neural Computation* **7**, 624–638.

Bishop, C. M. (1994). Mixture density networks. Technical Report NCRG/4288. Neural Computing Research Group, Aston University.

Bishop, C. M. (1995). *Neural Networks for Pattern Recognition*. Clarendon Press, Oxford.

Bishop, C. M. & Qazaz, C. S. (1995). Bayesian inference of noise level in regression. In F. Fogelman-Soulié & P. Gallineri, eds. *Proceedings of the International Conference on Artificial Neural Networks 1995 (ICANN 95)*. EC2 & Cie, Paris, pp. 59–64.

Breiman, L. (1996). Bagging predictors. *Machine Learning* **24**, 123–140.

Collett, D. (1991). *Modelling Binary Data*. Chapman & Hall, London.

de Bruijn, N. G. (1970). *Asymptotic Methods in Analysis*. North-Holland, Amsterdam.

Dobson, A. J. (1990). *An Introduction to Generalized Linear Models*. Chapman & Hall, London.

Draper, D. (1995). Assessment and propagation of model uncertainty (with discussion). *Journal of the Royal Statistical Society, Series B* **57**, 45–97.

Dudewicz, E. J. & Mishra, S. N. (1988). *Modern Mathematical Statistics*. John Wiley, New York.

Dybowski, R. (1997). Assigning confidence intervals to neural network predictions, Technical report. Division of Infection (St Thomas' Hospital), King's College London.

Dybowski, R. & Gant, V. (1995). Artificial neural networks in pathology and medical laboratories. *Lancet* **346**, 1203–1207.

Efron, B. (1979). Bootstrap methods: another look at the jackknife. *Annals of Statistics* **7**, 1–26.

Efron, B. & Gong, G. (1983). A leisurely look at the bootstrap, the jackknife, and cross-validation. *The American Statistician* **37**, 36–48.

Efron, B. & Tibshirani, R. J. (1993). *An Introduction to the Bootstrap*. Chapman & Hall, New York.

Everitt, B. S. & Hand, D. J. (1981). *Finite Mixture Distributions*. Chapman & Hall, London.

Geisser, S. (1993). *Predictive Inference: An Introduction*. Chapman & Hall, New York.

Gemen, S. Bienenstock, E. & Doursat, R. (1992). Neural networks and the bias/variance dilemma. *Neural Computation* **4**, 1–58.

Gilks, W. R., Richardson, S. & Spiegelhalter, D. J. (eds.) (1996). *Markov Chain Monte Carlo in Practice*. Chapman & Hall, London.

Goldberg, P. W., Williams, C. K. I. & Bishop, C. M. (1998). Regression with input-dependent noise: a Gaussian process treatment, Technical Report NCRG/98/002. Neural Computing Research Group, Aston University.

Hauck, W. W. (1983). A note on confidence bands for the logistic response curve. *The American Statistician* **37**, 158–160.

Heskes, T. (1997). Practical confidence and prediction intervals. In M. Mozer, M. Jordan & T. Petsche, eds., *Advances in Neural Information Processing Systems 9*. MIT Press, Cambridge, MA, pp. 176–182.

Hinton, G. E. (1989). Connectionist learning procedures. *Artificial Intelligence* **40**, 185–234.

Hogg, R. V. & Craig, A. T. (1995). *Introduction to Mathematical Statistics*. Prentice Hall, Englewood Cliffs, NJ.

Holst, H., Ohlsson, M., Peterson, C. & Edenbrandt, L. (1998). Intelligent computer reporting 'lack of experience': a confidence measure for decision support systems. *Clinical Physiology* **18**, 139–147.

Hosmer, D. W. & Lemeshow, S. (1989). *Applied Logistic Regression*. Wiley, New York.

Kyburg, H. E. & Pittarelli, M. (1996). Set-based Bayesianism. *IEEE Transactions on Systems, Man and Cybernetics* **26**, 324–339.

Lee, P. M. (1997). *Bayesian Statistics: An Introduction*, 2nd edn. Edward Arnold, London.

MacKay, D. J. C. (1991). Bayesian method for adaptive models. PhD thesis, California Institute of Technology.

MacKay, D. J. C. (1992a). The evidence framework applied to classification networks. *Neural Computation* **4**, 720–736.

MacKay, D. J. C. (1992b). A practical Bayesian framework for back-propagation networks. *Neural Computation* **4**, 448–472.

Neal, R. M. (1996). *Bayesian Learning for Neural Networks.* Lecture Notes in Statistics Series No. 118. Springer-Verlag, New York.

Nix, D. A. & Weigend, A. S. (1995). Learning local error bars for nonlinear regression. In G. Tesauro, D. Touretzky & T. Leen, eds., *Advances in Neural Information Processing Systems 7 (NIPS *94).* MIT Press, Cambridge, MA, pp. 489–496.

Penny, W. D. & Roberts, S. J. (1997). Neural network predictions with error bars. Research Report TR-97-1, Department of Electrical and Electronic Engineering, Imperial College, London.

Press, W. H., Teukolsky, S. A., Vetterling, W. T. & Flannery, B. P. (1992). *Numerical Recipes in C,* 2nd edn. Cambridge University Press, Cambridge.

Qazaz, C. S., Williams, C. K. I. & Bishop, C. M. (1996). An upper bound on the Bayesian error bars for generalised linear regression. Technical Report NCRG/96/005. Neural Computing Research Group, Aston University.

Robbins, H. & Munro, S. (1951). A stochastic approximation method. *Annals of Mathematical Statistics* **22**, 400–407.

Ross, S. (1988). *A First Course in Probability,* 3rd edn. Macmillan, New York.

Santner, T. J. & Duffy, D. E. (1989). *The Statistical Analysis of Discrete Data.* Springer-Verlag, New York.

Spiegelhalter, D. J. & Lauritzen, S. L. (1990). Sequential updating of conditional probabilities on directed graphical structures. *Networks* **20**, 579–605.

Tibshirani, R. (1996). A comparison of some error estimates for neural network models. *Neural Computation* **8**, 152–163.

Townsend, N. W. & Tarassenko, L. (1997). Estimation of error bounds for RBF networks. In *Proceedings of the 5th International Conference on Artificial Neural Networks.* IEE, Stevenage, pp. 227–232.

Tresp, V., Ahamad, S. & Neuneier, R. (1994). Training neural networks with deficient data. In J. Cowan, G. Tesauro & J. Alspector, eds., *Neural Information Processing Systems 6,* Morgan Kaufmann, San Mateo, CA, pp. 128–135.

Williams, C. K. I. (1999). Prediction with Gaussian processes: from linear regression to linear prediction and beyond. In M. Jordan, ed., *Learning in Graphical Models.* MIT Press, Cambridge, MA, pp. 599–621.

Wonnacott, R. J. & Wonnacott, T. H. (1985). *Introductory Statistics,* 4th edn. John Wiley, New York.

Wonnacott, T. H. & Wonnacott, R. J. (1981). *Regression: A Second Course in Statistics.* John Wiley, New York.

Wright, W. A. (1999). Neural network regression with input uncertainty. Technical Report NCRG/99/008. Neural Computing Research Group, Aston University.

Part IV

Ethics and clinical prospects

14

Artificial neural networks: practical considerations for clinical application

Vanya Gant, Susan Rodway and Jeremy Wyatt

Introduction

The past nine years have seen a steady increase in the number of publications concerning artificial neural networks (ANNs) in medicine (Figure 14.1). Many of these demonstrate that neural networks offer equivalent if not superior performance when compared with other statistical methods, and in some cases with doctors, in several areas of clinical medicine. Table 14.1 gives a by no means exhaustive list of academically driven applications, which are notable for their breadth of potential application areas. Despite this academic research portfolio demonstrating success, we know of very few examples of an ANN being used to inform patient care decisions, and few (if any) have been seamlessly incorporated into everyday practice. Furthermore, we know of no randomized clinical trial (RCT) examining the impact of ANN output on clinical actions or patient outcomes. This is in sharp contrast to the 68 RCTs published since 1976 assessing the impact of reminders and other decision support systems, none of them ANNs, on clinical actions and patient outcomes included in Hunt et al.'s (1998) systematic review.

To check whether our personal experience is reflected in the literature, we conducted a search of the Medline bibliographic database in all languages for the period January 1993 to March 2000 using the Medical Subject Headings term 'Neural-networks- (computer)'. Using the Silver Platter software, this yielded 3101 articles. When filtered using the Medline Publication Type = 'clinical-trial', this number plummeted 50-fold to 61 articles. We examined the 61 abstracts of these articles for any evidence that the output of the ANN had been given to clinicians or others to guide real patient care decisions, or quality improvement activities such as comparative audit. Despite their classification as a clinical trial, all of the studies were carried out on retrospective data, with none suggesting any clinical use of the ANN output. We also tried other publication types including 'controlled clinical trial', 'randomized controlled trial' and 'clinical trial phase III'. No article describing clinical use was found. Filtering the 3101 ANN articles using

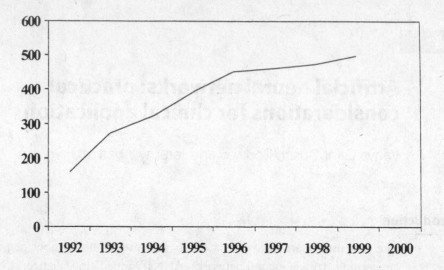

Figure 14.1. The increasing publication rate for neural network applications in medicine.

this last term yielded just one article (0.03% of total), which turned out to be a reanalysis of data collected during a completed RCT. Such a search strategy would normally have a sensitivity of 50–60% for RCTs (McKibbon et al. 1990). Thus we believe there are 0–1 articles published on Medline since 1993 describing the clinical use of ANN outputs, let alone a rigorous randomized study. We note, however, the large number of publications, both from the original group and from independent third parties, on the capabilities of the PAPNET system, described elsewhere in this book (Chapters 2 and 3). To our knowledge this is the sole example of ANN technology that has not only been assessed in both retrospective and prospective trials, but also implemented in patient care pathways, either as a commercial service or as an 'in-house' technology for the originating pathologists. To date, however, no prospective study specifically examining its impact on patient care or outcomes has been published.

Notwithstanding this anomaly, the potential for ANNs in medicine continues to grow with each new sphere of application, covering not only the areas of prediction of clinical states at some future date (life vs. death, relapse from treated cancer), but also the assessment of likelihood of disease from both 'hard' inputs (such as biochemical profiles), as well as more complex datasets (electroencephalogram waveforms, tracking eye movements, clinical imaging). It is notable that ANNs seem particularly successful as analysers of visual information, whether obtained from light microscopes (histopathology, cytology) or radiological equipment (ventilation perfusion and positron emission tomography scans).

So why have we not seen their implementation?

We believe that the very plasticity of ANNs as regards not only their internal architecture but also their adaptability to different data sets is also their Achilles' heel. It is exactly these extraordinarily wide ranging novel potential applications that bring with them equally novel and complex considerations of not only *where* they fit in the clinical decision-making algorithm, but also how ethically and legally *acceptable* their implementation might be. These considerations can be interpreted as important obstacles standing in the way of such devices becoming commonplace in clinical practice, which is traditionally dominated by decisions made by human clinicians. More specifically, the obstacles arise from a lack of defined criteria in several spheres of operation, such as their position in the decision-making process, uncertainty concerning their role, the lack of a support infrastructure, difficulties with evaluation of performance, and the ethical and legal issues that flow therefrom. All these conspire to make any process designed to address the necessary homologation through official national and international bodies (such as the Medical Devices Agency and the European In Vitro Diagnostic Medical Devices Commission) difficult and tortuous. This chapter addresses these specific areas of difficulty. We describe legal issues in the context of the UK legal system, although it is likely that most of the points we raise would apply at least in its broad principles to most, if not all, national legal structures. We conclude by suggesting some criteria that must be met for successful clinical application.

Data refinery and decision-taking: some examples illustrating uncertainty of role

Consider a clinician making a decision from patient data, such as a pathologist examining a biopsy specimen down the microscope to decide whether cancer is present or not. The eye and brain are besieged by a mass of raw visual data that must be preprocessed and filtered. The first stage in this data-processing is to abstract relevant features (Figure 14.2). For example, the pathologist will filter the raw visual data to abstract features such as 'nuclear pleomorphism' or 'penetration though the basement membrane'. The hallmark of experienced pathologists – and radiologists – is that they recognize significant features instantly and reliably from images. If questioned about how they achieve this, some may be able to provide an explanation, often a post hoc rationalization. However, most will admit that it is simply a learned skill, defying explanation – the 'paradox of expertise' (Dreyfus & Dreyfus 1988). The same is true for a cardiologist listening for a fourth heart sound or a psychiatrist determining whether a patient has insight or not.

It is not enough, however, simply to recognize features; these need to be interpreted or assembled to support decision-making before the clinician takes an

Table 14.1. Several recent applications of neural networks to different areas of clinical medicine

Subject (Ref.)	Comparator	Result
Assessment of need for neurosurgery in trauma (Li et al. 2000)	Logistic regression, radial basis function (RBF) and multilayer perceptron (MLP) ANN	ANN outperformed logistic regression model for need to operate; MLP superior to RBF
Prediction of coronary artery stenosis from angiographic records (Mobley et al. 2000)	None	Identifies additional patients who in retrospect did not need angiography
Prediction of schizophrenia from eye-tracking dysfunction (Campana et al. 1999)	Discriminant analysis	Back-propagation neural network analysis of eye tracking performance correctly classified more patients as schizophrenic than did discriminant analysis
Detection of suicidal tendency from patient files (Modai et al. 1999)	Logistic regression	Back-propagation neural networks were very successful at predicting serious suicidal tendency and isolated several discriminant factors not detected by logistic regression
Prediction of bladder cancer reoccurrence from clinical data (Qureshi et al. 2000)	Assessment by clinicians	Neural networks outperformed clinicians' successful prediction rate
Prediction of survival after breast cancer from histology data (Lundin et al. 1999)	Logistic regression	Neural networks were consistently more accurate in survival prediction than was logistic regression. Performance was particularly impressive for 15-year follow up, even without access to information concerning original lymph node status
Description of extent and severity of myocardial perfusion defects measured using SPET scintigrams (Lindahl et al., 1999)	Assessment by clinicians	Neural networks and clinicians correctly classified the scintigrams 70% of the time
Prediction of relapse of prostatic carcinoma after prostatectomy from histology and clinical data (Potter et al. 1999)	Logistic regression, Cox regression	Genetically engineered neural networks consistently outperformed other statistical methods and offered the best predictive performance
Classification of mammogram lesions as benign or malignant (Huo et al. 1999)	None	Neural networks were found to rely heavily on a single radiographic feature for decision. Performance was improved when combined with a hybrid one-step rule-based method

Table 14.1. (*cont.*)

Subject (Ref.)	Comparator	Result
Classification of early renal transplant rejection from histological features (Furness et al. 1999)	Logistic regression, conventional histopathological reporting	Neural networks predicted rejection better than logistic regression and 'expert' histopathologists
Prediction of the likelihood of pulmonary embolism from ventilation-perfusion scans (Scott 1999)	Clinical assessment of scans; 'gold standard' pulmonary angiography	Neural network predictive performance was superior to that of clinicians in prediction of embolism in cases with normal chest X-rays
Detection of invisible coronary artery surgical anastomotic errors from graft flow data in mongrel dogs (Cerrito et al. 1999)	Surgeon's visual assessment	Neural networks interpreted graft flow characteristics and detected anastomotic errors more consistently than did the surgeon's assessment at the time of the minimally invasive surgery
Prediction of mortality following intracerebral heamorrhage (Edwards et al. 1999)	Logistic regression	Neural networks correctly classified 100% of patients as alive or dead using demographic and radiological criteria, as opposed to a value of 85% for logistic regression
Prediction of creatinine clearance in HIV-infected patients using clinical and laboratory data (Herman et al. 1999)	Five other established mathematical models for this prediction	Neural networks performed better than all five equations
Detection of prostatic carcinoma using clinical and prostatic ultrasonic data (Ronco & Fernandez 1999)	Logistic regression	Predictive capability of neural networks was superior to logistic regression in terms of both positive and negative predictive values
Prediction of obstructive sleep apnoea (OSA) from 23 clinical criteria (Kirby et al. 1999)	None	Neural networks had a 98.9% positive predictive value for OSA, and did not misclassify (i.e. 'miss') patients with moderate to severe OSA
Prediction of tacrolimus blood levels in liver transplantation patients (Chen et al. (1999)	None	Neural networks predicted tacrolimus blood levels precisely using patient variables
Prediction of breast carcinoma from mammographic and patient history data (Lo et al. 1999)	Clinical radiologists	Neural networks consistently outperformed radiologists, and performed even better when patient age was incorporated

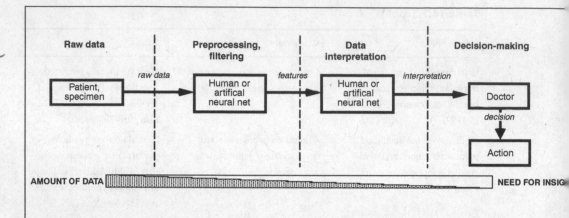

Figure 14.2. The clinical 'data refinery'.

action. In our example, pathologists must assign both a diagnosis (e.g. melanoma) and a stage (e.g. Clarke's level III) before a surgeon can operate. Far from being intuitive and data driven, this process uses rather few data – the abstracted features – and is heavily dependent on explicit, often written, rules, conventions and definitions.

As Figure 14.2 suggests, either of these two stages in the clinical 'data refinery' can be carried out by a human or an artificial neural net. However, given that there is a greater need for insight as one moves from preprocessing and filtering to interpretation and decision-making, the balance favours the human towards the right hand side, and leaves most opportunities open for ANN on the left. This is supported too by the fact that rules for humans become more difficult as the data they are interpreting become increasingly complex; human performance is perhaps more variable when rules are unclear. There is accordingly much less chance of (and need for) an explicit model. Thus it seems that ANNs can perhaps be safely substituted for humans for low level data-filtering tasks, assuming they can be shown in rigorous, reliable experiments at least to match the performance of expert humans, and to output the features that humans need for later processing. This role is exactly the kind of niche that the best-known clinical ANN, PAPNET (Boon et al. 1995), has fulfilled.

With such a concept in mind, we discuss two examples of potential applications for ANNs in the clinical arena. These specific examples are used to illustrate the different positions that ANNs can take up in the chain of information to decision-making; neither is in routine clinical use. The third example illustrates how PAPNET was implemented in 'real life', after having found its 'niche', and how the structure within which it is placed provides safeguards generally considered acceptable by all.

ANN interpretation of images: VQ scans as an example

One of the drivers for ANN development in clinical science has always been that the data sets produced by the physical measurement technology of biological systems are complex. Such complexity makes direct human interpretation very difficult, giving any decision a built-in element of *uncertainty*. Such uncertainty implies that human decisions following data interpretation must be expressed in the context of limits of confidence. This is the case for radionuclide ventilation–perfusion scans for the diagnosis of suspected pulmonary embolism. The scans shown in Figure 14.3 illustrate the problem of interpretation facing nuclear medicine physicians, whose scans have been described on occasion as 'nebulograms from the Department of Unclear Medicine'. The appearance of these images contrasts sharply with the more explicit 'gold standard' pictures produced by alternative but more invasive technology such as computed tomography (CT) pulmonary angiography, also shown for the sake of comparison.

The diagnosis of pulmonary embolism from such scans carries with it very important clinical decisions; needless administration of anticoagulant agents is potentially lethal, and conversely witholding treatment with anticoagulants in proven cases of embolism may be similarly lethal. In practice, these scans are read by trained physicians, who are free to report them using a variety of terms implying certainty (or not). Accordingly, reports are issued often couched in terms such as 'definite', 'likely', 'unlikely', 'non-diagnostic', 'no definite evidence'. Some physicians prefer to report the scans in terms of betting odds that the scan does *not* show embolism ('there is a four-to-one chance that this scan is normal . . .'). By so doing the clinician imparts more or less confidence in the primary (essentially all-or-none) diagnosis of embolism or no embolism. These practices are accepted and acceptable; although interestingly it might be argued that to be too didactic (and sometimes wrong) in one's reporting style is to open the door to criticism in the courts in those cases where the interpretation of the scan is subsequently discovered to be incorrect.

What makes these practices legally acceptable is the defence available in a civil action for negligent failure to act with appropriate care. This defence is based on the view that a responsible body of opinion would act in the same way. Thus a range of acceptable performance or approach is permissible in the human-decision making model. We would nevertheless hope that the 'driver' for softening reports with terms implying probability rather than certainty relates to a justified and carefully considered limit to the diagnostic quality of the scan (as perceived by human interpretation), rather than a fear of subsequent litigation.

(a)

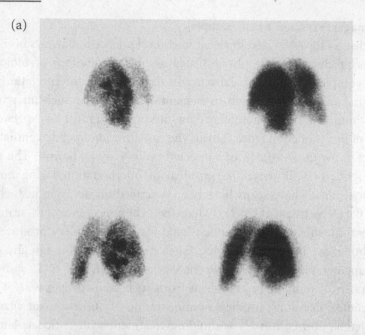

(b)

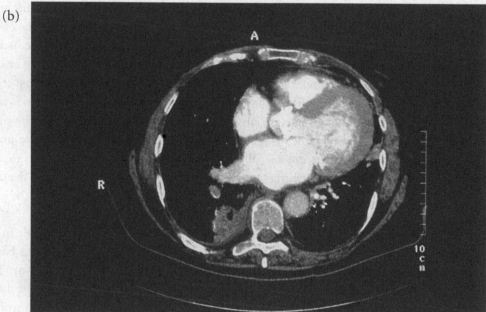

Figure 14.3. (a) Ventilation–perfusion (VQ) (Tc99m-Technegas and Tc99m-Maa) scan showing a triple matched perfusion abnormality in the right lower lobe inferoposteriorly. Right posterior oblique images are shown with ventilation on the left and perfusion on the right panel. (b) Computed tomography pulmonary angiogram showing a peripheral wedge infarction in the right lower lobe and a filling defect in an adjacent right lower lobe segmental pulmonary artery. (Figures very kindly supplied by Dr Brian Neilly, Department of Nuclear Medicine, Glasgow Royal Infirmary, Scotland.)

The human decision-maker

In law the human decision-maker is judged by the comparable actions of his or her peers.

In the field of clinical negligence, a breach of the duty of care to a patient is judged by measuring the action of the clinician against the standard reasonably to be expected from a practitioner in the same field. Although this is often referred to as the 'Bolam test', the case of *Bolam* v. *Friern Hospital Management Committee* [1957] 2 All ER 118 in fact referred to the 'ordinary skill of an ordinary competent man exercising that particular art'. The 'ordinary skill' test was that which had been propounded in the earlier decision in *Hunter* v. *Hanley* [1955] SC 200. There it was said that 'The true test for establishing negligence in diagnosis or treatment on the part of a doctor is whether he has been proved to be guilty of such failure as no doctor of ordinary skill would be guilty of if acting with ordinary care.'

As the law has evolved, the issue of reasonableness has entered into this test. Lord Scarman in *Siddaway* v. *Governors of Bethlem Royal Hospital* [1985] AC 871 worded the test thus: 'A doctor is not negligent if he acts in accordance with a practice accepted at the time as proper by a reasonable body of medical opinion even though other doctors adopt a different practice.' It is now generally accepted that a particular practice is judged objectively against the hypothetical reasonably competent practitioner.

Conversely, the defence to an allegation of negligence is that a body of opinion would have acted in the same way. One of the best-known statements of this principle is the speech of Lord Scarman in *Maynard* v. *West Midlands Health Authority* [1984] 1 WLR 634: 'It is not enough to show that there is a body of competent professional opinion which considers that theirs was a wrong decision, if there also exists a body of professional opinion, equally competent, which supports the decision as reasonable in the circumstances.' In various cases this test has been referred to as 'responsible', 'distinguished' and 'respectable'.

The human agent is, therefore, afforded a certain amount of leeway to reflect the range of acceptable approaches to a problem where either legitimate differences of opinion can exist or where it is accepted that the problem solver is inherently fallible.

The interesting point behind such apparent leniency is that it originates, essentially, from confidence in the decision-maker and his or her training. So an expert in a particular field may be relied upon *because* he or she has followed accepted and acceptable training pathways and demonstrated continued excellence by good results.

If we translate this to a machine model, considerable difficulties ensue.

In the first place, there is formidable suspicion in relation to any model that replaces human reasoning, intuition and insight. Where such a model actually challenges or betters human reasoning, our cynicism is heightened unless we can satisfy ourselves that the mechanics of the reasoning are so perfectly created as to be infallible. For example, we will pit our wits against a chess computer program or will rely upon a global positioning system because either we have confidence in the method by which the conclusion is reached or we know that we can, if we wish, test the result by some other means.

Contrast an ANN. Only two points are potentially amenable to measurement and confidence. In the first place, strict parameters can be set for the detailed and accurate training of the ANN. Secondly, if the end result can be measured or checked against known data, confidence can be instilled in the accuracy of the answer provided by the ANN. The missing link, of course, is the mechanism by which the ANN reaches this result.

When, in this context, machine takes over from human, mistakes or variety of interpretation are no longer acceptable and will not serve as a legal justification for a frankly incorrect prediction.

The additional complication is the inability to 'compare' the deductions of an ANN with other ANNs in the same field. ANNs are trained only for a specific task. There is nothing comparable. It follows that, in the law of negligence, reliance upon the deduction of the ANN will arguably present a fresh problem. Such a problem will arise because ANNs are unlikely to be afforded any leeway, unlike that which is permitted to their human counterparts employed on the same decision-making task.

Obstacles to ANN replacing human beings in interpretation of VQ scans

With the above in mind, it is easier to understand the obstacles in the way of ANNs replacing human beings in the interpretation of VQ scans.

Several publications demonstrate that ANNs can be trained in this context *and* their successful diagnostic performance subsequently measured against an unrelated dataset (such as that of Scott (1999)). As set out above, the law accepts that radiologists may not always be right, and are not necessarily required to perform faultlessly.

Validation of the ANN in this context should be related to the performance of human observers, or to a better-defined endpoint or 'gold standard'. In this case the results of the (more invasive) pulmonary angiogram, where radio-opaque dye is injected directly into the pulmonary circulation, offer the requisite 'gold standard', against which both the doctors and the ANN can be compared. The original training set should, if at all possible, contain such gold standard data, as otherwise the network would perform only as well as the radiologists. There remains a fundamental problem, however, with this particular ANN application. The ANN is here acting not only as a data filter but also as a diagnostic device, offering an interpretation of the data. The final human decision-making is therefore to accept or reject the ANN's conclusion of the significance of the scan in question. We consider that this step should continue to be essential; the best solution here would be for the radiologist to examine the scans *in the light of the ANN's decision*. The ANN in this role should therefore be that of an 'adviser' rather than a diagnostician, and the final decision as to the scan's significance is ultimately a human one.

ANN interpretation of clinical data – mortality in the critically ill

This example of the potential for ANNs in the clinical arena illustrates several points that are much more difficult to embrace in an ethical and legal sense. Dybowski et al. (1996) demonstrated that an ANN could predict mortality in the critically ill by using selected physiological parameters of organ function and patient demographics as input fields. Whilst prediction accuracy was not perfect, it was superior to that obtained by logistic regression. The ANN here acted as a data refinery, producing an output that could be interpreted in many different ways, and used for many different purposes. The authors pointed out that the ANN was designed with the specific purpose of gaining insight into those factors associated with poor prognosis. Thus the role of the ANN was defined as a means to an end, namely insight into critical illness and death.

The work of another group, using different statistical techniques, but also predicting mortality in the critically ill was unfortunately interpreted as a possible means of allocating increasingly scarce resources to those patients whose probability of death (as measured by their system) was lower. Much criticism from public and professional bodies ensued. Whilst both systems were valuable as data refinery tools for research into those elements responsible for mortality, the perceived difference between these two systems designed for identical data sets and desired outputs was therefore one of the *role* or the *purpose* to which they were put. This is not difficult to understand in the ethical context of the doctor's overwhelming duty to act in the best interests of his or her patient. This is a duty in relation to the specific patient and not the patient body as a whole. So, in the example above, the prediction of mortality for the purpose of allocating scarce resources would place the needs of the general above the needs of the specific patient. Patient A, deprived of treatment as a result of a prediction of mortality, would have a cast iron claim for negligence during the period of absent medical care and the fact that he died (in accordance with the prediction of the ANN) would act as no defence to the action by his family. In the same example, however, the ANN prediction could arguably be used to support the contention that the patient would have died in any event.

The example illustrates well the increasing difficulties facing ANN implementation when these are used more at the 'decision-making', rather than the 'data-refining' end of the clinical management spectrum. The further towards the decision-making end of the spectrum the ANN is placed, the less acceptable it is for decisions to stand alone.

ANN in 'real life': the PAPNET system

This system is described in detail in Chapter 3. Briefly, the system consists of two ANNs capable of recognizing those abnormal elements in Papanicolaou-stained cervical smears that are associated with cancer. The early stages of cervical cancer are curable, and cervical smears offer the possibility of detecting these at a stage that results in cure. National screening cervical programmes place an enormous burden on cytology laboratories, which have to employ large numbers of trained technicians. A technician's job consists of examining every cell in each smear (numbered in their thousands) to detect those few cells characteristic of early cancer. This job is time consuming, repetitive, and tedious. PAPNET is designed to receive stained microscope slides, scan all the formed elements of the slide, and interpret cells or groups of cells as normal, or not. Abnormal areas are then digitally photographed, together with their exact xy coordinates on the slide; these pictures are referred to as 'tiles'. The pathologist will review these 'tiles', and can choose to return to that precise area of the slide using a suitably designed microscope fitted with a motorized microscope stage. The system therefore analyses data at the 'input' end, and does not attempt to 'decide' anything other than taking the pathologist to areas that it has classified as abnormal. The system therefore sits at the 'data refinery' end of the diagnostic equation, by filtering out non-diagnostic noise and enriching those elements with diagnostic potential. It is designed to *replace* the initial manual screening process, for which it has been shown to be at least as, and probably slightly more, effective and robust than its human counterparts in both retrospective and prospective studies. Some studies have suggested that the system offers a lower false negative rate than do its human counterparts, implying that it 'misses' malignancy less often than cytologists do. In such closely monitored trial situations, therefore, the system appears very attractive. Many European laboratories began to avail themselves of the PAPNET service, feeling increasingly confident that the cells which the system was isolating and presenting were indeed the most abnormal ones on the smear. The role played by the ANN-driven system was therefore very well defined. Its excellent performance in this strictly defined role had been demonstrated beyond question; this was also considered acceptable because interpretation of the images was still ultimately human. Despite this apparently bright future, the system is now no longer commercially available. Firstly, the commercial manufacturer charged a considerable fee-per-test, which for some laboratories could not be recouped by increased efficiency. Secondly, their marketing tactics allegedly implied that cancers might be 'missed' by the inferior performance of cytologists as primary screeners. This statement was not surprisingly received with much hostility by the American pathology community. Finally, the company subsequently went into liquidation. It should be noted that it was not possible to buy the system and install it in individual laboratories; slides had to be sent to the company's laboratories, where they were analysed and sent back with a digital tape containing the tiles ready for review. This was presumably done in order to retain control of the system and its internal workings. The significance of this in a legal context is discussed below.

Required evaluation

Much has been written (Wasson et al. 1985; Wyatt & Spiegelhalter 1990; Wyatt & Altman 1995; Friedman & Wyatt 1998; Altman & Royston 2000) about how to design and conduct a rigorous evaluation of a classification tool, including:

The selection of representative test cases.
The need for separate test sets of data distinct from those used to train the ANN.
The need not only for good discrimination (low false positive and false negative rates against a reliable and valid gold standard) but also for good calibration.

Within this uncomplicated framework an ANN can be objectively trained by 'real-life' data and have experience of potentially thousands of events with a known, measurable and measured outcome. Training efficiency can be tested using an unrelated data set (again with known outcomes), and performance can therefore be directly validated in terms of sensitivity and specificity against a retrospective gold standard. This exercise can (and should) be repeated in a prospective manner to ensure consistency of performance over time.

There is less recognition, however, of the need for, and methods of, conducting field trials into the impact of the classification tool on clinical decisions, actions and patient outcomes.

Once a tool such as an ANN has adequate discrimination and calibration, it is necessary to test its benefit as a decision aid, i.e. how much it improves unaided decisions. For example, if the decisions about choice of drugs taken by doctors are already optimal, an ANN with 100% diagnostic accuracy may not help. Only a field trial of the impact of providing the ANN output on clinical decisions can determine how much the doctors will use the ANN, how much they will allow its output to influence their decisions, and how much this will change their patient care actions. Again, there are studies published concerning how to avoid the many biases and pitfalls they pose (Wyatt & Spiegelhalter 1991) but, as described earlier, there is little evidence that the developers of ANNs have so far taken the plunge.

Table 14.2. Cumulative performance criteria and evaluation requirements of predictive tools as the role of the model is extended

Role of prognostic model	Performance criteria (cumulative)
Guiding health policy/management	Broad predictive accuracy ($\pm 50\%$)
Guiding biomedical research	Accounts for most experimental results
	Able to support 'what if' queries
Teaching students	Number of alternative scenarios supported
	Clinical plausibility of scenarios
	Able to generate explanations
Guiding the care of groups of patients (CQI)	High accuracy for groups of patients
	Covers the majority of case types
	Valid across institutions/states
	Modest data requirements
Grading patient outcomes in clinical trials	Good accuracy on each case
	Sensitive to important differences in patient state
	Reliable in different hands
Guiding choice of low risk tests or treatment in individual patients	Able to identify atypical cases
	Reasonably calibrated probabilities
	Good discrimination per case
	Explicit model with explanations
Guiding high risk choices in individuals	Well-calibrated probabilities
	High discrimination per case

This may be partly because of concern over ethical or legal issues. It may also be because the requirements for performance and quality are cumulative as one progresses down the list of possible roles for predictive models (Table 14.2), so that complex and searching preliminary evaluations are required before reaching the stage of testing the impact of an ANN on clinical decisions in a field trial.

Necessary support infrastructure

Once again, the very plasticity of ANNs represents their Achilles' heel. A crude analogy here is the plasticity of human beings. Humans wishing to practice medicine have to be trained, and then have to prove competence by passing examinations, and by satisfying statutory authorities that they remain competent with time – a process referred to as Continuous Medical Education (CME). Similarly, if they wish to enter the diagnostic disciplines, higher examinations set by statutorily appointed bodies are necessary. In the UK these disciplines are governed by the Royal Colleges (of Pathology, Radiology, etc.).

These mechanisms provide perceived safeguards for the quality of human decision-making, thereby attempting to protect patients from substandard levels of care. Because of the omnipresent spectre of human error, however, these mechanisms can be regarded only as the best available and do not pretend to ensure patients against the possibility of medical malpractice.

We have illustrated examples in this chapter of systems that are, in theory at least, capable of making equally important diagnostic decisions. The publications concerning the success of ANNs, driven by academics, demonstrate that (in an academic setting) such systems can perform equally well if not better than human beings. This lack of implementation therefore reflects not so much their capability, but rather more uncertainty about the universal structure within which they can be assessed, monitored, endorsed, and implemented in a way acceptable to clinicians and patients alike.

For this reason, we suggest that the application of ANNs might be loosely placed within the structure appropriate for pathologists. If ANNs became routine diagnostic tools for the clinician, with no reference back to a body of opinion that might identify faults in the conclusions reached, there is a danger of complacent reliance on the ANN to the exclusion of other diagnostic procedures or even common sense. Although the current reliability and performance of ANNs is in some circumstances exceptional, and there is no reason to doubt that this will not remain so, no structure exists to ensure that this should remain so. Pathologists are trained in Good Laboratory Practice; this is the reason why clinicians can, and do, rely, on the answers to the tests they perform on their patients. The 'black-box' nature of the networks themselves also serves to increase feelings of uncertainty about whether such devices are to be used in critical areas of health care. Unlike established diagnostic and medical equipment such as microscopes, CT scanners, biochemistry autoanalysers, and ventilators, such devices are not amenable to engineering maintenance. It is, however, abundantly clear that they need to be 'monitored' for correct use, performance, internal consistency, and may also need regular 'upgrades' in the form of (perhaps) retraining on larger or more appropriate data sets. Without such monitoring, these devices are very unlikely to be endorsed either by health care organizations, or by patients.

As regards ANNs whose role has been designed as data-refining devices, we suggest that their implementation cannot proceed because of the lack of endorsement and approval by any statutory authority.

The UK Royal College of Pathologists oversees and governs those doctors who have been charged with providing quality and excellence in diagnostic laboratory skills (such as histopathology, chemical pathology, immunology, haematology, and microbiology). Clinicians whose performance is endorsed by such statutory bodies responsible for the principles of Good Laboratory Practice and Continuous

Medical Education are accepted and acceptable in an ethical and legal sense. Implicit in this statement are the concepts of 'policing' performance and protecting the public from those clinicians whose performance becomes substandard for whatever reason.

ANNs created by, and borne out of, academic curiosity, have no such umbrella organization to represent them. They currently have neither identity nor ethical and legal framework within which they can be legitimately incorporated into clinical decision-making. The fact that they are 'black boxes' is probably of no consequence, as human beings are accepted as decision-makers in the absence of easily definable reasons (see the paradox of the expert, above).

The most promising area for ANNs in medicine consists of their ability to act as 'data refineries' for large and complex data sets; their ability to make decisions based on the experience of thousands of individual records is particularly attractive. A correctly trained network containing the post hoc experience of the clinical features and outcome of, say, 10 000 patients is a potentially very valuable clinical tool. We suggest that there must be a regulatory body for the assessment, maintenance, and supervision of such tools.

The traditional diagnostic pathology disciplines are currently not able to embrace such novel technology based in mathematics. It is therefore difficult to see how to integrate ANNs within recognized pathology specialities, although many practices and procedures in pathology could be applied to ANNs. One can envisage, therefore, the necessity for the development of Departments of, for example, Neural Networking and Decision Support within health care organizations. The aim would be to promote the development of, and design and implement the strategies for, the maintenance and quality control aspects of network applications. Such departments would have to work together with clinicians to initiate proper systems for the integration and use of ANNs in the clinical arena. A link with pathologists would also seem logical, as they are familiar with the concept of quality control, which is central to the safe continuing existence of an ANN.

It is difficult to begin to assess the true value of ANNs on clinical practice as no RCT data exist specifically examining this; it may be that no such trials have been performed because the behaviour, design, and role of ANNs do not fit easily, for both ethical and legal reasons, into any existing statutory regulatory structure.

Until such a regulatory structure exists, no progress can be made. It should not be the remit of academics, industry, or both, who are responsible for such networks, to implement these systems. Furthermore the plasticity (and therefore room for error through incorrect usage) of ANNs implies that clinicians should equally not be charged with being guardians of such technology. There are examples where much simpler technology has been incorrectly used by doctors outside the normal 'safety envelope' provided by statutory bodies such as the Royal College of Pathologists, and litigation has ensued.

Until this fundamental problem is resolved we see no way whereby the advantages of ANNs can be exploited for the benefit of the individual patient; some of these concepts are explored in the following section concerning their legal status.

Some legal aspects of ANN implementation

What is the legal definition of ANN?

For reasons that will be outlined briefly in this chapter, the manner in which ANNs are used, as well as the purposes to which they may be put, will lead to specific legal outcomes, which we will discuss.

ANNs begin their life as mathematical models 'trained' for a specific purpose. Because the creator of the ANN already knows the application to which he or she intends the ANN to be put, this analysis of legal ramifications may appear to place the cart before the horse. As we will show, however, the manner in which the law will determine liability for faulty outcomes will probably have the effect of itself dictating the areas in which ANNs will be most widely used.

The 'black box' concept

We are not aware of any legal precedents that have considered the medical applications of ANNs nor sought to give legal definition. The law has considered the issue of computer technology, both software and hardware, and articles and papers abound in relation to artificial intelligence and computer-aided decision-making. The concept of ANNs, however, is novel in the following respects:

Although involving hardware and software, the inner workings of individual ANNs are difficult to visualize (the 'black-box' problem (see Hart & Wyatt 1990)).

The ultimate commercial producer of the ANN is, in practice, unlikely to release the source code for the structure to the endpoint user for fear of piracy and replication.

The accuracy of the results from ANNs can be measured only against known parameters. In other words, this is not equivalent to a machine, tool or equipment where the results stand for themselves. For example, an electron microscope or a thermometer can be relied upon *because* the manner by which the result is arrived at is known.

Why is this important?

The practical future of ANNs must lie in their potential commercial value. The beneficiary of such use in medical applications is the patient.

To render the use of ANNs commercially viable, the patient population at which they are aimed is likely to be high and probably worldwide.

Thus, in terms of legal liability for any failure in the ANN system, in legal terms the patient is likely to fall into the category of 'third party'. In other words the patient is unlikely to be a direct party to any contract involving the use of ANNs.

In law, the direct relationship in this context would be governed by a contract. For the patient to have an effective remedy should he or she be harmed by any fault in the system, the usual remedy would be through strict liability of the manufacturer of a product or through negligence.

Product liability

Most jurisdictions entertain the concept that the manufacturer of faulty goods is strictly liable to an end-user for any damage caused by such faults.

In European and UK law, this liability has been reduced to legislation.

Under the Consumer Protection Act 1987,[1] which was implemented under the European Product Liability Directive, the patient has the opportunity to make a direct claim against the 'producer' of a defective 'product' for any damage caused by such defects. Because the claimant does not have to prove negligence or breach of contract, this is a remedy arising out of what is known as strict liability.

In the context of widespread use of ANNs by hospital or health Trusts and medical institutions, it would plainly be in their interests to direct any litigation away from themselves and against the creator of the specific ANN.

The first question, therefore, arises: is an ANN a product in the legal sense?

A product is defined in the 1987 Act as 'any goods or electricity and . . . includes a product which is comprised in [sic] another product whether by virtue of being a component part or raw material or otherwise'.

The definition of defect is set out in Section 3 of the Act. A relevant defect is one that affects the safety of the product. In the context of ANNs used for health benefits to patients, any defect is likely to come within the definition.

It follows that if an ANN is defined as a machine or computer hardware, it would undoubtedly qualify as a product and come within the provisions of the Act.

If, on the other hand, ANNs are defined as comparable to software, the Act would not bite. In reality the actual ANN includes both software and hardware. Any defect in the software that has an effect upon the performance of the machine itself would be a defect within the meaning of the Act.

In a third scenario, if the ANN remains with the manufacturer and the Trust is only sending specimens and receiving reports (albeit reports generated by the ANN) such reports will not conform to the definition of a product. In the

PAPNET application, for example, the slides were sent to the company's laboratory. In such a situation, as long as it can be shown that it is the fault in the ANN itself that has led to an inaccurate or incorrect report, it should still be open to the patient, harmed by an incorrect report, to sue the manufacturer directly if it can be shown that it is a defect in the ANN rather than later human intervention that has caused his or her damage.

If ANNs are defined as products, then the Act provides that the producer of the ANN will be liable for *any* damage caused *wholly or partly by a defect in a product*. Such liability will also fall upon anyone *holding himself or herself out to be the producer* of the product or anyone who has imported the product into a European member state from outside the member states in order to supply it to another in the course of business.

As long as the Trust or medical institution does not come within the definition of someone *holding himself out to be the producer*, then liability will rest with the original manufacturer of the ANN. Whether or not the Trust or user holds himself or herself out as a producer may be significant in the context of the proposal to set up internal Departments of (for example) Neural Networking and Decision Support. A department with the necessary skills to police the quality control aspects of the ANN may expose itself to liability as the producer of the same. It would be iniquitous if something that could be of considerable financial and medical benefit were disregarded because of such difficulties and the potential for exposure to litigation may simply be the price that has to be paid for such scientific advancement.

A further area in which a Trust or user might find itself exposed to strict liability for any errors in the ANN is found in the provisions of Section 2(3) of the Act. This section provides that any *person who supplied the product* to the person suffering damage is liable for the damage if he or she cannot provide the person who has suffered damage with the identity of the producer.

In order for the Trust/user to avoid liability under this section it will be necessary to argue that the purpose to which the ANN was put did not involve the supplying of the product. The Trust/user ought in any event to be easily able to identify the producer.

There are defences provided by the Act. In Section 4(1), anyone sued under the Act is provided with a defence if the *state of scientific and technical knowledge at the relevant time was not such that a producer of products of the same description as the product in question might be expected to have discovered the defect if it had existed in the products while they were under his or her control*.

This so-called 'state of the art' defence poses numerous conundrums in the context of ANNs. In the first place there may in fact be only one producer of ANNs for a particular application. Would such a producer be able to rely upon the state of knowledge of a producer of ANNs in a different field? In the second place, there is the whole issue of the inability of any producer to know 'how' the ANN works or what deductive process it employs to produce a result. In real terms, no producer could ever be expected to discover a defect in the ANN itself.

Contract

Whether regarded as products or not, it is axiomatic that any defects in ANNs could give rise to serious legal consequences. The contractual framework within which the ANN is put to practical use is likely to be of central importance in establishing who pays for any eventual damage.

The relationship between the original creator and the end-user of an ANN will normally be governed by one or a series of contracts. It should, therefore, be possible for the Trust/user to protect itself against exposure to huge damage claims by the inclusion of carefully worded terms. In those circumstances it should not matter whether the contract is for the actual supply of the ANN itself (for use internally in a department) or for the provision of test results. It ought also to be possible for the manufacturer to obtain insurance in respect of any defects in the ANN.

The end result of a faulty ANN used in a medical context is likely to be damage in the form of personal injury to a patient or patients. In English law, personal injury has historically been defined as 'any disease and any impairment of a person's physical or mental condition'.

Various statutes limit or control the extent to which a party to a contract can exempt himself or herself from liability by reference to a term of that contract and Section 2 of the Unfair Contract Terms Act 1977[2] prohibits limitation or exclusion of liability for death or personal injury arising from negligence. Negligence is defined in the Act as the breach:

(a) of any obligation arising from the express or implied terms of a contract to take reasonable care or exercise reasonable skill in the performance or a contract;
(b) of any common law duty to take reasonable care or exercise reasonable skill (but not any stricter duty)

Since it is anticipated that the most likely reason for a failure in an ANN will arise from negligent training or some act or human error, an exclusion clause in these terms ought not to be effective.

Section 2 will always apply in relation to actions for personal injury. Circumstances may arise, however, in which the loss suffered by the Trust/user is purely economic.

In this instance, Section 2 does not apply to a contract relating to 'the creation or transfer of a right or interest in any patent, trade mark, copyright, registered design, technical or commercial information or other intellectual property . . .'.

It appears that Section 2 is thought to apply to software but that the requirement of reasonableness will have to be met. The Act imposes such a requirement and sets out five guidelines. These cover the relative strengths of bargaining position between the parties: whether a customer was induced to enter into the contract, whether the customer ought to have known of the existence and extent of the exclusion clause, where the exclusion clause is dependent upon a condition not being complied with, whether compliance with the condition was practicable, and whether the goods were manufactured, processed or adapted to the special order of the customer.

A case of importance in this regard is *St Albans City and District Council* v. *International Computers Ltd* [1997] FSR 251. This was a case concerning an error in software supplied by the defendant for the purpose of assessing the level of community charge. The error led to the charge being set too low and large financial losses ensued. There was plainly a breach of contract but the defendant sought to rely upon limitation clauses in the agreement, which set their liability at £100 000.

The judge at first instance decided that the limitation clause was unreasonable. This decision was upheld by the Court of Appeal. The decision focused upon the relative bargaining power of the parties. The courts were clearly influenced by the fact that one was a multinational company and the other a relatively impecunious local authority.

The case shows that limitation clauses can, in principle, apply to software but it is also interesting to note (by analogy) that there would be considerable force in an argument that such a clause would be unenforceable in relation to ANNs. The producer of the ANN is likely to be a large, profit-making organization and the user a relatively impecunious Trust. The bargaining position argument would be bound to be employed by such a Trust in this jurisdiction. The case reinforces the need for expert legal advice in drawing up and entering into the contract as well as the need for prudence on the part of the producer of the ANN in obtaining adequate insurance to cover potential claims.

Negligence

The background to allegations of negligence in clinical practice have been discussed above. Any fault in the ANN will be likely to lead to harm to patients who are not in a contractual relationship with the originator of the ANN. If the patient cannot sue under the product liability provisions, the next ready route is an action in negligence *either* against the manufacturer *or* the health care provider.

Can the patient sue the manufacturer of the ANN?

In the world of software design, the original author would be unlikely to be held responsible to the whole world, even though it could be said to be foreseeable that a fault could lead to loss or damage.

The famous words of Cardozo C. J. in *Ultramares Corporation* v. *Touche* [1931] 174 N.E., a New York Court of Appeal decision often cited with approval by English courts, still held good and the law sets its face against liability 'in an indeterminate amount for an indeterminate time to an indeterminate class'.

In order to succeed in showing that the manufacturer of the ANN owes a duty to the patient, the latter must be proved to come within a defined class of people who must have been in the manufacturer's contemplation. This is the legal concept of *proximity*. The landmark decision on this point is that of the House of Lords in 1991 in *Caparo Industries plc* v. *Dickman* [1990] 2AC 605. This was a case about the liability of auditors for negligent misstatements in their report upon which shareholders relied to their financial detriment, but it has redefined the test for establishing the existence of duty of care situations.

The test to be applied involves reasonable foreseeability that damage will be suffered, the existence of proximity in the relationship between the parties and whether it is fair, just and reasonable to impose a duty.

The ANN will be aimed at a specific purpose and thus an identifiable class of people who could foreseeably suffer injury as a consequence of defects. It is likely, therefore, that even with an application employed in a national screening process, the cohort of screened patients would be deemed to come within a finite class that ought to have been in the contemplation of the ANN creator.

It follows that any person injured as a consequence of a fault in an ANN is likely to be able to claim in negligence against the original manufacturer.

In practice, of course, the first line of attack for an injured patient will probably be to sue the Trust or medical institution responsible for his care. Exposure to the threat of such a burden of litigation could be a serious disincentive to such Trusts to use ANNs. For this reason, the terms of the contract between the ANN manufacturer and the user and the judicious inclusion of appropriate indemnities will be of central importance if national institutions are to be encouraged to employ ANNs in any context.

Limitations on the practical application of ANNs

This leads on to the essential consideration of the limitation of the applications of ANNs. Because the actual methods by which results are reached can never be analysed, it is all the more important that ANNs are applied in circumstances where their continuing accuracy can be assessed by reference to fixed parameters. Thus, in the field of cervical screening, for example, random quality control checks can be made by physically examining the smears assessed by the ANN.

This is also important in situations where a 'grey area' of liability emerges. If it is not plain and obvious that a Trust or user should avoid liability on any of the grounds set out above, the Trust defence to the patient will lie in the reasonableness of its reliance on the ANN.

The doctor/patient relationship is essentially defined by the obligation of the doctor to act in the best interests of his or her patient. This is supplemented by the requirement to obtain the consent of the patient in relation to treatment and procedures.

In the use of ANNs in many of the contexts suggested, the consent of the patient will not be a requirement. Thus, in large-scale screening applications, the patient will probably be unaware of the use of ANNs. If, however, disaster struck and there was no 'producer' to whom liability could attach, would the Trust inevitably be doomed to compensate any injured victims?

Here the first practical effect of the law on limiting the arenas in which ANNs could sensibly be applied comes into play. In the screening example, if the Trust was able to show that its use of ANNs was reasonable, was in the best interests of the patient, that there were effective systems in place to check the continued accuracy of the ANN, and there were no reasons to suspect errors, then an arguable defence to a claim emerges.

Contrast this with the use of ANNs in more experimental situations. To take an extreme example, the ANN could be used as a predictor for the efficacy or otherwise of a particular expensive treatment in a particular patient. For the reasons set out above, a defence based upon an argument that this is beneficial to the patient community as a whole will fail. Such an application will necessarily deprive particular patients of treatment they would otherwise have received.

Reliance on the ANN to the exclusion of personal judgement in such a situation would almost certainly be indefensible. The only way in which such an application could properly be applied would be with the express knowledge and valid consent of the patient.

These considerations underline the points already made. The use of the ANN is unlikely to be extended beyond data refinery or adjunct to decision-making (in the same way as a textbook) until the law develops and recognizes how to deal with the complications more sophisticated applications present.

Conclusions: criteria for medical use of ANNs

Table 14.3 illustrates the strengths and weaknesses of ANNs in relation to other methods of data classification. These are judged by the five criteria of accuracy, generality, clinical credibility, ease of development, and clinical effectiveness. This interface between ANNs and clinical need is also discussed by Wyatt (2000). The table demonstrates the drawbacks of ANNs in several of these criteria, at least

Table 14.3. Criteria for predictive tools and comparison of the ability of three predictive technologies to satisfy them

Criterion	Specific requirement	Artificial neural nets	Explicit statistical models	Knowledge-based systems
1. Accuracy	Accurate discrimination	✓	✓	?
	Well-calibrated probabilities	×	✓?	×
2. Generality	Valid when transferred to other sites	?	?	?
	Model can be adjusted to reduce overoptimism	×	✓	?
3. Clinical credibility	Model's structure apparent, explanations available	×✓?	✓	
	Ability to browse the system's 'knowledge'	×	✓	✓
	Simple to calculate predictions	×	✓?	×
	Ability to display 'common sense'	×	×	?
4. Ease of development	Avoids need for large, prospective verified database	×	×	✓?
	Avoids need for skilled personnel	?	?	×
	Ability to encode clinical policy, systematic review results, etc.	×	×	✓
	Ability to encode aetiology, disease mechanisms, etc.	×	✓	✓
	Ability to learn from experience	✓	✓	×
5. Clinical effectiveness	RCT evidence of impact on clinical process, patient outcome[a]	×	✓	✓

From Wyatt & Altman 1995.
[a]RCT, randomized clinical trials; data from Hunt et al. 1998.

some of which relate to insufficient experience with their actual performance in the field and in well-defined randomized clinical trial settings. Progress therefore will depend on a careful assessment of ANN performance in tightly controlled situations, under a tightly controlled set of parameters. The following section suggests outline protocols for the assessment and possible ultimate adoption of ANNs in clinical situations.

A suggested outline framework for the application of ANNs in clinical practice

The following is a six-point protocol, which it is suggested should be adopted in relation to the clinical use of ANNs in any setting:

1. The use must always be for the intention of benefit to the individual patient rather than to the patient body as a whole. The use of ANNs to determine outcome for the purpose of saving money or allocating resources should be prohibited.
2. The use of an ANN in a specific diagnostic or predictive area, and the advantages accrued therefrom, must always be justified by appropriately conducted randomized clinical trials.
3. The parameters deciding where to set ANN sensitivity and specificity must be determined for each and every specific application, as must the design and power calculations necessary for the clinical trial. These parameters depend upon both the implications of using the technology (the clinical importance of the output of the ANN) and, in the case of screening, the prevalence of the disease in the population to be screened. Such decisions should be made up of a nationally appointed panel of clinicians and statisticians with experience in this area.
4. ANNs should be used only in locations where there is direct access to expertise in their design, implementation and quality control.
5. ANNs must be used only within a structure of well-defined and established 'Good Network Practice', supervised by statutory bodies to act as regulators of continued quality performance.
6. ANNs may be used at the discretion of the treating clinician in circumstances in which the veracity of the data provided is not capable of being checked against known scientific data at that time. In such circumstances their use shall be restricted to those patients or volunteers who have been fully informed of the use of the same and provided with such information as enables such patient volunteers to provide valid consent to their use.

Acknowledgements

The authors thank Doug Altman, Centre for Statistics in Medicine, Oxford, and David Spiegelhalter, MRC Biostatistics Unit, Cambridge, for constructive discussion and criticism of many of the concepts presented in this chapter.

NOTES

1. Distinctions in the Act relating to different parts of the UK are not relevant to this chapter.
2. This Act applies to England, Wales and Northern Ireland for contract terms and otherwise and to Scotland for contract terms alone.

REFERENCES

Altman, D. G. & Royston, P. (2000). What do we mean by validating a prognostic model? *Statistics in Medicine* 19, 453–473.

Boon, M. E., Kok, L. P. & Beck, S. (1995). Histologic validation of neural network-assisted cervical screening: comparison with the conventional procedure. *Cell Vision* 2, 23–27.

Campana, A., Duci, A., Gambini, O. & Scarone, S. (1999). An artificial neural network that uses eye-tracking performance to identify patients with schizophrenia. *Schizophrenia Bulletin* 25, 789–799.

Cerrito, P. B., Koenig, S. C., VanHimbergen, D. J., Jaber, S. F., Ewert, D. L. & Spence, P. A. (1999). Neural network pattern recognition analysis of graft flow characteristics improves intraoperative anastomotic error detection in minimally invasive CABG. *European Journal of Cardiothoracic Surgery* 16, 88–93.

Chen, H. Y., Chen, T. C., Min, D. I., Fischer, G. W. & Wu, Y. M. (1999). Prediction of tacrolimus blood levels by using the neural network with genetic algorithm in liver transplantation patients. *Therapeutic Drug Monitor* 21, 50–56.

Dreyfus, H. & Dreyfus, S. (1988). *Mind over Machine.* Free Press, New York.

Dybowski, R., Weller, P., Chang, R. & Gant, V. A. (1996). Prediction of outcome in critically ill patients using artificial neural network synthesized by genetic algorithm. *Lancet* 347, 1146–1150.

Edwards, D. F., Hollingsworth, H., Zazulia, A. R. & Diringer, M. N. (1999). Artificial neural networks improve the prediction of mortality in intracerebral hemorrhage. *Neurology* 53, 351–357.

Friedman, C. & Wyatt, J. (1998). *Evaluation Methods in Medical Informatics.* Springer-Verlag, New York.

Furness, P. N., Levesley, J., Luo, A., Taub, N., Kazi, J. I., Bates, W. D. et al. (1999). A neural network approach to the biopsy diagnosis of early acute renal transplant rejection. *Histopathology* 35, 461–467.

Hart, A. & Wyatt, J. (1990). Evaluating black boxes as medical decision-aids: issues arising from a study of neural networks. *Medical Informatics* 15, 229–236.

Herman, R.A., Noormohamed, S., Hirankarn, S., Shelton, M. J., Huang, E., Morse, G. D. et al. (1999). Comparison of a neural network approach with five traditional methods for predicting creatinine clearance in patients with human immunodeficiency virus infection. *Pharmacotherapy* **19**, 734–740.

Hunt, D. L., Haynes, R. B., Ha, S. E. & Smith, K. (1998). Effects of computer-based clinical decision support systems on physician performance and patient outcomes: a systematic review. *Journal of the American Medical Association* **280**, 1339–1346.

Huo, A., Giger, M. L. & Metz, C. E. (1999). Effect of dominant features on neural network performance in the classification of mammographic lesions. *Physics in Medicine and Biology* **44**, 2579–2595.

Kirby, S. D., Eng, P., Danter, W., George, C. F., Francovic, T., Ruby, R. R. et al. (1999). Neural network prediction of obstructive sleep apnea from clinical criteria. *Chest* **116**, 409–415.

Li, Y. C., Liu, L., Chiu, W. T. & Jian, W. S. (2000). Neural network modeling for surgical decisions on traumatic brain injury patients. *International Journal of Medical Informatics* **57**, 1–9.

Lindahl, D., Palmer, J. & Edenbrandt, L. (1999). Myocardial SPET: artificial neural networks describe extent and severity of perfusion defects. *Clinical Physiology* **19**, 497–503.

Lo, J. Y., Baker, J. A., Kornguth, P. J. & Floyd, C. E., Jr (1999). Effect of patient history data on the prediction of breast cancer from mammographic findings with artificial neural networks. *Academic Radiology* **6**, 10–15.

Lundin, M., Lundin, J., Burke, H. B., Toikkanen, S., Pylkkanen, L. & Joensuu, H. (1999). Artificial neural networks applied to survival prediction in breast cancer. *Oncology* **57**, 281–286.

McKibbon, K. A., Haynes, R. B., Walker Dilks, C. J., Ramsden, M. F., Ryan, N. C., Baker, L. et al. (1990). How good are clinical Medline searches? A comparative study of end-user and librarian searches. *Computers in Biomedical Research* **23**, 583–593.

Mobley, B. A., Schechter, E., Moore, W. E., McKee, P. A. & Eichner, J. E. (2000). Predictions of coronary artery stenosis by artificial neural network. *Artificial Intelligence in Medicine* **18**, 187–203.

Modai, I., Valevski, A., Solimish, A., Kurs, R., Hines, I. L., Ritsner, M. & Mendel, S. (1999). Neural network detection of files of suicidal patients and suicidal profiles. *Medical Informatics and Internet Medicine* **24**, 249–256.

Potter, S. R., Miller, M. C., Mangold, L. A., Jones, K. A., Epstein, J. I., Veltri, R. W. et al. (1999). Genetically engineered neural networks for predicting prostate cancer progression after radical prostatectomy. *Urology* **54**, 791–795.

Qureshi, K. N., Naguib, R. N., Hamdy, F. C., Neal, D. E. & Mellon, J. K. (2000). Neural network analysis of clinicopathological and molecular markers in bladder cancer. *Journal of Urology* **63**, 630–633.

Ronco, A. L. & Fernandez, R. (1999). Improving ultrasonographic diagnosis of prostate cancer with neural networks. *Ultrasound Medicine and Biology* **25**, 729–733.

Scott, J. A. (1999). Using artificial neural network analysis of global ventilation–perfusion scan morphometry as a diagnostic tool. *American Journal of Roentgenology* **173**, 943–948.

Wasson, J. H., Sox, H. C., Neff, R. K. & Goldman, L. (1985). Clinical prediction rules: applications and methodological standards. New England Journal of Medicine **313**, 793–799.

Wyatt, J. (1995). Nervous about artificial neural networks? *Lancet* **346**, 1175–1177 (editorial).

Wyatt, J. C. (2000). Knowledge for the clinician. 1. Clinical questions and information needs. *Journal of the Royal Society of Medicine* **93**, 168–171.

Wyatt, J. C. & Altman, D. G. (1995). Prognostic models: clinically useful, or quickly forgotten? *British Medical Journal* **311**, 1539–1541.

Wyatt, J. & Spiegelhalter, D. (1990). Evaluating medical expert systems: what to test and how? *Medical Informatics* **15**, 205–217.

Wyatt, J. & Spiegelhalter, D. (1991). Field trials of medical decision-aids: potential problems and solutions. In P. Clayton, ed., *Proceedings of the 15th Symposium on Computer Applications in Medical Care*, Washington. McGraw Hill Inc., New York, pp. 3–7.

Index

Note: page numbers in *italics* refer to figures and tables; 'n' suffix refers to notes